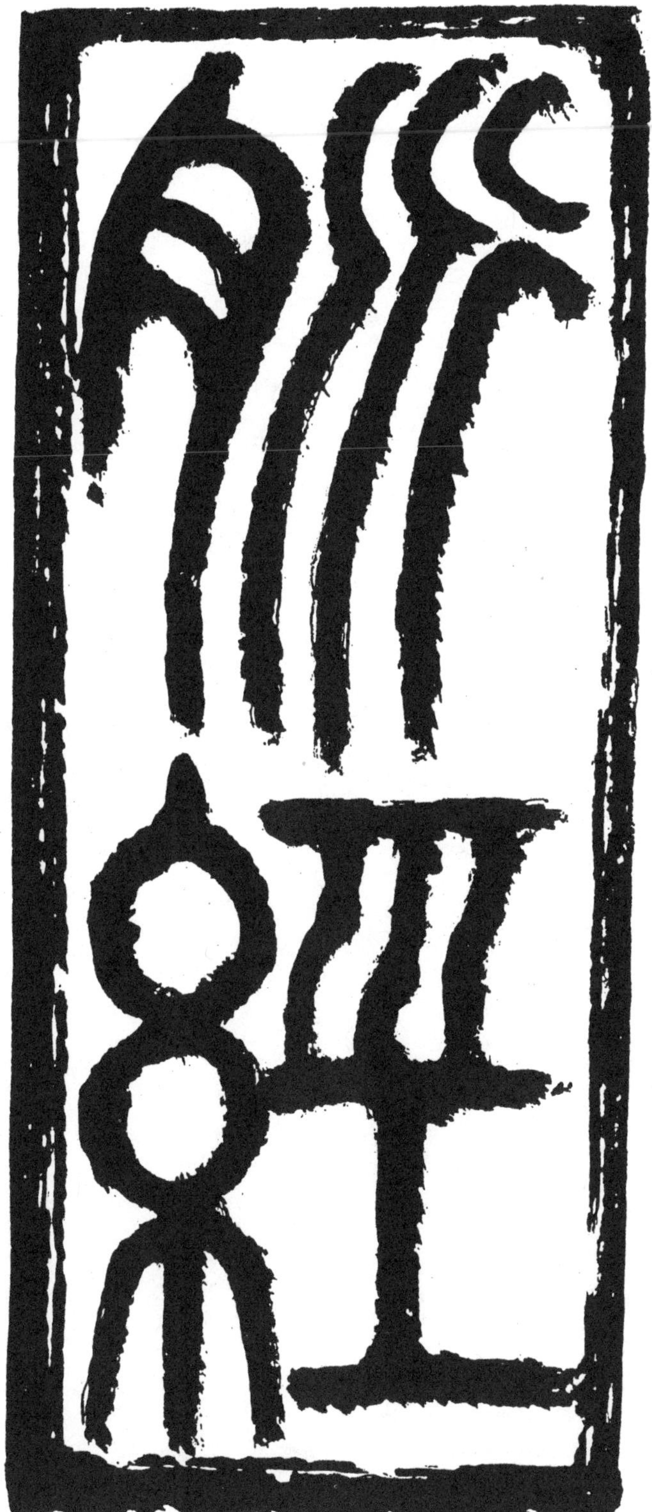

脈
經

The
Pulse
Classic

A Translation of the *Mai Jing* by Wang Shu-he

translated by
Yang Shou-zhong

BLUE POPPY PRESS

Published by:
BLUE POPPY PRESS
A Division of Blue Poppy Enterprises, Inc.
4804 SE 69th Avenue
Portland, OR 97206

First Edition, January, 1997
Second Printing, January, 2002
Third Printing, January, 2007
Fourth Printing, February, 2008
Fifth Printing, July, 2009
Sixth Printing, August, 2010
Seventh Printing, February, 2012
Eighth Printing, August, 2013
Ninth Printing, February, 2015
Tenth Printing, September, 2015
Eleventh Printing, November, 2017
Twelfth Printing, July, 2018
Thirteenth Printing, December, 2019
Fourteenth Printing, March, 2020
Fifteenth Printing, November, 2020
Sixteenth Printing, July, 2023

ISBN 0-936185-75-9
ISBN 978-0-936185-75-0

LC 96-86688

COMP Designation: A denotative translation.

20 19 18 17 16

Printed at Frederic Printing, Aurora, CO

Translator's Foreword

Wang Shu-he's *Mai Jing (Pulse Classic)* is the oldest surviving book specifically on pulse examination in the Chinese medical literature. Although the *Nei Jing (Inner Classic), Nan Jing (Classic of Difficulties)*, and *Shang Han Lun/Jin Gui Yao Lue (Treatise on Cold Damage/Essentials of the Golden Cabinet)* contain discussions of Chinese pulse examination, the *Mai Jing* is, as its name states, the classic of Chinese pulse examination. Written some time in the second century CE, the majority of great Chinese doctors in the centuries immediately after Wang all acknowledged that their learning of the theories and techniques of pulse examination was based on the foundation laid by Wang Shu-he. For instance, Wang Tao, the author of the *Wai Tai Mi Yao (Secret Essentials of the External Tower)*, and Chao Yuan-fang, the author of the *Zhu Bing Yuan Hou Lun (Treatise on the Origins & Symptoms of Various Diseases)*, both incorporated parts or the whole of the *Mai Jing* in their own writings. Sun Si-miao's *Qian Jin Fang (Formulas [Worth] a Thousand [Pieces of] Gold)* likewise includes parts of this venerable classic. In the Tang and Song dynasties, the study of the *Mai Jing* was an obligatory course in the curriculum of the imperial medical academy along with the *Su Wen (Simple Questions), Ling Shu (Spiritual Pivot), Zhen Jiu Jia Yi Jing (The Systematic Classic of Acupuncture & Moxibustion)*, and a small number of other medical classics.

As time went by, however, this work was gradually overshadowed by other books on the pulse, nearly all of which were, in fact, derivations of the *Mai Jing*. This is because, with the passage of time, the language in which this book was written was too arcane and hard to decipher even for readers living in premodern times hundreds of years ago. Everyone admitted that none of these popular books, many of which were oversimplified and contained wrong information, compared to this magnum opus. Nevertheless, due to the difficulty of reading the *Mai Jing* in the original, they preferred to neglect this brilliant work, to be misled by inferior authors. Happily, even in those times when this erroneous tendency prevailed, there were outstanding medical figures who never relaxed their efforts in the study and research of this work and who repeatedly raised their voices to direct the pubic's attention to the historical and practical significance of this great classic.

In recent years, the government of the People's Republic of China gathered a convocation of learned TCM scholars from across the country in order to carry out large scale research on the most worthy old Chinese medical classics. Chinese scholars on the mainland are very critical when it comes to categorizing an old work as a classic. The *Zhou Hou Fang (Behind the Elbow Formulary)* by Ge Hong is a very valuable medical work, having significantly influenced the development of

TCM, but few Chinese scholars call it a classic. Among the great number of surviving premodern medical texts, the scholars of this national convocation selected only eleven works as classics to be designated as priorities for scholarly research. The *Mai Jing* is one of these eleven preeminent Chinese medical classics, the *creme de la creme* of the ancient Chinese medical literature. So far, Blue Poppy Press has published three of these eleven classics: the *Zhen Jiu Jia Yi Jing (The Systematic Classic of Acupuncture & Moxibustion)*, Hua Tuo's *Zhong Zang Jing (The Classic of the Central Viscera)*, and now the *Mai Jing*.

About Wang Shu-he

Wang Shu-he was once the chief doctor of the royal family's private medical center. In feudal China it was said, "Every inch of land within the borderlines was the property of the emperor, and everything, including the inhabitants on it, was part of the wealth of the royal family." Thus the attending physician of an emperor was naturally the best medical worker throughout the land of the Son of the Heaven.

In regard to Wang's life history, very little is known, not even his family background. We know only that he lived a little earlier than Huang-fu Mi, the author of the *Jia Yi Jing (The Systematic Classic)*, who lived from 215-282 CE.

Fragmentary references dispersed throughout the literature suggest that Wang Shu-he was expert in nearly every branch of Chinese medicine and acupuncture and also in Chinese literature. One story says that he was particularly well-known for his diagnosis. Once he came across a funeral procession with a coffin from which fresh blood was leaking. He stopped the procession and asked to examine the dead body in the coffin. According to Chinese custom, it was a gross offence to the dead if the coffin was uncovered. Nevertheless, Wang insisted, declaring with confidence that the person inside was still alive. The coffin was opened. Inside was a birthing woman who, it turned out, had fallen faint during a difficult labor with the child still in the womb. Wang immediately performed needling for the dead. Shortly after, the woman was resuscitated. After another round of emergency treatment, a child was delivered alive.

Although Wang's main contribution to Chinese medicine is his *Mai Jing*, he is also praised and remembered for his collation of the works by Zhang Zhong-jing: the *Shang Han Lun (Treatise on Cold Damage)* and the *Jin Gui Yao Lue (Essentials of the Golden Cabinet)*. If it were not for Wang's efforts as editor, these two other preeminent Chinese medical classics might not exist at all today, let alone in the form we have them. In fact, there are two different versions of the *Mai Jing*. One of the two consists of these works by Zhang Zhong-jing in addition to a multitude of other formulas as well as all the contents of the current version of the *Pulse Classic*. This is evidence that, before Wang's editing and collation, these works by Zhang Zhong-jing existed as merely ill-organized and fragmentary bits of instruction scattered here and there.

About this edition

This translation was primarily prepared from the *Mai Jing Jiao Zhu (The Collated & Annotated Pulse Classic)* by Shen Yan-nan, published by the People's Health & Hygiene Press, Beijing, 1991. However, the translator has had to repair many typographical errors in this Chinese version of the *Mai Jing*. Therefore, if there reader were to compare that Chinese version with this English version, there are a number of places where this English version is at variance with the *Mai Jing Jiao Zhu* version. The translator made these corrections after checking several other versions of the *Mai Jing*.

As mentioned above, this book is written in a very terse and cryptic style. Often it is difficult to decide how to understand the particular meaning of generic terms like yin and yang which are used in many different ways in different places in the text. For instance, in one place, yin refers to the deep level of the pulse, while, in another, it implies a choppy pulse quality. Somewhere else, it refers to the cubit position in particular, while it is also used to mean the pulse at the wrist as a whole. If, as translator, I had simply used the word yin in every one of these instances, the reader would have no way of understanding what the author actually meant. Therefore, I have, in certain instances, in order to facilitate the understanding of the text, substituted the meaning for such cipher-like, generic words rather than the word itself.

The reader should also take special note of my translation of the name of the pulse at the wrist and its three positions. The wrist pulse is called the qi opening (*qi kou*) in traditional Chinese medicine, but it is also commonly called the inch opening (*cun kou*). This creates a problem because the distal most position of its three positions is also called the qi opening or, more frequently, the inch opening. This can be quite confusing even to a well-versed Chinese scholar, and proper handling of these terms is crucial to a work on the pulse. Because not every reader has either the time or the expertise to decide whether a reference to the inch opening means the pulse as a whole or its most distal position in particular, I have attempted to provide a uniform treatment to clarify this issue. Thus every time the pulse at the wrist is meant, I have rendered this as either the qi or inch opening, while the distal position of the pulse at the wrist is simply referred to as the *cun*. I believe this approach can be justified by the following fact that the three divisions of the wrist pulse are properly called the *cun kou, guan shang,* and the *chi zhong. Guan shang* literally means on or above the *guan* or bar, while *chi zhong* means in or within the *chi* or cubit. That is to say, the final word of both these terms is a particle. Therefore, the final word in the term *cun kou, i.e. kou,* can also be taken as a particle and, thus, in translation, can be dispensed with when necessary in order to clarify the meaning.

Another point that deserves attention is the insertion in parentheses of the words "the Yellow Emperor" and "the master." Just as in many old Chinese classics, this book takes the form of a series of questions and answers. However, it is not always clear just who the interlocutors are in the majority of chapters. There is reason to think that all the materials in this book were derived from other, now unidentifiable sources. Hence there is no way to verify who the speakers were. Where I have assumed that it is the Yellow Emperor who is speaking in places this is not specified, I have placed this name in parentheses.

As for editorial insertions in order to make the text more readable and intelligible, those that are in parentheses are the translator's insertions, while those within brackets are annotations made by some unknown, previous editors of the original Chinese text. Sometimes such annotations by previous Chinese editors are helpful to Western readers and sometimes they are not. In my opinion, lengthy expositions on the etymology of a Chinese word is, in most cases, not particularly useful to the Western reader. Therefore, in order to keep this translation from becoming too voluminous, I have omitted annotations by previous Chinese editors which I felt would have little significance to the target audience of this edition.

The terminology and methodology used in this translation is based upon Nigel Wiseman and Ken Boss' *Glossary of Chinese Medical Terms and Acupuncture Points,* Paradigm Publications, Brookline, MA, 1990 with updates and emendations as contained in Nigel Wiseman's *English-Chinese Chinese-English Dictionary of Chinese Medicine,* Hunan Science & Technology Press, Changsha, 1995. Formulas are identified by their Chinese names written in Pinyin followed by their English names in parentheses. Ingredients in these formulas are identified first in Latinate pharmacological nomenclature followed by Pinyin in parentheses. The main sources for the identifications of medicinal ingredients used in preparing this work were Bensky and Gamble's *Chinese Herbal Medicine: Materia Medica;* Hong-yen Hsu's *Oriental Materia Medica: A Concise Guide;* and the Shanghai Science & Technology Press's *Zhong Yao Da Ci Dian (A Dictionary of Chinese Medicinals).*

Because the *Mai Jing* was published in columns read from top to bottom and from right to left and because the epigrammatic lines in the *Mai Jing* were commonly set off as independent paragraphs for ease of memorization, the reader will note that large sections of this edition consist of one and two sentence paragraphs. Rather than running these together, we have decided to print them in the groupings they occur in the People's Health & Hygiene Edition, Beijing, 1982 edition. Thus readers can more fully experience for themselves the terse and epigrammatic nature of this classic. On the next page is a reprint of a page from this edition showing how these lines are listed in a very brief and concise manner.

Yang Shou-zhong
Tangshan, Hebei, PRC

病人面青目黃者，五日死。
病人著床，心痛短氣，脾竭內傷，百日復愈，能起傍徨，因坐於地，其亡倚床，能治此者，可謂神良。
病人面無精光，若土色，不受飲食者，四日死。
病人目無精光及牙齒黑色者，不治。
病人耳目及顴頰赤者，死在五日中。
病人耳目鼻口有黑色起入于口者，必死。
病人黑色出於額上髮際，下直鼻脊兩顴上者，亦死在五日中。
病人黑氣出於天中，下至年上，顴上者，死。
病人及健人黑色若白色起入目及鼻口，死在三日中。
病人及健人面忽如馬肝色，望之如青，近之如黑者，死。
病人面黑目直視，惡風者，死。
病人面黑脣青者，死。
病人面青脣黑者，死。
病人面黑，兩脇下痛，不能自轉反者，死。
病人面回回直視，肩息者，一日死。
病人頭目久痛，卒視無所見者，死。
病人陰結陽絕，目精脫，恍惚者，死。
病人陰陽絕竭，目眶陷者，死。
病人眉系傾者，七日死。
病人口如魚口，不能復閉，而氣出多不反者，死。
病人口張者，三日死。
病人脣青人中反者，三日死。
病人脣反人中滿者，死。
病人脣口忽乾者，不治。
病人脣腫齒焦者，死。
病人陰陽俱竭，其齒如熟小豆，其脈駃者，死。
病人齒忽變黑者，十三日死。
病人舌卷卵縮者，必死。
病人汗出不流，舌卷黑者，死。
病人髮直者，十五日死。
病人髮如乾麻，善怒者，死。
病人髮與眉衝起者，死。
病人爪甲青者，死。
病人爪甲白者，不治。
病人手足爪甲下肉黑者，八日死。
病人榮衛竭絕，面浮腫者，死。
病人卒腫，其面蒼黑者，死。
病人手掌腫，無文者，死。
病人臍腫反出者，死。
病人陰囊莖俱腫者，死。
病人脈絕口張足腫，五日死。
病人足趺上腫，兩膝大如斗者，十日死。
病人臥，遺尿不覺者，死。
病人尸臭者，不可治。
肝病皮黑，肺之日庚辛死。
心病目黑，腎之日壬癸死。
脾病脣青，肝之日甲乙死。
肺病頰赤目腫，心之日丙丁死。

Foreword to the Collated *Pulse Classic*

Under an imperial edict, we humble subjects have been commissioned to collate various ancient medical classics and formulary works. Among those to be collated and edited is the *Pulse Classic* compiled by Wang Shu-he. Shu-he was from Gaoping[1] and lived in the Western Jin.[2] He was a reserved person of deep thinking particularly bent on writing. He was profoundly versed in the (medical) classics and formularies, profound in the study of the techniques of physical examination, and erudite in the ways of life-cultivation. His life story can be found in the *Ming Yi Zhuan* (*Biographies of Distinguished Medical Figures*) written by Gan Bo-zong[3] of the Tang dynasty.

As one will see, this work includes discussions of yin and yang and the exterior and interior. It defines the three positions and the nine indicators (of the pulse), dividing the pulse into the *ren ying* (*i.e.*, the *cun* at the left hand), the *cun* opening (*i.e.*, the *cun* at the right hand), and the spirit gate (*i.e.*, the *chi*). It analyses the twelve channels, the twenty-four vessel qi, and the eight extraordinary vessels in order that diseases of the five viscera and six bowels, the triple burner, and the four seasons may thus be diagnosed. Hence this work is well-organized, like a net well laid out with a headrope. It enables the reader to know the internal by examining the external and to see life in death. It contains most detailed and comprehensive information, all of which can be learned and applied to practice.

Since its language is economical, how can (this book) cover a most extensive range of topics? During the compilation of this book, besides the *Huang Di Nei Jing* (*The Yellow Emperor's Inner Classic*) which cannot be exhaustive, inevitably having some oversights and omissions, Shu-he

---

[1]   *I.e.*, an ancient county in present Shanxi Province.

[2]   This dynasty lasted from 215-316 CE.

[3]   A literary man living in the Tang dynasty (618-907 CE) about whose life little is known.

also based his work on the methodologies of Bian Que,[4] (Zhang) Zhong-jing,[5] and Yuan Hua (*i.e.,* Hua Tuo),[6] while rejecting all sorts of absurd, heterodox, or other unjustified doctrines. If this were not such a valuable work, how could it have proved itself in practice to be free from any mistakes as small as a hair during over a thousand years of circulation? Moreover, the mechanisms of the pulse are fine and subtle. The pulse images are difficult to differentiate, and, apart from this, there is the confusing problem that several different pulse images may appear simultaneously or that several different diseases may exhibit the same type of pulse. Relying merely on the feeling under the fingers cannot fully expose that which is covert and hidden (in the body). For that reason, this work gives an all-embracing description of vacuity and repletion indicated by the form and the signs (other than the pulse) and elaborates on the interrelationships between sound, color, and the pulse. It is by cross-referencing all of these to determine life from death that unfailingly leads to correct diagnosis without a single mistake. This is a proven fact.

Because the Jin court was forced to move eastward across the river,[7] the country was split into south and north and an eventful epoch followed. (Since then,) few people have been able to spare the time (to study) works on life-cultivation, and what those handful of people who, nevertheless, were imparted medicine had access to is of questionable (value) or erroneous in practice. Therefore, the truth (embodied in this work) is now in such danger of being lost to the (medical) dao that no one short of a saint is able to collate and correct this work. Fortunately, His Majesty fosters the compassion of loving lives like Great Shun,[8] treasures the (medical) writings which

---

[4] Bian Que was originally a legendary divine physician of remote antiquity. This name is also given to the most distinguished medical figure of the Warring States period, Qin Yue-ren, who was the supposed author of the *Nan Jing* (*Classic of Difficulties*).

[5] Zhang Zhong-jing (circa 150-219 CE) was one of the most outstanding of all Chinese medical scholars. His *Shang Han Lun* (*Treatise on Cold Damage*) is universally acknowledged as the pioneer work on Chinese internal medicine.

[6] Hua Tuo, style-name Yuan Hua, is believed to be the inventor of drug anesthesia and the founder of surgery in China.

[7] As a result of the invasion of northern tribes, the Jin court was forced to move its capital southeast in 316 CE. Its territory was accordingly reduced by half and its jurisdiction was confined to the areas south of the Yangtze River.

[8] Great Shun, or simply Shun, was the second of the first three semi-legendary emperors of Chinese history. He is remembered for his generosity and humanity.

amount to norms of (social) order laid by the Divine Yu,[9] and intends to put into practice his charitable heart of administering blessings (to his subjects). Being alive to the profound significance of protection from disease, His Majesty has handed out this ancient book to be collated anew. Thus, we humble subjects have each tried to make the best of our learning, to seek out all the variant versions of (this text) available, and, based on the classics, have made judgement as to what should be retained and what should be removed. This judgement has never been done on the basis of our personal predilections.

The versions (of *The Pulse Classic*) which have been in circulation are largely three different editions. One version includes the *Bing Yuan (Disease Origins)* by Chao Yuan-fang[10] of the Sui dynasty as its tenth book. One only has to compare these two works in terms of their time of compilation to see that this version betrays itself as a forgery.[11] Another version divides the fifth book into two parts and augments the number of books and chapters by drawing parts from other places (of the work). Scrutiny of the texts reveals that this version is also groundless. A study of the above two versions fails to prove their authenticity. Each of them can be valued as a prize by their keepers only!

During our collation of this work, we made reference to those texts related to the pulse in the *Su Wen (Simple Questions)*, the *Jiu Xu (Nine Ruins)*,[12] the *Ling Shu (Spiritual Pivot)*, the *Tai Su (Pristine*

---

[9]   Yu was the last of the first three semi-legendary emperors of Chinese history. He was distinguished for his ability to rule the country and particularly for his harnessing of the Yellow River. Before this, it had been constantly flooding and bringing about disasters.

[10]   *Bing Yuan (Disease Origins)* is the shortened title of the *Zhu Bing Yuan Hou Lun (Treatise on the Origins & Symptoms of Various Diseases)*. This is a magnum opus on pathogenesis and the signs and symptoms of diseases. The author, Chao Yuan-fang (550?-630? CE), was the director of the imperial medical academy.

[11]   Since Chao Yuan-fang lived after Wang Shu-he, it is impossible for Wang to have drawn upon anything from Chao.

[12]   *I.e.,* an ancient version of the *Ling Shu (Spiritual Pivot)*.

Simple)[13], the *Nan Jing* (*Classic of Difficulties*),[14] the *Jia Yi* (*Systematic Classic*),[15] and the works by (Zhang) Zhong-jing as well as the *Qian Jin Fang* (*Thousand [Taels of] Gold Formulas*)[16] and the *Yi* (*The Wing*).[17] We have removed redundant repititions, filled in lacunae, and changed the order of the chapters in order to arrange the same subjects under the same headings. The number of books remains the same, that is, ten, with a total of 97 chapters. (This newly collated edition) is published in the hope that readers may be able to know the internal by examining the external and to see life in death without the need of drinking the water from the Upper Pool.[18]

Gao Bao-heng, Chacellor of the Royal Academy

Sun Qi, Minister of Land Reclamation

Lin Yi, Chief of the Imperial Secretariat

---

[13] *I.e.,* the *Huang Di Nei Jing Tai Su* (*The Yellow Emperor's Inner Classic: Pristine Simple*) in full. This is an annotated version of the *Su Wen* (*Simple Questions*) edited by Yang Shang-shan in the Tang dynasty.

[14] This is a magnum opus credited to Bian Que but written in the late Han dynasty. It deals with five phase theory as it applies specifically to acupuncture and particularly to the five transport points. It also contains a number of chapters on the examination of the pulse at the wrist.

[15] *I.e.,* the *Huang Di Zhen Jiu Jia Yi Jing* (*The Yellow Emperor's Systematic Classic of Acupuncture & Moxibustion*) in full. This was compiled by Huang-fu Mi (215-282 CE) and has been acclaimed for centuries as the most authentic work in the field of acupuncture. An English version has been published by Blue Poppy Press Inc.

[16] *I.e.,* the *Bei Ji Qian Jin Fang* (*The Thousand [Taels of Gold] Formulas for Emergency*) in full. This was compiled by the great Chinese medical scholar, Sun Si-miao (581-682 CE).

[17] *I.e.,* the *Bei Ji Qian Jin Fang Yi Fang* (*The Companion Book to the Thousand [Taels of] Gold Formulas for Emergency*) in full, also compiled by Sun Si-miao.

[18] This is an allusion to a story about Bian Que. Once Bian Que attended a party in his honor and the host treated him to water from the Upper Pool. After drinking this water, he suddenly acquired a special ability to see the internal organs of people and his medical skills were consequently greatly enhanced.

Preface to *The Pulse Classic*

Wang Shu-he, Director of the Imperial Medical Academy, Jin dynasty

The mechanisms of the pulse are fine and subtle, and the pulse images are difficult to differentiate. The bowstring and the tight, the floating and the scallion-stalk confusingly resemble one another. They may be readily distinct at heart (*i.e.*, their verbal definition may have been memorized), but it is difficult for the fingers to distinguish them. If a deep pulse is taken as a hidden one, the formula and treatment will never be in the right line. If a moderate pulse is taken as a slow one, crisis may crop up instantly. In addition, there are cases where several different kinds of pulse images appear all at once or several different categories of disease may exhibit the same type of pulse.

Life hangs on the practice of medicine. Even the most excellent of physicians, (Yi) He[1] and Bian Que, had to deliberate (before they arrived at a correct diagnosis. Zhang) Zhong-jing was truly judicious and clear-minded, but he (nevertheless) had to examine the form and signs (other than the pulse). If there was even a shred of doubt, he studied every factor to get confirmation. In his *Shang Han ([Treatise] on Cold Damage)*,[2] for example, there are admonitions about *Cheng Qi Tang* (Support the Qi Decoction)[3] recording the necessity of questioning about the lower burner before treating retching and vomiting.[4] The writings left by the predecessors are pregnant with such far-reaching imports that only a few in later generations have been able to practice them, and the

---

[1] Yi He, an outstanding physician of the Qin kingdom in the Spring and Autumn period, lived around the 6th century BCE. He was the first person to advance the theory of the movements of the six qi.

[2] This is a work by Zhang Zhong-jing specializing in the treatment of febrile disease. It is the *locus classicus* of the theory of treating based on six apsect pattern discrimination.

[3] There are several different kinds of *Cheng Qi Tang* (Support the Qi Decoction), the common ones being *Da* (Major), *Xiao* (Minor), and *Tiao Wei* (Balance the Stomach). Nevertheless, all are applied to the *yang ming* pattern of cold damage. Before prescribing any of these, one must be certain of the existence of internal repletion.

[4] Retching and vomiting can be treated in different ways. If due to repletion in the upper burner, for example, they should be treated with ejection. But if they are ascribed to the lower burner, that treatment is categorically incorrect.

arcana transmitted in the old classics are too abstruse and enigmatic to be divulged. Therefore, later students have been kept in the dark about the ins and outs (of the study of the pulse), and, alleging that the old classics are fallacious, they all egotistically vaunt their own competency. The result is that their treatments turn mild maladies into mortal diseases and inveterate infirmities into hopeless cases. Indeed there are such examples.

Now I have collected the essential and pithy discussions on the pulse from Qi Bo[5] down to Hua Tuo and have compiled these into ten books in which the origins and causes of the hundreds of diseases are handled in order of category with the comprehensive inclusion of sound, color, pattern, and pulse sign. I have drawn on and kept the various teachings of Wang (Sui), Ruan (Bing), Fu, Dai, Ge (Hui), Lu (Guang), and Zhang (Miao).[6] If one makes a careful and thorough study of this present work, probing into its subtleties, one may become a match to the ancient sages and there will be no premature death in the future.

---

[5] Qi Bo was a minister of the legendary Yellow Emperor specializing in medicine.

[6] All the persons mentioned in this sentence were accomplished physicians before the author.

Contents

BOOK NINE

BOOK TEN

BOOK ONE

Collated & edited by Honorary Minister Without Portfolio,
Curator of the Imperial Library,
Imperial Courier, and Senior Army Protector,
Lin Yi *et al.*

Chapter One

The Secrets of the Shapes & Images of the Pulses Under the Fingers
[24 Types]

The floating pulse is a pulse potent when felt with no pressure applied but impotent when felt with pressure applied.

The scallion-stalk pulse is a floating pulse, large but soft. It is empty in the middle but solid at the sides when pressure is applied. [It is said in another version to be a pulse absent directly under the (feeling) fingers but present at the sides.]

The surging pulse is a very large pulse [floating and large in another version] under the fingers.

The slippery pulse is a pulse coming and going fluently, running unobstructedly. It resembles the rapid pulse [floating yet forceful in another version; rolling like water in still another version].

The rapid pulse is a pulse coming and going abruptly and urgently[1] [beating 6-7 times in one respiration in another version; named an advancing (pulse) in yet another version].

The skipping pulse is a pulse coming and going rapidly with occasional interruption but having the ability to recover.

The bowstring pulse is a pulse absent when felt with no pressure applied but like a bowstring when felt with pressure applied [in another version, like a fully drawn bowstring and firm when pressure is applied; in yet another version, defined as floating and tight].

The tight pulse is an inflexible pulse like a tensely drawn rope [said in another version to feel irregular like a turning rope].

The deep pulse is a pulse impotent when felt with no pressure applied but potent when felt with pressure applied [said in another version to be absent unless heavy pressure is applied].

---

[1] The word *ji* or urgent in this context is difficult to translate succinctly. It refers to a pulse that is tight and bowstring but is also rapid like a racing pulse.

The hidden pulse is a pulse imperceptible till the fingers touch the bone with extremely heavy pressure [said in another version to be hardly (felt) pulsating under the fingers; in still another version, to be impotent when pressure is applied and absent when pressure is released; said in yet another version to be known as a deep pulse not emerging in the *guan*].

The drumskin [suspected to be firm instead] pulse, which is somewhat like the deep pulse, is replete, large, and long as well as a little bowstring. [The *Qian Jin Yi (Thousand [Taels of] Gold Wing)*[2] has the firm pulse instead of the drumskin.]

The replete pulse is a large and long pulse as well as a little strong, impressing stiffly on the (feeling) fingers [said in another version to be palpable at both the superficial and the deep levels].

The faint pulse is a very fine, soft pulse possibly bordering on expiry, sometimes there and sometimes not [said in another version to be small; in still another to be quick under the fingers; in yet another to be floating and thin; in still another to come almost to an end when pressure is applied].

The choppy pulse is a fine and slow pulse, coming and going with difficulty and scattered or with an interruption but the ability to recover [said in another version to be floating and short; in still another version to be short with interruption or scattered].

The fine pulse is a little larger pulse than the faint pulse, a pulse constantly present yet thin.

The soft pulse is a very soft pulse as well as floating and thin [said in another version to be absent when pressure is applied but potent when pressure is released; in still another version to be small and soft; soggy instead of weak in yet another, where the soggy pulse is said to be like the clothes in water which are reachable only to a gentle hand].

The weak pulse is a very soft, deep, and fine pulse bordering on expiry under the (feeling) fingers when pressure is applied [said in another version to be impalpable unless pressure is applied and absent when pressure is released].

The vacuous pulse is a slow, large, and limp pulse, impotent when felt with pressure applied and giving the (feeling) fingers an impression of wide hollowness.

The dissipated pulse is a large yet scattered pulse. The dissipated pulse is an indication of qi

---

[2] See note 17 to the Preface by Gao Bao-heng *et al.*

repletion but blood vacuity, presence (*i.e.,* repletion) in the exterior but absence (*i.e.,* vacuity) in the interior.

The moderate pulse[3] is also a pulse slow in coming and going but a little faster than the slow pulse [said in another version to be floating and large but soft, equally floating in the yin and yang (*i.e.,* the *cun* and *chi*)].

The slow pulse is a pulse that beats three times for one respiration, very slow in coming and going [said in another version to be impotent when felt with no pressure applied but firm throughout when pressure is applied; in still another version to be firm throughout when pressure is applied but absent when pressure is released].

The bound pulse is a pulse slow in coming and going with occasional interruption but the ability to recover. [A pulse slow in coming when pressure is applied with occasional interruption is called the yang bound pulse. That which is stirring with interruption at first, small and rapid later, without the ability to recover, and stirring when pressure is relieved is called the yin bound pulse.]

The interrupted pulse is a pulse with regular interruption and inability to recover itself, resuming to beat (only after a long pause). The bound pulse is prognosticative of survival but the interrupted one of death.

The stirring pulse is a pulse that appears merely in the *guan,* a pulse with no ends, as large as a bean[4] stirring and rotating in a small way. [The *Shang Han Lun (Treatise on Cold Damage)* says: "Contention between yin and yang is called stirring. A stirring (pulse) in the yang (*i.e.,* superficial level) points to sweating, while a stirring (pulse) in the yin (*i.e.,* deep level) points to generation of heat (internally) with a cold body and aversion to cold. A rapid pulse that is perceptible only in the *guan* with no ends in the upper or lower position (*i.e.,* the *cun* or *chi*) and which is as large as a bean stirring and rotating in a small way is called a stirring pulse."]

---

3   To a Chinese, a *huan mai* or moderate pulse connotes both a non-impetuous pulse image, thus suggesting freedom from disease, but also a pulse which is a little slow and which usually does indicate a pathological condition.

4   Recently, sections of the *Mai Jing* have been unearthed in the Dun Huang Grottoes. Because they date from the Tang dynasty, they are considered more authentic than other extant versions which were all published later. In those sections it says "like a soybean" in place of the phrase "as large as a bean." To the translator, the Dun Huang version sounds more logical because the description is of the stirring image rather than of the size of the pulse. "No ends" in this context means that the pulse is impalpable in the *cun* and *chi.*

The floating and scallion-stalk [suspected to be surging] pulses are similar to one another. The bowstring and tight are similar to one another. The slippery and rapid are similar to one another. The drumskin and replete are similar to one another. [The *Qian Jin Yi* says, "The firm and replete are similar to one another".] The deep and hidden are similar to one another. The faint and choppy are similar to one another. The limp and weak are similar to one another. The moderate and slow are similar to one another [the soft and slow are similar to one another].

_______________ Chapter Two _______________
Choosing Between Morning & Evening
in Examining the Pulse

The Yellow Emperor asked:

Why is the pulse usually examined in the early morning?

Qi Bo answered:

Early in the morning, the yin qi is not yet stirred up, while the yang qi is not yet dissipated. No food has yet been taken. The channels and vessels are not yet exuberant, and the vessel networks are harmonious and in equilibrium. The blood and qi are not yet out of order. Therefore, (morning) is the appropriate (time) for pulse examination. Later than that time, it is not proper. [The *Qian Jin* agrees (with this explanation). The *Su Wen* and *Tai Su* say, "(Therefore, it is easy) to identify the faulty pulse (in the morning)."]

While examining the changes of the pulse, one should look into the bright essence (*i.e.*, the eyes), study the five colors, and observe the surplus and insufficiency of the five viscera, the strength and weakness of the six bowels, and exuberance and debility of the constitutional form. Cross-referencing all of these helps decide between life and death.

The Delineation of the Boundaries Between the Three Passes[1] & What These Pulse Images Govern

From the fish's margin[2] to the prominent bone[3], one *cun* proximal to the bone [which is conspicuous], is named the *cun* opening. From the *cun* to the *chi* is called the Cubit Marsh (*Chi Ze*). This is why (the pulse here) is spoken of as the *chi cun*.[4] (The position) proximal to the *cun* but distal to the *chi*, it is named the *guan*. It serves as the dividing line between emerging yang and submerging yin.[5] Emerging yang takes three shares and submerging yin also takes three shares.[6] Therefore, it is said that there are three yin and three yang. Yang is engendered in the *chi* but presents itself in the *cun*, while yin is engendered in the *cun* but presents itself in the *chi*. The *cun*

---

[1] A pass is a passageway for qi to go through, and, in this context, the three passes specifically refer to the three positions or divisions of the wrist pulse. One should note that the term *cun* opening or simply the *cun*, derived from the word meaning inch, may refer either to the wrist pulse as a whole or to the position distal to the *guan* division of the pulse. It also deserves note that the *chi*, derived from the word meaning foot as a unit of measurement, sometimes refers to the position proximal to the *guan* and sometimes to the whole distance from the *guan* to Cubit Marsh (*Chi Ze*, Lu 5).

[2] The fish's margin is the thenar eminence.

[3] This is the radial styloid process.

[4] The term *chi cun* is synonymous with the *cun* opening or the wrist pulse. The implication is that, if one measures from thenar eminence to the point Cubit Marsh, one *cun* is left after ruling off one *chi*. From the fish's margin to Cubit Marsh is 11 body inches or 1.1 *chi*. The *cun* opening takes up 1.9 *cun*.

[5] Here, yang is spoken of as emerging because it governs uprising or, in other words, the upper part of the body. Yin is spoken of as submerging because it governs downbearing or, in other words, the lower part of the body. In terms of the pulse, by analogy, the *chi* is yin where yang qi is supposed to be engendered, and the *cun* is yang where yin qi is supposed to be engendered. That is to say, yang qi starts in the *chi* but causes pulsation in the *cun*, while yin qi is generated in the *cun* but presents itself in the *chi*. In addition, the *chi* is called the lower as opposed to the *cun* which is called the upper. In terms of traditional Chinese medicine, the lower is synonymous with the internal, while the upper is synonymous with the external. Thus the concepts of emerging and submerging are easily accessible.

[6] There is a pun here in relation to the word share which implies division. Therefore, the word group "three shares" can be understood as the three divisions or positions of the wrist pulse. A share can be large or small. The yin qi and yang qi may thus take up a different share (of pulse qi?) depending on the particular physical and pathological condition so that the pulse gives varying pictures in terms of yin and yang in the three positions.

rules the upper burner, including the head, the skin and hair, and as far as the hands. The *guan* rules the middle burner, including the abdomen and the lumbar region. (And) the *chi* rules the lower burner, including the lower abdomen to the feet.

Chapter Four
Discriminating the Yin & Yang of the *Chi Cun* & the Measurement of the Circuits of the Constructive & Defensive

Since all the twelve channels each have their own pulsating vessels, why is the *cun* opening alone selected as the indicator for deciding (the conditions of) the five viscera and six bowels, death and life, and auspicious and ominous endings?

The answer is as follows: The *cun* opening is the grand rendezvous of the vessels. It is the pulsating vessel of the hand *tai yin*. In humans, during an exhalation, the pulse beats twice and the qi moves three *cun*. During an inhalation, the pulse beats twice more and the qi moves three *cun* more. During a whole process of respiration with the interval (in between breaths), the qi moves six *cun*. In humans, during a day and night, there are 135,000 respirations and (thus) qi travels 50 circuits around the body. During the time when the water in the clepsydra drops 100 gradations, the constructive and the defensive (qi) travel 25 circuits in yang and the same number of circuits in yin, making a whole cycle. Therefore, after 50 circuits, they return and gather at the hand *tai yin*. The *tai yin* means the *cun* opening which is the ending and beginning (place of the qi) of the five viscera and six bowels. For that reason, the *cun* opening is justifiably chosen (as the indicator).

There is a term *chi cun* in relation to the pulse. Why is it so termed?

The answer is as follows: The *chi cun* is the grand, important rendezvous of the vessels. From the *guan* to the Cubit Marsh (*Chi Ze*, Lu 5) is the sphere of the *chi* (cubit region), a place ruled by yin. From the *guan* to the fish's margin is the sphere of the *cun*, a place ruled by yang. Thus, taking off one *cun*, there is one *chi* left. Taking off one *chi*, there is one *cun*[1] left. (Practically, however,) yin

---

[1] See note 2 in the immediately preceding chapter.

occupies one *cun* in the *chi*, while yang takes up nine *fen* in the *cun*. The total length (of the pulse) from the beginning to the end is one *cun* and nine *fen*. Therefore it is called *chi cun*.

As regards the pulse, there are excess and inadequacy, overwhelming of yin and yang over one another, pouring and spillage,[2] and block and repulsion.[3] What do they mean?

The answer is as follows: Distal to the *guan*, that which beats is yang. This pulse ought to appear nine *fen* long and floating. If it exceeds (that length), it is technically called excess, and minus (that length), it is technically called inadequacy. It follows that (a pulse) reaching up to the fish's margin is known as spillage, a result of external block with internal repulsion.[4] This is a pulse of overwhelming yin. Proximal to the *guan*, that which beats is yin. This pulse ought to appear one *cun* long and deep. If it exceeds (that length), it is technically called excess, and minus (that length), it is technically called inadequacy. It follows that (a pulse) reaching into the *chi* (cubit region) is known as pouring, a result of internal block with external repulsion.[5] This is a pulse of overwhelming yang. There is reason to say that pouring and spillage are true visceral pulses.[6] In presence of them, people may die even if not (seemingly) diseased.

---

2 The distal position, *i.e.*, the *cun* is called the upper, while the *chi* is the lower. Therefore, if the pulse outreaches the *cun* position, this is analogous to water spilling over the brim, whereas when the pulse exceeds downward from the *chi*, it is likened to water pouring down.

3 This means that yin or yang becomes hyperactive and form block and repulsion one to the other.

4 This implies that yang qi is trapped in the exterior by exuberant yin qi.

5 This implies that yin qi is repulsed and stalled in the exterior by yang qi which takes up the interior.

6 The true visceral pulse is a pulse lacking in stomach qi. Stomach qi is that which modifies and moderates the pulse in any season. For example, the bowstring pulse is the liver pulse. In a liver problem, a bowstring pulse which is devoid of any quality of moderateness is a true visceral pulse and is an ominous sign. This means that it is lacking stomach qi, and having stomach qi is main prognosticative indicator in Chinese medicine.

The Method of Favorable & Unfavorable (Indications) in Pulse Examination (*Vis à Vis*) Large or Small, Long (*i.e.*, Tall) & Short, Male & Female Persons

When examining the pulse, it is necessary to take into consideration whether the person is large or small, long or short, and whether their nature's qi is moderate or impetuous. If the pulse, whether slow or quick, large or small, long or short, is in agreement with the form and nature of the person, it is auspicious. Otherwise it is ominous. The three positions of the pulse are inclined to be equal in size. For example, if the person is small, a female, or thin, the pulse is (accordingly) small and limp. If a child between four and five years has a pulse which beats 8 times per respiration and is fine and rapid, it is auspicious.

[The *Qian Jin Yi* says: "A large person with a thin pulse, a thin person with a large pulse, a happy person with a replete pulse, a misery-stricken person with a vacuous pulse, a quick temper with a moderate pulse, a moderate nature with an impetuous pulse, a robust person with a thin pulse, a thin person with a large pulse, all these are ominous, and ominous (conditions) are difficult to treat. Those opposite to the above is propitious. Propitious (conditions) are easy to treat. The pulses in females are inclined to be more soggy and weaker than in males. In children between four and five years of age, the pulse is fast, beating 8 times per respiration. For males, the left (pulse) being larger is favorable, while for females the right being larger is favorable. In corpulent persons, the pulse is deep and in thin persons, it is floating."]

__________Chapter Six__________

The Application of Light & Heavy Pressure in Feeling the Pulse

Examination of the pulse demands the application of light or heavy pressure. What does this imply? The answer is as follows: Initially, the pulse should be felt with a pressure amounting to the weight of three soybeans. This pressure penetrates the skin and hair and (reflects) the lungs. A pressure amounting to the weight of six soybeans reaches the blood vessels and (reflects) the heart. A pressure amounting to the weight of nine soybeans reaches the muscles and flesh and (reflects) the spleen. A pressure amounting to the weight of twelve soybeans reaches the level of the sinews and (reflects) the liver. (Finally,) press to the bone and then release the pressure. If then the pulse comes impetuously, this indicates the kidneys. This is what is meant by light and heavy pressure.

Chapter Seven

Yin & Yang and Favorable & Unfavorable (Conditions of) the Five Viscera & Six Bowels Ruled by the Six Pulses on Both Hands

The *Mai Fa Zan (A Panegyric on the Method of Pulse [Examination])*[1] says that the liver and heart (qi) emerge on the left hand, the spleen and lung (qi) on the right, and (the qi of) both the kidneys and life gate emerge in the *chi*. The ethereal soul (*hun*), corporeal soul (*po*), the grain and the spirit[2] all have their reflections in the *cun* opening. The left (pulse) rules and reflects the offices and the right rules and reflects the mansions.[3] (A pulse) larger on the left is favorable in males, while (a pulse) larger on the right is favorable in females. One *fen* distal to the *guan* is the governor of the human

---

[1]   This is a long-lost ancient medical classic on the pulse.

[2]   *Hun* refers to the liver and *po* to the lungs. Grain refers to the stomach qi or the spleen. The spirit is equivalent to the heart.

[3]   Concerning this reference to offices and mansions, there are different interpretations. The translator believes that the most plausible one has to do with the fact that, in Chinese culture, the left is believed to be superior to or more respectable than the right. Therefore, the viscera that the left pulse reflects are offices, while the viscera reflected by the right pulse are mansions. This point is made clear by the following comparison:
Heart (fire)-lung (metal); liver (wood) -spleen (earth); kidney (water)- life gate (ministerial fire).
The pairs are arranged in order of the *cun-guan-chi*, and the first viscus of each pair corresponds with a position on the left hand, while the second is relegated to the right hand.

life.[4] The left is called the *ren ying* (man's prognosis) and the right is the qi opening.[5] The spirit gates, which are located proximal to the *guan*, are decisive in prognosis. If a person exhibits no pulse in either of these positions, the disease will end in death without any possibility of recuperation.[6] The various channels all express their damage and reduction in their corresponding parts (of the pulse. One should) examine yin and yang and make certain which of them is first affected and (which is) later (affected). A yin disease should be treated through the offices, and a yang disease through the mansions.[7] Facing an unusual evil,[8] one should try to search out its location. If a careful study leads to knowledge (of the location), then once the needle is inserted, the disease will be cured.

The heart is assigned to the *cun* on the left hand, distal to the *guan*. The channel (of the heart) is the hand *shao yin* which stands in an interior/exterior relationship with the hand *tai yang*. (The heart) is united with the small intestine which is a bowel. (These two channels) meet in the upper burner at a point named Spirit Court (*Shen Ting*, GV 24). This is located five *fen* below Tortoise Tail (*Gui Wei*, GV 1) [Turtledove Tail, *Jiu Wei*, GV 15].[9]

The liver is assigned to the *guan* on the left hand. Its channel is the foot *jue yin* which stands in an interior/exterior relationship with the foot *shao yang*. (The liver) is united with the gallbladder

---

[4]   Because the *cun* on the left and right hands rule the heart and the lungs respectively and these are the most important viscera in terms of qi and blood, they are called the governor of life. "One *fen* distal to the *guan*" refers to the *cun*.

[5]   One should take special note that here the terms qi opening and *ren ying* are defined in a different way from the conventional concept. Here the qi opening refers to the *cun* of the right pulse, while the *ren ying* refers to the left *cun* of the wrist pulse rather than the pulse in the neck.

[6]   The spirit gates refer to the *chi* positions on both hands. Because the *chi* pulse indicates the kidneys and the life gate, both of which are vital to life, the pulses here merit particular attention. According to Wang Shu-he, the presence or absence of life qi can be determined mainly by the *chi* pulse. He called this the root of life.

[7]   Here it may be more reasonable to define offices as viscera and mansions as bowels.

[8]   Unusual evil here refers to any evil (qi).

[9]   Neither Spirit Court (*Shen Ting*, GV 24) nor Tortoise Tail (*Gui Wei*, GV 1) has anything to do with the channels mentioned in this passage. Therefore an error is suspected in the text. The note in brackets may be right. That is, the point may well be Turtledove Tail (*Jiu Wei*, GV 15).

12

which is a bowel. (These two channels) meet in the middle burner at a point named Bladder Gate (*Bao Men*), three *cun* bilateral to Supreme Granary (*Tai Cang*, CV 12).[10]

The kidneys are assigned to the *chi* on the left hand, proximal to the *guan*. Their channel is the foot *shao yin* which stands in an interior/exterior relationship with the foot *tai yang*. (The kidneys) are united with the urinary bladder which is a bowel. (These two channels) meet in the lower burner at a point located to the left of Origin Pass (*Guan Yuan*, CV 4).

The lungs are assigned to the *cun*, distal to the *guan* on the right hand. Their channel is the hand *tai yin* which stands in an interior/exterior relationship with the hand *yang ming*. (The lungs) are united with the large intestine which is a bowel. (These two channels) meet in the upper burner at a point named Mansion for Respiration located at Cloud Gate (*Yun Men*, Lu 2).

The spleen is assigned to the *guan* on the right hand. Its channel is the foot *tai yin* which stands in an interior/exterior relationship with the foot *yang ming*. (The spleen) is united with the stomach which is a bowel. (These two channels) meet in the middle burner at a point between the spleen and the stomach, named Camphorwood Gate (*Zhang Men*, Liv 13). This is located one and a half *cun* anterior to the (last) free rib.

The kidneys are assigned to the *chi* on the right hand, proximal to the *guan*. Their channel is the foot *shao yin* which stands in an interior/exterior relationship with the foot *tai yang*. (The kidneys) are united with the urinary bladder which is a bowel. (These two channels) meet in the lower burner at a place located to the right of Origin Pass (*Guan Yuan*, CV 4). The left (*chi*) is ascribed to the kidneys, while the right to the infant door which is also called the triple burner.[11]

---

[10] Here is a problem similar to that pointed out in note 9 above. Bladder Gate (*Bao Men*, CV 4) is far apart from Supreme Granary (*Tai Cang*, CV 12).

[11] It is suspected that this last passage has become garbled to the point that some points in it are quite confusing.

The Great Method of Distinguishing Visceral & Bowel Diseases (*Vis à Vis*) Yin & Yang Pulses

How can the pulse give information about the disease of the viscera and bowels? The answer is as follows: The rapid (pulse) points to the bowels, while the slow (pulse) indicates the viscera. A rapid pulse shows existence of heat and a slow pulse shows generation of cold. The various yang (pulses) are indications of heat, while the various yin (ones) are indications of cold. The diseases of the viscera and the bowels are thus made known and distinguished. [The bowels are yang. So their (disease) pulses are rapid. While the viscera are yin. So their (disease) pulses are slow. Yang moves slowly, but, when there is disease, it moves rapidly. Yin moves rapidly, but, when there is disease, it moves slowly.][1]

A pulse arriving large and floating is the lung pulse. A pulse arriving deep and slippery like a stone is the kidney pulse. A pulse arriving like a bowstring is the liver pulse. A pulse swift in coming but slow in retreating is the heart pulse. A pulse (image) which ought to but does not appear indicates disease.[2] Disease may lie deep or shallow, but one should know the way how the evil is contracted.

---

[1] Understanding why the pathological pulse of the bowels is rapid and the pathological pulse of the viscera is slow has been a controversial question for centuries. However, classification of the various pulse qualities into yin and yang categories is instructive, and it is taken as the headrope for grasping the complicated system of the pulse.

[2] This sentence implies that, in a certain season, a typical pulse is expected. In summer, for example, the pulse should be surging. If it is not, disease is indicated.

The Great Method of Distinguishing
Yin & Yang Pulses

There is a yin-yang approach to the pulse. What is it? The answer is as follows: Exhalation is (the affair of) the heart and lungs, and inhalation is (the affair of) the kidneys and liver. Between exhalation and inhalation, is (the affair of) the spleen which receives the flavor of grains, and its pulse is in the center.[1] A floating (pulse) is yang, while a deep (pulse) is yin. Yin and yang are thus defined.

(The pulses of) the heart and the lung are both floating. Then how to distinguish them? The answer is as follows. A pulse not only floating but large and dissipated is the heart pulse, while a pulse not only floating but short and choppy is the lung pulse.

(The pulses of) the kidneys and the liver are both deep. Then how to distinguish them? The answer is as follows. A firm and long pulse is the liver pulse; the kidney pulse is soft when pressure is applied but comes replete when the fingers are lifted. The spleen lies in the central country; so its pulse is in the center. [The *Qian Jin Yi* says, "Slow, moderate and long is the spleen pulse."] This is the yin-yang approach (to the pulse).

There are pulses of exuberant yang but vacuous yin or of exuberant yin but vacuous yang. What are they like? The answer is as follows. (A pulse) reduced (in force) and small at the superficial level but replete and large at the deep level is justifiably known as exuberant in yin but vacuous of yang. (A pulse) reduced and small at the deep level but replete and large at the superficial level is justifiably known as exuberant in yang but vacuous of yin. This is what is meant by vacuity and repletion of yin and yang (in terms of the pulse).

It is stated in the classic[2] that there are pulses of one yin with one yang, one yin with two yang,

---

[1]   Besides the sense of being located in the middle position of the wrist pulse, the phrase, in the center, may have either of two other meanings. One meaning is neither floating nor deep. The other is that the pulse has a moderate quality. Moderateness is typical of the spleen-stomach pulse. This quality should always be manifest as a modifier of a pulse image peculiar to a certain season or a certain viscus.

[2]   This refers to the *Nan Jing (The Classic of Difficulties)*.

or one yin with three yang, and pulses of one yang with one yin, one yang with two yin, or one yang with three yin. Does such a statement mean that in the *cun* opening there are six pulses beating simultaneously? The answer is as follows. When the classic states this, (it does not mean that) there are six pulses beating simultaneously. It refers to floating, deep, long, short, slippery, and choppy (pulse images). The floating is yang, the slippery is yang, and the long is yang. The deep is yin, the choppy is yin, and the short is yin. That which justifies the reference of one yin with one yang is that the pulse arrives deep yet slippery. One yin with two yang speaks of a pulse arriving deep, yet slippery and long. One yin with three yang speaks of a pulse arriving floating, slippery, and long but occasionally deep. That which justifies the reference of one yang with one yin is that the pulse arrives floating but choppy. One yang with two yin speaks of a pulse arriving long but deep and choppy. One yang with three yin speaks of a pulse arriving deep, choppy, and short but occasionally floating. One can make a favorable or unfavorable prognosis of a disease in light of the position of the involved channel (in the wrist pulse).

In terms of the pulse, the large is yang, the floating is yang, the rapid is yang, the stirring is yang, the long is yang, and the slippery is yang. The deep is yin, the choppy is yin, the weak is yin, the bowstring is yin, and the faint is yin. These are composed of three yin and three yang (pulses).[3] A yin pulse appearing in a yang disease is adverse, ruling death. A yang pulse appearing in a yin disease is favorable, ruling life (*i.e.*, survival).

Distal to the *guan* is yang, while proximal to the *guan* is yin. If the pulse in the yang (position) is rapid, ejection of blood is indicated. If the pulse in the yin is rapid, diarrhea is indicated. If the pulse in the yang (position) is bowstring, headache is indicated. If the pulse in the yin is bowstring, abdominal pain is indicated. If the pulse in the yang (position) is faint, exuding of sweat is indicated. If the pulse in the yin is faint, loose stools are indicated. If the pulse in the yang (position) is rapid, sores grow at the mouth. If the pulse in the yin is rapid as well as faint, there must be aversion to cold and vexation and agitation with inability to sleep.

When yin is subjugated to yang,[4] mania arises. When yang is subjugated to yin, withdrawal arises. If a yang (pulse) is ever found, this is ascribed to the bowels, while a yin (pulse) if ever

---

[3] The pulse is divided into three positions, and each of the three may present a distinctive image of yin-yang quality. Thus there are three yin and three yang.

[4] Yin here means the *chi* position, while yang refers to the *cun*. A deep pulse, for example, is a yin pulse. This is most commonly felt in the *chi* (yin) in normal cases. If the *cun* (yang) presents a deep pulse, then this is called yang subjugated by yin, while subjugation of yin by yang is the just reverse.

found is ascribed to the viscus. In the absence of yang,[5] inversion arises. In the absence of yin,[5] retching arises. If the pulse in the yang (position) is faint, there is inability to exhale. If the pulse in the yin (position) is faint, there is inability to inhale. When there is inadequacy of respiration, there is shortness of qi in the chest. (One should) examine disease in light of this yin and yang (approach).

If the pulse is floating, large, and racing in the *cun*, this is called yang within yang. The diseases include the bitterness (*i.e.*, suffering) of distressing fullness, body heat, headache, and heat inside the abdomen.

If the pulse is deep and fine in the *cun*, this is called yin within yang. The diseases include the bitterness of susceptibility to sorrow, melancholy, aversion to people's voice, diminished qi, occasional (spontaneous) sweating, inhibited yin qi, and inability to lift the arms.

If the pulse is deep and fine in the *chi*, this is called yin within yin. The diseases include the bitterness of aching pain in the lower legs, inability to stand for long, debilitated yin qi, dribbling of urine at the end of voiding, and damp, itchy genitals.

If the pulse is slippery, floating, and large in the *chi*, this is called yang within yin. The diseases include the bitterness of lower abdominal pain and fullness, inability to void urine, pain arising inside the genitals on voiding, and analogous trouble with defecation.

If the pulse is firm and long in the *chi* but absent from the *guan*, this is yin interfering with yang. The person's bitterness includes heaviness of the lower legs and lower abdominal pain radiating to the lumbar region.

If the pulse is strong and large in the *cun* but absent from the *chi*, this is yang interfering with yin. The bitterness includes upper and lower back pain, injured genitals, and cold in the feet and lower legs.

Wind brings damage to yang, while cold to yin. In a disease of yang nature, yin may be unaffected, while in a disease of yin nature, yang is involved. (Therefore,) yang disease is easy to treat and yin disease is difficult. (If a disease) lies between the stomach and the intestines, it can be treated by means of harmonizing with medication. If the disease lies in the channels and vessels, acupuncture and moxibustion can effect a cure.

---

[5] Absence of yang refers to a pulse which is impalpable in the *cun* (yang) position, while absence of yin refers to a pulse which is impalpable in the *chi* (yin) position.

Chapter Ten

A Discussion of Vacuity & Repletion

There are three kinds of vacuity and repletion in humans. What are they? The answer is as follows: There is vacuity and repletion of the pulse, vacuity and repletion of disease, and vacuity and repletion of manifestations. In terms of vacuity and repletion of the pulse, that which arrives soft is a vacuous pulse, while that which is firm is a replete one. In terms of vacuity and repletion of disease, that which causes exit is vacuity, while that which invades is repletion.[1] That with ability to talk is vacuity, while that with no speech is repletion.[2] That slow (in advancing) is vacuity, while that swift (in advancing) is repletion. In terms of vacuity and repletion of manifestations, itching is a sign of vacuity, while pain of repletion. Pain in the exterior with ease of the interior shows external repletion with internal vacuity. Pain in the interior with ease of the exterior shows internal repletion with external vacuity. These are what is meant by vacuity and repletion.

(The Yellow Emperor) asked:

What do vacuity and repletion mean?

(Qi Bo) answered:

Exuberance of evil qi is repletion, and retrenchment of essence qi is vacuity. What is dual repletion? So-called dual repletion means great heat disease. Since the qi is hot and the pulse is full, this is called dual repletion.

(The Yellow Emperor) asked:

What is meant by repletion of both the channels and the vessel networks and how to treat them?

(Qi Bo) answered:

---

[1] That which causes exit refers to an exhausting illness. In this case, essence and qi are forced out of the body in such a disorder. An invading problem means invasion of exogenous evils.

[2] A disease with ability to talk implies a chronic one, while a disease in which the patient is silent is more often an acute disease where replete evils have rendered the patient voiceless or deprived them of the ability to speak.

Repletion of both the channels and the vessel networks is shown by an urgent pulse in the *cun* opening with the cubit (skin) relaxed. (In this case,) both the channels and the vessel networks should be treated. It follows that slipperiness is favorable, while roughness is unfavorable.[3] Vacuity and repletion can be determined by analogy to similar things. If the five viscera and the bones and flesh are slippery and smooth, a long life may be maintained.

———————————————————

[3] Slipperiness here means that the wrist pulse is slippery and the cubit skin well lubricated, while roughness means that the wrist pulse is choppy and the cubit skin rough and coarse.

———————————Chapter Eleven———————————
Sequential & Rebellious, Counter & Natural, Latent & Hidden Pulses

(The Yellow Emperor) asked:

In terms of the pulse, restraint may be called sequential, rebellious, counter, or natural. What does this mean?

The master answered:

If the water phase restrains fire (or) the metal phase restrains wood, this is called sequential. If the fire phase restrains water (or) the wood phase restrains metal, this is called rebellious. If the water phase restrains metal (or) the fire phase restrains wood, this is called counter. If the metal phase restrains water (or) the wood phase restrains fire, this is called natural.

The classic says that the pulse can be latent or hidden. Then in which viscus is (the evil) hidden when (a pulse) is spoken of as latent? The answer is as follows. (Latency) means that yin and yang restrain reciprocally and may have to hide in one another. When the pulse located in the yin (*i.e.*, the *chi*) presents contrarily a yang image, this is yang restraining yin. Even though the pulse may be occasionally deep, choppy, and short, this is but yin hidden within yang. If the pulse in the yang (*i.e.*, the *cun*) presents contrarily a yin image, this is yin restraining yang. Even though it is occasionally floating, slippery, and long, this is but yang hidden within yin.

A double yin pulse reflects withdrawal. A double yang pulse reflects mania.[1]

Yin desertion leads to illusion of ghosts; yang desertion to blindness.[2]

---

[1] A double yin pulse refers to two yin pulse images, for instance a short and vacuous pulse, manifesting in both the *chi* and *cun*, while a double yang pulse refers to two yang pulse images, for example a large and surging pulse, appearing in both the *chi* and *cun*.

[2] Yin desertion is severe loss of essence, while yang desertion is severely injured and exhausted yang qi.

_____________Chapter Twelve_____________
Discrimination of the Miscellaneous Pulses of Catastrophic Oddness and Fear & Apprehension

(The Yellow Emperor) asked:

What is the pulse of murderous evil?

The master answered:

If the pulse is bowstring, tight, choppy, slippery, floating, or deep, these six (pulse images) point to murderous evils which are capable of causing disease in various channels.

(The Yellow Emperor) asked:

(I) was once perplexed by someone asking how a tight pulse arises.

The master answered:

Suppose there is sweat collapse (*i.e.*, massive perspiration) or vomiting (due to) cold in the lungs, the pulse will become tight. Suppose there is coughing due to drinking cold water, the pulse will become tight. Suppose there is diarrhea due to vacuity cold in the stomach, the pulse will become tight.

(The Yellow Emperor) asked:

(A pulse) emerging swiftly followed by falling is called slippery.[1] What does this imply?

The master answered:

Falling is pure yin, while emerging is righteous yang. When yin and yang are in harmony and cooperate, the pulse is slippery.

(The Yellow Emperor) asked:

What is meant by a catastrophic odd pulse?

The master answered:

Suppose a person is ill. (A physician) perceives a pulse of the *tai yang* (pattern),[2] and the pulse is in congruity with the disease pattern and signs. Accordingly, a decoction is prepared, but when (the physician) comes back with the prepared decoction, the patient is observed to have drastic vomiting or diarrhea with the illness of abdominal pain. (The physician) may say, "I didn't see this pattern when I first came to examine the pulse." Now (the condition) has become strange. This is spoken of as catastrophic oddness. If one asks what has caused this vomiting and diarrhea, then the answer may be that (the patient) has taken some medicinals before and they are just now starting up (the new trouble). Therefore, a catastrophic oddness is given rise to.

(The Yellow Emperor) asked:

What kind of pulse will appear when a person is diseased by fear and apprehension?

The master answered:

The pulse feels as if touching a thread. It beats continuously without a break, and (the patient) has a white face of desertion color.

(The Yellow Emperor) asked:

What sort of pulse will appear when one is ashamed?

The master answered:

---

[1] In this context, the slippery pulse should be understood as a normal pulse.

[2] The *tai yang* pattern is the first stage in a cold damage disease, mainly manifesting as aversion to cold, fever, rigidity of the nape of the neck, headache, a floating pulse, and thin, white tongue fur.

The pulse is invariably floating and weak, and the face looks suddenly (*i.e.*, sometimes) white and suddenly red.

(The Yellow Emperor) asked:

What kind of pulse will appear if one has not drunk water (for a long time)?

The master answered:

The pulse will inevitably become choppy and the lips and mouth dry.

Sluggish speech suggests wind. Head-shaking while speaking suggests internal pain. Sluggish movement suggests exuberance of exterior (evils). Leaning forward while sitting suggests shortness of breath. Sitting with one leg extended suggests pain in the lower back. Protecting the stomach as if keeping an egg in the case of internal repletion is invariably (a reflection of) heart pain. If the person yawns while the physician is feeling his pulse, (the patient) is free of disease. If the sick person stretches [groans in another version] while his pulse is being felt, he is free of disease.

If (the patient) lies facing the wall, but does not rise up in a start, just casting a squint [looking up in another version] when they hear the physician come or if (they) falter and swallow down saliva while their pulse is being felt, they are feigning being ill. As long as the pulse is tranquil all the time, one can declare this is a very severe illness requiring administration of emetics and purgatives. (Together with medication,) needling or moxaing tens of or a hundred points will send him to recovery.

————————Chapter Thirteen————————
The Method (of Discriminating) the Miscellaneous Slow, Rapid, Long & Short Pulses

The Yellow Emperor asked:

I have learned the pulse examination method in relation to the stomach qi, the triple burner of the hand *shao yang*, the four seasons, and the five phases. People say that the pulse is (also) classified into three yin and three yang and, (in light of them,) one may know the presence or absence of disease. Through externally feeling the pulse, one may acquire a knowledge of the internal, (judging by) the largeness and smallness of the *chi* and *cun*. I would like to hear about this.

Qi Bo answered:

Within the *cun* opening, there is the division of superficial and deep levels, the proximal and distal positions, and the left and right sides. The essentials (of determining) vacuity or repletion, life or death all lie within the *cun* opening.

A (pathological) pulse reveals a repletion evil if (the pulse) arises from its antecedent (phase), a vacuity evil if it arises from its posterior (phase), a murderous evil if it arises from its restraining (phase), and a slight evil if it arises from its restrained (phase).[1] The evil may (also) be a righteous one if (the viscus) is diseased by its own.[2]

External binding (of evils) gives rise to the illness of *yong*[3] swelling, and internal binding (of evils) to the disease of *shan* conglomeration.[4] If the pulse becomes occasionally urgent, there is a disease right in the heart. This is concretion qi. If the pulse is racing, it points to wind. If the pulse is slippery, it points to a disease of food (accumulation). If the pulse is slippery and agitated, it points to a disease of heat. If the pulse arrives choppy, it points to a disease of cold dampness. The *dao* of the normal and abnormal pulses cannot be discussed among the populace (;they should only be imparted to the worthy).

---

[1] When speaking of the five phases, the child, for example water, is called the antecedent in terms of metal, the mother. Thus an illness of lung metal transmitted from kidney water, for example, should be replete in nature. Conversely, an illness of kidney water transmitted from lung metal should be vacuous in nature.
If an illness of a viscus, for example liver wood, is transmitted from its restraining viscus, lung metal, then the illness is called a murderous evil and is understood to be a grave trouble. On the contrary, if the illness of liver wood is transmitted from spleen earth, *i.e.*, the phase restrained by liver wood, the disorder is but a slight ailment.
The above interrelationships between the five phases can also be applied to the pulse. Judging by the pulse, if there is heart trouble as evidenced by a surging pulse and if disease has been transmitted from liver wood, then this is a repletion evil.

[2] The term, righteous evil, implies merely that pathogens are limited to the viscus where they have originally arisen.

[3] *Yong* is a general term for an acute, localized, suppurative, inflammatory lesion of the skin and subcutaneous tissues or of the internal organs.

[4] Masses in the lower abdomen are known as *shan* in males but conglomerations in females. They are usually accompanied by pain.

The master explained:

Respiration is a yardstick for the pulse. If the pulse is at first felt to be racing in coming but slow in departing, this shows that (the qi) exits racing but enters slowly.[5] This reveals internal vacuity but external repletion. If the pulse is at first felt to be slow in coming but racing in departing, this shows that (the qi) exits slowly but enters racing. This reveals internal repletion but external vacuity.

A rapid pulse is ascribed to the bowels and a slow pulse to the viscera. A long, bowstring pulse shows there is an illness in the liver. If the pulse is small with shortage of blood, disease is located in the heart. [Bian Que says, "A large and surging pulse points to illness arising from the heart."] If the pulse is hard in the lower (*i.e.*, the *guan*) but vacuous in the upper (*i.e.*, the *cun*), there is disease in the spleen and stomach. If the pulse is slippery and slightly floating, there is disease in the lungs. If the pulse is large and hard, there is disease in the kidneys. [Bian Que says, "If the pulse is small and tight..."] A slippery pulse shows abundant blood but scanty qi. A choppy pulse shows scanty blood but abundant qi. A large pulse shows abundance of both blood and qi.

It is also said that if a pulse arrives large and hard, there is a repletion of both blood and qi. If it arrives small, both blood and qi are scanty. Again, it is said that if a pulse arrives fine and faint, there is a vacuity of both blood and qi. A deep, fine, slippery, and racing pulse indicates heat. A slow and tight pulse indicates cold. [It is said in another version that a rapid, slippery, (or) surging pulse indicates heat; a choppy, slow, deep, (or) fine pulse indicates cold.] If the pulse is exuberant, slippery, and tight, there is disease in the external and it is heat. If the pulse is small, replete, and tight, there is disease in the internal and it is cold. A small, weak, and choppy pulse tells of an enduring disease, while a slippery, floating, and racing pulse tells of a disease of recent onset.

If the pulse is slippery and floating, the sick person is suffering from external heat and migratory wind giving pricking pain. If rheum exists (in addition), this is difficult to treat. If the pulse is deep and tight, there is heat in the upper burner and cold in the lower (burner). If cold is (further) contracted, there will instantly arise diarrhea. If the pulse is deep and fine, there is cold in the lower burner giving rise to frequent voidings of urine and, from time to time, there is the bitterness of gripping pain (in the lower abdomen), dysentery, and pressure in the rectum. If the pulse is floating and tight as well as slippery and straight, there is heat externally and cold internally with inability to urinate and defecate.

---

[5] The pulse when it is rising is yang, while the pulse while it is falling is yin. These correspond respectively to the entrance and exiting of the pulse qi. It follows that exiting of the pulse qi, *i.e.*, yang, and entrance of the pulse qi, *i.e.*, yin, are matched with the exterior and the interior. Furthermore, as rapidity is an indication of repletion, whereas slowness reveals vacuity, a pulse which is slow in coming but quick in leaving shows internal vacuity and external repletion.

If the pulse is surging, large, tight, and urgent, the disease is advancing rapidly in the external. The bitterness includes heat in the head with *yong* swelling. If the pulse is thin, small, tight, and urgent, the disease is advancing rapidly in the center manifesting as *shan* conglomeration, gatherings and accumulations, and pricking pain in the abdomen due to cold (internally). If the pulse is very deep, arriving straight but coming to a stop suddenly, the disease is blood (stasis) inside the intestines. If the pulse is very deep and becomes dissipated half way, (this shows) concretions developing from eating cold (food). If the pulse arrives straight but becomes dissipated (and/or) expired half way, there is the disease of wasting thirst [disease of diffusing pain in another version]. If the pulse is very deep and unable to reach the *cun* distally, just faltering (in the *guan* and *chi*) and then coming to a stop, there is disease in the muscles and flesh. This is called lingering cadaver.[6] If the pulse twists to the left and is very deep, there is qi concretion due to yang (evils gathered) in the chest. If the pulse twists to the right and is unable to reach the *cun*, there are flesh concretions internally. If the pulse goes on without a break like a string of pearls and is unable to reach the distal position, there is wind cold in the large intestine which lies deep and persistent. If the pulse goes on (like a string of pearls) yet pauses (occasionally) and is limp in the *cun*, there is heat bound and persisting in the membranes of the small intestine. If the pulse comes forward striking (forcefully) against its right and left sides, there is disease in the blood vessels. (The pathogen is) dead coagulated blood. If the pulse strikes against its right and left sides in the proximal position, there is disease in the sinews and bones. If the pulse is large in the distal position and small in the proximal, this shows headache and visual dizziness. If the pulse is small in the distal position but large in the proximal, this shows chest fullness and shortness of breath. If the pulse is present in the upper (*i.e.*, the *cun*) but absent from the lower (*i.e.*, the *chi*), the (sick) person ought to suffer from vomiting. If not, (the sick person) will die. If the pulse is absent from the upper but present in the lower, there is nothing to worry about, although there is indeed some trouble.

Since the pulse is the mansion of blood, the qi is in a good state if the pulse is long, but diseased if the pulse is short. A rapid pulse points to heart vexation; a large one to advance of disease. If the pulse is exuberant in the upper, there is shallow breathing. If it is exuberant in the lower, there is qi distention. A regularly interrupted pulse indicates debilitated qi. A fine pulse suggests diminished qi [slippery instead of fine in the *Tai Su*].[7] A choppy pulse suggests heart pain. If the

---

[6] This is a pattern of pathogens lingering in the flesh. In a fit, the patient will suffer from distention, fullness, and pricking pain in the chest and abdomen accompanied by gasping for breath and qi attacking the flanks and surging up into the chest and heart. This condition is so named because the fit recurs repeatedly and makes the patient suffer a lot.

[7] This is a very old version of the *Nei Jing* (*Inner Classic*) collated and annotated by Yang Shang- shan living between the Sui and Tang dynasties.

pulse is rolling impetuously like a gushing spring, the disease is not only advancing but is dangerous. If the pulse is obscure and sluggish and goes off like an abruptly severed string, death will ensue. If the pulse is short and urgent, the disease is in the upper (part of the body). If it long and slow, the disease is located in the lower. If it is deep as well as bowstring and urgent, the disease is in the internal. If it is floating as well as large and surging, the disease is in the external. If it is replete, the disease is in the internal. If it is vacuous, the disease is in the external. The distal position is ascribed to the exterior; the proximal to the interior. A floating pulse is ascribed to the exterior, and a sinking one to the interior.

Chapter Fourteen
A Discussion on How Diseases Arise in Normal Persons

How can one know in spring whether a disease is contracted? Absence of the liver pulse.[1] In summer, absence of the heart pulse suggests contraction of disease. In autumn, absence of the lung pulse suggests contraction of disease. In winter, absence of the kidney pulse suggests contraction of disease. In the last month of each of the four seasons, absence of the spleen pulse suggests contraction of disease.[2]

Take liver disease. One may contract it if one travels westward or eats chicken. It will start up in the season of autumn. It is contracted on the days of *geng* or *xin*.[3] Aquatic food in the house will

---

[1] The liver pulse is bowstring. The heart pulse is racing. The lung pulse is floating and soft. The kidney pulse is sunken or deep. And the spleen pulse is moderate. The liver is associated with spring; the heart with summer, etc. In each season, the presence of the pulse of a corresponding viscus is an indication of health. In spring, for example, the pulse should be somewhat bowstring in normal persons. If it is not, the liver pulse is said to be absent.

[2] Each of the five viscera except the spleen is supposed to govern one of the four seasons, while the last month of each season is allotted to the spleen for it to govern. In these last months of each seasons, one should feel the spleen pulse which is characterized by its moderateness.

[3] These Chinese words are the names of the ten Heavenly Stems. Each of these ten stems are correlated to one of the days in the ten day cycle of the traditional Chinese calendar. Because the tens stems are divided into the five phases, two days out of each ten are ascribed to the same phase. Thus disease may arise on either of the two days associated with the phase in question. The five phase ascriptions of the ten stems

cause death (in such cases). The appearance of a woman may bring disaster. In cases other than the above, (the disease) may be contracted as a result of acquisition of gold or silver objects.[4]

Take spleen disease. One may contract it if one travels eastward or eats pheasant, hare meat, or the fruits of various trees. In cases other than the above, it ought to start up in the season of spring. It is contracted on the days of *jia* or *yi*.[3]

Take heart disease. One may contract it if one travels northward or eats pork or fish. In cases other than the above, it ought to start up in the season of winter. It is contracted on the days of *ren* or *gui*.[3]

Take lung disease. One may contract it if one travels southward or eats horse or deer meat. In cases other than the above, it ought to start up in the season of summer. It is contracted on the days of *bing* or *ding*.[3]

Take kidney disease. One may contract it if one travels to the central (region) or eats beef or produce from the ground. In cases other than the above, it ought to start up in the long summer (*i.e.*, the last month of summer). It is contracted on the days of *wu* or *ji*.[3]

If one finds a king's (*i.e.*, exuberant) pulse, it should be found in the house of the sheriff. If one finds a minister's (*i.e.*, harmonious) pulse, it should be found in a house where a wedding or celebration is held. If one finds a fetal (*i.e.*, pregnant) pulse, it should be found in the house where birth will be given. If one finds a prisoner's pulse, it should be found in the house of a prisoner. If one finds a termination pulse, the patient has had enduring disease in the past but will recover without treatment. If one finds a death pulse, it will be found in the house of bereavement. It is caused by affection by mourning.

---

is as follows: *Jia/yi* = wood/ liver; *bing/ding* = fire/heart; *wu/ji* = earth/spleen; *geng/xin* = metal/lungs; *ren/gui* = water/kidneys

Everything in the phenomenal world is correlated with the five phases, including the directions of the compass and various types of meat, grains, and vegetables. Therefore, the directions of the compass and meats and vegetables mentioned in these parallel passages are those associated with the diseased phase: Metal, west, autumn, chicken; wood, east, spring, pheasant; water, north, winter, pork; fire, south, summer, horsemeat; earth, center, longsummer, beef.

Based on the generating and restraining inter-relationships among the five phases, one can easily understand the logic behind such statements as to what kind of disease arises or ends in death on what day.

[4] In the *cun* or the distal position, the pulse presents a yin image, for example deep and/or fine.

How can one know if a person becomes ill from lying in the open? There appears yin in yang.[5]

How can one know if a person has become ill in summer? Various yang intrude into yin.[6]

How can one know if a person has been poisoned by food or drink? No yang is perceived at the superficial level. (That means the pulse) is too faint and fine to be observed (at the superficial level). Yet there is a yin pulse.[7]

If (the pulse) comes and goes racing, this image reflects water qi toxins.

If the pulse is slow, toxins have been obtained by eating dry (solid) food.

---

[5] In the yang, *i.e.*, the *cun*, there is a pulse of yin nature, for example deep and/or fine.

[6] In the yin position, *i.e.*, the *chi*, there appears a pulse of yang nature, for instance large and/or floating.

[7] A normal pulse should be full and beat evenly at both the superficial and deep levels. If one can only feel the pulse at a deep level, then one can say there is only yin left.

_____________ Chapter Fifteen _____________
Determining Through the Pulse if a Disease is About to be Cured or is Difficult to Relieve

(The Yellow Emperor) asked:

When a sick person is on the mend, recuperation can be determined through feeling the pulse. How to identify the pulse?

The master answered:

If the *cun*, *guan*, and *chi* are equally large or small, slow or racing, floating or sinking, in spite of lingering cold and heat, this pulse is balanced in terms of yin and yang and suggests healing on its own. When a person is ill, if the *cun* opening pulse and the *ren ying* pulse[1] are the same in terms of their size and depth, the disease is difficult to cure.

---

[1] The *ren ying* pulse refers to the pulse felt lateral to the Adam's apple in the neck. This pulse is an indication of yang and the exterior, while the *cun* opening pulse reflects yin and the interior. In normal cases, these two pulses should be different in strength, size, etc.

BOOK TWO

Collated & edited by Honorary Minister Without Portfolio,
Curator of the Imperial Library,
Imperial Courier and Senior Army Protector,
Lin Yi *et al.*

A Discussion of the Twenty-four Qi of the Yin & Yang Pulses in the Three Passes[1]

Yang expiry[2] in the *cun* distal to the *guan* on the left hand is absence[2] of the small intestine pulse. The bitterness (*i.e.*, suffering) includes umbilical *bi*[3] and *shan* conglomerations in the lower abdomen. In the months when (the small intestine) is the king,[4] cold qi will surge up into the heart. Needle the channel of the hand heart governor (*i.e.* the hand *jue yin*) to treat yin.[5] The (point of) the heart governor (to be needled) is located in the transverse crease proximal to the palm [*i.e.*, Great Mound, *Da Ling*, Per 7].

Yang repletion[6] in the *cun* distal to the *guan* on the left hand points to repletion of the small intestine. The bitterness includes urgent *bi* [acute pain in another version] below the heart, heat

---

[1] The three passes refer to the *cun, guan,* and *chi* positions of the wrist pulse. Counting the two hands, there are thus six pulses or pulse positions. Since each pulse position may present four images, *i.e.* yang expiry, yang repletion, yin expiry, and yin repletion, there are altogether 24 pulse images (qi).

[2] Yang expiry is a very weak and faint pulse when felt at the superficial level. One should note that the *cun* on the left hand corresponds to the small intestine/heart. The superficial level is yang as compared to the deep level which is yin. Therefore, since the bowels are yang compared to the viscera being yin, it makes sense in this system that the superficial level (yang) corresponds to the bowel (yang), while the deep level (yin) corresponds to the viscus (yin). Therefore, absence of a visceral pulse means a very weak and faint pulse at the deep level in that position and refers to the viscus which corresponds to the deep level at that *cun, guan,* or *chi* position.

[3] This refers to umbilical pain due to qi block.

[4] Each viscus with its associated bowel is supposed to govern a season. For example, autumn corresponds to metal, and, therefore, during the fall, the lung qi prevails over the other visceral qi. Thus, in the three months of autumn, the qi of the lungs and the large intestine is the king. One should also note that the word king or royal is a homophone with the word exuberance which is used instead of king in certain contexts later in this work. The months of exuberance of the other viscera or bowels can be determined in the same manner. As to the small intestine, its months of exuberance are the three months of summer, the season corresponding to fire.

[5] This implies no more than one should treat a yin channel. Nevertheless, it should be noted that the condition is yang in nature, *i.e.*, it involves a bowel, the small intestine.

[6] Yang repletion is reflected by a strong and solid pulse at the superficial level.

in the small intestine, and yellow or dark-colored urine. Needle the hand *tai yang* channel to treat yang.[7] (The point of) the *tai yang* (to be needled) is located in a depression of the base joint on the ulnar side of the little finger [*i.e.*, the point Back Ravine, *Hou Xi*, SI 3].

Yin expiry[8] in the *cun* distal to the *guan* on the left hand is absence of the heart pulse. The bitterness includes tormenting pain below the heart, heat in the palms, frequent vomiting, and sores and ulceration in the mouth. Needle the hand *tai yang* channel to treat yang.

Yin repletion in the *cun* distal to the *guan* on the left hand points to repletion of the heart. The bitterness includes the existence of water qi below the heart which is initiated by anxiety and indignation. Needle the channel of the hand heart governor to treat yin.

Yang expiry in the *guan* on the left hand is absence of the gallbladder pulse. The bitterness includes pain in the knees, a bitter taste in the mouth, dim vision, apprehension as if seeing ghosts, susceptibility to fright, and weakness. Needle the foot *jue yin* channel to treat yin. (The point) is located in the web of the big toe [*i.e.*, Going Between, *Xing Jian*, Liv 2]. Or needle the three hairs region (of the great toe).

Yang repletion in the *guan* on the left hand points to repletion of the gallbladder. The bitterness includes tightness in the abdomen with restlessness and fidgeting of the body. Needle the foot *shao yang* channel of the gallbladder to treat yang. (The point) is located 1 *cun* proximal to the base joint of the second toe of the foot. [It should be the toe next to the small toe, the point being Foot On the Verge of Tears, *Zu Lin Qi*, GB 41.]

Yin expiry in the *guan* on the left hand is absence of the liver pulse. The bitterness includes dribbling urinary block, enuresis, difficult speech, evil qi in the lateral costal regions, and frequent vomiting. Needle the foot *shao yang* channel to treat yang.

Yin repletion in the *guan* on the left hand points to repletion of the liver. The bitterness includes pain in the flesh and cramps often arising on movement. Needle the foot *jue yin* channel to treat yin.

Yang expiry in the *chi* proximal to the *guan* on the left hand is absence of the urinary bladder pulse. The bitterness includes counterflow frigidity (of the extremities). In females, there is

---

[7]   See note 5 above.

[8]   Yin expiry or absence of a pulse is reflected by a very weak, faint pulse when felt at the deep level.

menstrual irregularity and, in the months when (the bladder) is the king,[9] menstrual block. In males, there is seminal emission and dribbling after voiding urine. Needle the foot *shao yin* channel to treat yin. (The point) is located on the pulsating vessel below the medial malleolus [*i.e.*, Great Ravine, *Tai Xi*, Ki 3].

Yang repletion in the *chi* proximal to the *guan* on the left hand points to repletion of the bladder. The bitterness includes counterflow frigidity (of the extremities) and the existence of evil qi giving rise to a contracting pain in the lateral costal region. Needle the foot *tai yang* channel to treat yang. (The point) is located in a depression on the lateral aspect of the small toe posterior to its base joint [*i.e.*, Bundle Bone, *Shu Gu*, Bl 65].

Yin expiry in the *chi* proximal to the *guan* on the left hand is absence of the kidney pulse. The bitterness includes heat in the soles of the feet, hypertonicity of the medial aspects of the thighs, and exhausted and scanty essence and qi. (All these) are due to taxation and fatigue. Needle the foot *tai yang* channel to treat yang.

Yin repletion in the *chi* proximal to the *guan* on the left hand points to repletion of the kidneys. The bitterness includes spirit abstraction, impaired memory, blurred vision, complete deafness, and ringing in the ears. Needle the foot *shao yin* channel to treat yin.

Yang expiry in the *cun* distal to the *guan* on the right hand is absence of the large intestine pulse. The bitterness includes diminished qi, the existence of water qi below the heart, and cough arising with the Beginning of Autumn. Needle the hand *tai yin* channel to treat yin. (The point) is located in the fish's border [*i.e.*, Great Abyss, *Tai Yuan*, Lu 9].

Yang repletion in the *cun* distal to the *guan* on the right hand points to repletion of the large intestine. The bitterness includes lancinating pain in the intestine as if stabbed by an awl or knife. The pain persists with no end. Needle the hand *yang ming* channel to treat yang. (The point) is located on the wrist [*i.e.*, Yang Ravine, *Yang Xi*, LI 5].

Yin expiry in the *cun* distal to the *guan* on the right hand is absence of the lung pulse. The bitterness includes shortness of breath, counterflow coughing, constriction of the throat, and counterflow belching. Needle the hand *yang ming* channel to treat yang.

Yin repletion in the *cun* distal to the *guan* on the right hand points to repletion of the lungs. The bitterness includes diminished qi, inflating fullness of the chest, and a contracting discomfort

---

9   The winter months are the months when the kidneys and the bladder are exuberant.

between the chest and shoulder. Needle the hand *tai yin* channel to treat yin.

Yang expiry in the *guan* on the right hand is absence of the stomach pulse. The bitterness includes acid regurgitation, headache, and cold in the stomach. Needle the foot *tai yin* channel to treat yin. (The point) is located one *cun* posterior to the base joint of the great toe [*i.e.*, Grandson of the Noble, *Gong Sun*, Sp 4].

Yang repletion in the *guan* on the right hand points to repletion of the stomach. The bitterness includes hidden accumulations [depressed binding in another version] in the intestines, no desire for food, and inability to disperse the food taken in. Needle the foot *yang ming* channel to treat yang. (The point) is located on the pulsating vessel on the foot [*i.e.*, Surging Yang, *Chong Yang*, St 42].

Yin expiry in the *guan* on the right hand is absence of the spleen pulse. The bitterness includes diminished qi, diarrhea, abdominal fullness, generalized heaviness, no desire to move the limbs, and frequent retching. Needle the foot *yang ming* channel to treat yang.

Yin repletion in the *guan* on the right hand points to repletion of the spleen. The bitterness includes something lying hard in the intestines and difficult defecation. Needle the foot *tai yin* channel to treat yin.

Yang expiry in the *chi* proximal to the *guan* on the right hand is absence of the infant door[10] pulse. The bitterness includes counterflow frigidity of the feet, sterility, vaginal discharge, infertility, and cold in the external genitalia. Needle the foot *shao yin* channel to treat yin.

Yang repletion in the *chi* proximal to the *guan* on the right hand points to repletion of the bladder. The bitterness includes lower abdominal fullness causing pain in the lower back. Needle the foot *tai yang* channel to treat yang.

Yin expiry in the *chi* proximal to the *guan* on the right hand is absence of the kidney pulse. The bitterness includes counterflow frigidity of the feet, (qi counterflowing) up into and causing pain in the chest, dreams of plunging into water and coming across ghosts, sleep fraught with incubi, and (dreams of) something black coming on people. Needle the foot *tai yang* channel to treat yang.

Yin repletion in the *chi* proximal to the *guan* on the right hand points to repletion of the kidneys.

---

[10] The infant door here is synonymous with the life gate. It is called child's gate since the life gate is specifically associated with the function of reproduction.

The bitterness includes pain in the bones, pain in the lumbar spine, and internal cold and heat. Needle the foot *shao yin* channel to treat yin.

Above are the pulses of the twenty-four qi.

Chapter Two
A Discussion of the *Ren Ying*, Spirit Gate & Qi Opening[1] Pulses

Heart Repletion

If the distal *cun* or *ren ying* pulse is replete in the *yin*[2] on the left hand, the hand *jue yin* channel[3] (is replete). The disease bitterness (*i.e.*, suffering) includes (qi) block, inhibited defecation, abdominal fullness, heaviness of the limbs, bodily heat (*i.e.*, fever), and tormenting stomach distention. (To treat this,) needle Three Li (*San Li*, St 36).

Heart Vacuity

If the distal *cun* or *ren ying* pulse is vacuous in the yin on the left hand, the hand *jue yin* channel[3] (is vacuous). The disease bitterness includes palpitations, fear, melancholy, pain in the cardiac and abdominal regions which is nondescript, the heart is as if (struck by) cold, and spirit abstraction.

Small Intestine Repletion

---

[1] The distal position of the wrist pulse is called the *cun* opening or the *cun* for short. However, on the right hand, this position is also sometimes called the qi opening, while on the left hand, the *ren ying*. This should not be confused with the pulse in the neck which also is called *ren ying*. The spirit gate is the *chi* position of the pulse.

[2] In terms of the pulse, yin and yang may be used to refer to the depth. In that case, yin means the deep level, while yang means the superficial level. It follows, therefore, that, in this chapter, what yin vacuity refers to is a vacuous pulse at the deep level, while yang repletion refers to a replete pulse at the superficial level.

[3] In the *Qian Jin (Thousand [Taels of] Gold)*, the hand *shao yin* is mentioned instead of the hand *jue yin*, and, in fact, the *Qian Jin* may be right on this point.

If the distal *cun* or *ren ying* pulse is replete in the yang on the left hand, the hand *tai yang* channel (is replete). The disease bitterness includes bodily heat, fever coming and going, vexation in spite of sweat exiting [refusing to exit in another version], fullness of the heart, generalized heaviness, and sores in the mouth.

Small Intestine Vacuity

If the distal *cun* or *ren ying* pulse is vacuous in the yang on the left hand, the hand *tai yang* channel (is vacuous). The disease bitterness includes hemilateral headache at the hairline and pain in the ear and cheek.

Repletion of Both the Heart & Small Intestine

If the distal *cun* or *ren ying* pulse is replete in both the yin and yang on the left hand, the hand *shao yin* and hand *tai yang* channels are both replete. The disease bitterness includes headache, bodily heat, difficult defecation, vexation and fullness in the cardiac and abdominal regions, and sleeplessness. This is caused by a water-grain repletion due to inability of the stomach to turn.

Vacuity of Both the Heart & Small Intestine

If the distal *cun* or *ren ying* pulse is vacuous in both the yin and yang on the left hand, the hand *shao yin* and hand *tai yang* channels are both vacuous. The disease bitterness includes downpour diarrhea, tormenting cold, diminished qi, cold of the limbs, and intestinal *pi*.[4]

Liver Repletion

If the *guan* pulse is replete in the yin on the left hand, the foot *jue yin* channel (is replete). The disease bitterness includes tightness and fullness below the heart, constant pain in the lateral costal regions, and irascibility with looking as if (always) angry.

Liver Vacuity

If the *guan* pulse is vacuous in the yin on the left hand, the foot *jue yin* channel (is vacuous). The disease bitterness includes tightness in the lateral costal regions, (alternating) cold and heat, fullness of the abdomen, no desire for food, abdominal distention, melancholy, and, in females, inhibited menstrual flow and pain in the loins and abdomen.

---

[4]   Intestinal *pi* refers to dysentery with copious blood in the stools.

Gallbladder Repletion

If the *guan* pulse is replete in the yang on the left hand, the foot *shao yang* channel (is replete). The disease bitterness includes qi fullness of the abdomen, failure of drink and food to descend, dry throat, heavy headedness and headache, aversion to cold as after a soaking, and pain in the flanks.

Gallbladder Vacuity

If the *guan* pulse is vacuous in the yang on the left hand, the foot *shao yang* channel (is vacuous). The disease bitterness includes dizziness, inversion, wilting, inability to move the toes, limp legs with inability to rise up from a sitting position, sudden collapse, yellowing of the eyes, seminal loss, and blurred vision.

Repletion of Both the Liver & Gallbladder

If the *guan* pulse is replete in both the yin and yang on the left hand, the foot *jue yin* and the foot *shao yang* channels are both replete. The disease bitterness includes stomach distention, counterflow retching, and inability to disperse food.

Vacuity of Both the Liver & Gallbladder

If the *guan* pulse is vacuous in both the yin and yang on the left hand, the foot *jue yin* and the foot *shao yang* channels are both vacuous. The disease bitterness includes spirit abstraction, deathlike inversion with inability to recognize people, confused vision, diminished qi, inability to speak, and susceptibility to fright.

Kidney Repletion

If the proximal *chi* or spirit gate pulse is replete in the yin on the left hand, the foot *shao yin* channel (is replete). The disease bitterness includes bladder distention and block and a dragging pain between the lateral abdomen and the lumbar spine.

If the *chi* or spirit gate pulse is replete in the yin on the left hand, the foot *shao yin* channel (is replete). The disease bitterness includes dry tongue, swollen throat, heart vexation, dry throat, occasional pain in the chest and flanks, dyspnea, cough, (spontaneous) perspiration, distention and fullness of the lower abdomen, rigidity of the upper and lower back, generalized heaviness, heat in the bones, yellow or dark-colored urine, irascibility, forgetfulness, heat and pain in the soles of the feet, a black complexion of the limbs, and deafness.

Kidney Vacuity

If the proximal *chi* or spirit gate pulse is vacuous in the yin on the left hand, the foot *shao yin* channel (is vacuous). The disease bitterness includes oppression of the heart, heaviness of the lower limbs, and swollen feet which are not able to touch the ground.

Urinary Bladder Repletion

If the proximal *chi* or spirit gate pulse is replete in the yang on the left hand, the foot *tai yang* channel (is replete). The disease bitterness includes (qi) counterflow fullness, pain in the low back, and inability to bend (the body) either forward or backward. (All this is due to) taxation.

Urinary Bladder Vacuity

If the proximal *chi* or spirit gate pulse is vacuous in the yang on the left hand, the foot *tai yang* channel (is vacuous). The disease bitterness includes tense sinews in the foot, abdominal pain sending a dragging discomfort to the upper and lower back, inability to bend or stretch (the back), cramps, aversion to wind, hemilateral withering, low back pain, and pain posterior to the lateral malleolus.

Repletion of Both the Kidneys & Urinary Bladder

If the proximal *chi* or spirit gate pulse is replete in both the yin and yang on the left hand, the foot *shao yin* and foot *tai yang* channels are both replete. The disease bitterness includes arched back rigidity, upturned eyes, qi surging up into the heart, pain in the spine, and inability to turn around by oneself.

Vacuity of Both the Kidneys & Urinary Bladder

If the proximal *chi* or spirit gate pulse is vacuous in both the yin and yang on the left hand, the foot *shao yin* and foot *tai yang* channels are both vacuous. The disease bitterness includes uninhibited urination (*i.e.*, frequent voidings), heart pain, cold in the back, and frequent fullness in the lower abdomen.

Lung Repletion

If the distal *cun* or qi opening pulse is replete in the yin on the right hand, the hand *tai yin* channel (is replete). The disease bitterness includes lung distention, sweat exiting like dew (drops), qi ascent counterflow dyspnea, and constriction of the throat with a desire to retch.

Lung Vacuity

If the distal *cun* or qi opening pulse is vacuous in the yin on the right hand, the hand *lui yin* channel (is vacuous). The disease bitterness includes diminished qi not enough for breath and a dry throat due to fluids not being (enough to) moisten.

Large Intestine Repletion

If the distal *cun* or qi opening pulse is replete in the yang on the right hand, the hand *yang ming* channel (is replete). The disease bitterness includes fullness of the abdomen, frequent dyspnea and cough, a red face, bodily heat, and a feeling of a kernel stuck in the throat.

Large Intestine Vacuity

If the distal *cun* or qi opening pulse is vacuous in the yang on the right hand, the hand *yang ming* channel (is vacuous). The disease bitterness includes (fullness) in the chest with dyspnea, rumbling in the intestines, thirst due to vacuity (of fluids), dry lips and mouth, tense eyes, susceptibility to fright, and white substances in the stools.

Repletion of Both the Lungs & Large Intestine

If the distal *cun* or qi opening pulse is replete in both the yin and yang on the right hand, the hand *tai yin* and *yang ming* channels are both replete. The disease bitterness includes headache, visual dizziness, fright mania, throat *bi*[5] pain, contracted arms, and inability to contract the corners of the mouth.

Vacuity of Both the Lungs & Large Intestine

If the distal *cun* or qi opening pulse is vacuous in both the yin and yang on the right hand, the hand *tai yin* and *yang ming* channels are both vacuous. The disease bitterness includes clamoring in the ears, frequently seeing bright lights, and fear and apprehension.

Spleen Repletion

If the *guan* pulse is replete in the yin on the right hand, the foot *tai yin* channel (is replete). The disease bitterness includes cold in the feet yet with heat in the lower legs, distention and fullness

---

[5] This is a general term for various troubles characterized by swollen throat.

of the abdomen, and vexation and agitation causing sleeplessness.

Spleen Vacuity

If the *guan* pulse is vacuous in the yin on the right hand, the foot *tai yin* channel (is vacuous). The disease bitterness includes outpour diarrhea, fullness of the abdomen, qi counterflow, a choleraic disorder of vomiting and diarrhea, jaundice, heart vexation causing sleeplessness, and rumbling in the intestines.

Stomach Repletion

If the *guan* pulse is replete in the yang on the right hand, the foot *yang ming* channel (is replete). The disease bitterness includes abdominal tightness and pain with heat [headache in the *Qian Jin*[6]], sweat refusing to exit as in warm malaria,[7] dry lips and mouth, frequent retching, breast *yong*, and swelling and pain in the supraclavicular fossae and the armpits.

Stomach Vacuity

If the *guan* pulse is vacuous in the yang on the right hand, the foot *yang ming* channel (is vacuous). The disease bitterness includes cold in the lower legs, sleeplessness, aversion to cold as after a soaking, tense eyes, abdominal pain, vacuity ringing in the ears, sometimes cold, sometimes hot, dry lips and mouth, and puffy swelling of the face and eyes.

Repletion of Both the Spleen & Stomach

If the *guan* pulse is replete in both the yin and yang on the right hand, the foot *tai yin* and *yang ming* channels are both replete. The disease bitterness includes distention of the spleen and abdominal tightness causing pain in the lateral costal regions, inability of the stomach qi to turn, difficult defecation which often turns into its opposite, diarrhea, abdominal pain, (qi) surging up into the lungs and liver and stirring up the five viscera so as to cause instant dyspneic rale, susceptibility to fright, bodily heat, sweat refusing to exit, throat *bi*, and scant essence.

---

[6] The *Bei Ji Qian Jin Yao Fang* (*Formulas [Worth] a Thousand [Taels of] Gold For Emergency*) in full by Sun Si-miao.

[7] Warm malaria is malaria which is characterized by heat followed by cold or absence of cold during an attack.

Vacuity of Both the Spleen & Stomach

If the *guan* pulse is vacuous in both the yin and yang on the right hand, the foot *tai yin* and *yang ming* channels are both vacuous. The disease bitterness includes a feeling of emptiness in the stomach, diminished qi not enough for breath, counterflow cold of the four limbs, and ceaseless outpour diarrhea.

Kidney Repletion

If the proximal *chi* or spirit gate pulse is replete in the yin on the right hand, the foot *shao yin* channel (is replete). The disease bitterness includes *bi*,[8] bodily heat, heart pain, contracting pain between the spine and the flanks, counterflow frigidity of the feet, heat, and vexation.

Kidney Vacuity

If the proximal *chi* or spirit gate pulse is vacuous in the yin on the right hand, the foot *shao yin* channel (is vacuous). The disease bitterness includes weakness and wilting of the feet and lower legs, aversion to wind and cold, a regularly interrupted, expiring pulse which pauses from time to time, cold feet, top-heaviness, unsteady steps in walking, distention and fullness of the lower abdomen, and (qi) surging up into the chest and flanks causing pain in the regions below the armpits.

Urinary Bladder Repletion

If the proximal *chi* or spirit gate pulse is replete in the yang on the right hand, the foot *tai yang* channel (is replete). The disease bitterness includes shifted bladder[9] with inability to void urine, dizziness, headache, distressing fullness, and rigidity of the spine and the back.

Urinary Bladder Vacuity

If the proximal *chi* or spirit gate pulse is vacuous in the yang on the right hand, the foot *tai yang* channel (is vacuous). The disease bitterness includes tremors of the muscles, tense sinews in the feet, and deafness (or impaired hearing) with aversion (of the ears) to wind and ringing in them as if wind was whistling.

---

[8] In its general sense, *bi* means block of the channels or vessel networks. However, in a narrow sense, it refers specifically to rheumatic complaints.

[9] This refers to acute umbilical pain with urinary block.

Repletion of Both the Kidneys & Urinary Bladder

If the proximal *chi* or spirit gate pulse is replete in both the yin and yang on the right hand, the foot *shao yin* and *tai yang* channels are both replete. The disease bitterness includes madness, heavy headedness, a contracting pain between the head and eyes, inversion, a desire to move about, upturned eyes, great wind,[10] and copious perspiration.

Vacuity of Both the Kidneys & Urinary Bladder

If the proximal *chi* or spirit gate pulse is vacuous in both the yin and yang on the right hand, the foot *shao yin* and *tai yang* channels are both vacuous. The disease bitterness includes heart pain, pressure in and inability to contract the rectum resulting in prolapsed rectum, frequent tormenting downpour diarrhea, cold center, and pain in both the kidneys and heart.

One theory says the kidneys have a right and left while there is only one urinary bladder. Nowadays in (clinical) practice, the left kidney is united with the urinary bladder, and the right kidney is united with the triple burner.

---

[10] As a generic term, great wind refers to any severe disease caused by wind. In this context, however, it specifically refers to leprosy.

Chapter Three
A Discussion of the Diseases Reflected by the Three Passes & Their Appropriate Treatments

If the *cun* pulse is floating, there is wind stroke manifesting as fever and headache. It requires taking *Gui Zhi Tang* (Cinnamon Twig Decoction)[1] and *Ge Gen Tang* (Pueraria Decoction),[2] needling Wind Pool (*Feng Chi*, GB 20) and Wind Mansion (*Feng Fu*, GV 16), and heating (the sick person)

---

[1] The ingredients of this formula include Ramulus Cinnamomi Cassiae (*Gui Zhi*), Radix Paeoniae Lactiflorae (*Shao Yao*), Rhizoma Zingiberis (*Jiang*), and Radix Glycyrrhizae (*Gan Cao*).

[2] The ingredients of this formula include Radix Puerariae (*Ge Gen*), Herba Ephedrae (*Ma Huang*), Fructus Zizyphi Jujubae (*Da Zao*), Ramulus Cinnamomi Cassiae (*Gui Zhi*), Radix Paeoniae Lactiflorae (*Shao Yao*), Rhizoma Zingiberis (*Jiang*), and Radix Glycyrrhizae (*Gan Cao*).

by making them face a fire while treating by rubbing with *Feng Gao* (Wind Paste)[3] to promote perspiration.

If the *cun* pulse is tight, there is the bitterness of headache and pain in the bones and flesh. This is cold damage and requires taking *Ma Huang Tang* (Ephedra Decoction)[4] to promote perspiration, needling Eyebrow Ascension (*Mei Chong*, Bl 3) and Temple Region (*Nie Ru*, GB 19), and treating by rubbing with *Shang Han Gao* (Cold Damage Paste).[5]

If the *cun* pulse is faint, there is the bitterness of cold and spontaneous external bleeding. This requires taking *Wu Wei Zi Tang* (Schisandra Decoction)[6] and rubbing with *Zhu Yu Gao* (Evodia Paste)[7] to promote perspiration.

If the *cun* pulse is rapid, there will be vomiting. This is the result of heat existing in the venter which fumes the chest. It requires taking certain medicinals for the purpose of emesis, needling Stomach Venter (*Wei Wan*, CV 12), and taking *Chu Re Tang* (Eliminate Heat Decoction).[8] If, on the seventh, eighth, or the tenth day of cold damage, heat settles in the center, giving rise to vexation, fullness, and thirst, it is appropriate to take *Zhi Mu Tang* (Anemarrhena Decoction).[9]

If the *cun* pulse is moderate, there is insensitivity of the skin due to wind cold in the muscles and flesh. This requires taking *Fang Feng Tang* (Ledebouriella Decoction),[10] ironing with a heated bag

---

[3] This is a paste made of Herba Glechomae Longitabae (*Feng Cao*).

[4] This formula is composed of Herba Ephedrae (*Ma Huang*), Ramulus Cinnamomi Cassiae (*Gui Zhi*), Semen Pruni Armeniacae (*Xing Ren*), and Radix Glycyrrhizae (*Gan Cao*).

[5] This is a paste made of Herba Vernoniae Cinereae (*Shang Han Cao*).

[6] This formula is composed of Fructus Schisandrae Chinensis (*Wu Wei Zi*), Radix Platycodi Grandiflori (*Jie Geng*), Radix Asteris Tatarici (*Zi Wan*), Radix Glycyrrhizae (*Gan Cao*), Radix Dipsaci (*Xu Duan*), Radix Rehmanniae (*Di Huang*), Cortex Radicis Mori Albi (*Sang Pi*), Caulis Bambusae In Taeniis (*Zhu Ru*), and Semen Phaseoli Calcarati (*Chi Xiao Dou*).

[7] This is a paste prepared from Fructus Evodia Rutecarpae (*Zhu Yu*).

[8] The translator has not been able to identify the ingredients in this formula.

[9] The ingredients of this formula include Rhizoma Anemarrhenae Aphodeloidis (*Zhi Mu*), Radix Paeoniae Lactiflorae (*Shao Yao*), Radix Scutellariae Baicalensis (*Huang Qin*), Cortex Tubiformis Cinnamomi Cassiae (*Guan Gui*), and Radix Glycyrrhizae (*Gan Cao*).

[10] This formula consists of Radix Ledebouriellae Divarticatae (*Fang Feng*), Radix Ligustici Wallichii (*Chuan Xiong*), Radix Angelicae Dahuricae (*Bai Zhi*), Radix Achyranthis Bidentatae (*Niu Xi*), Rhizoma Cibotii Barometsis (*Gou Ji*), Rhizoma Dioscoreae Hypoglaucae (*Bei Xie*), Rhizoma Atractylodis Macrocephalae (*Bai Zhu*), Radix Et Rhizoma Notopterygii (*Qiang Huo*), Radix Puerariae (*Ge Gen*), Radix Praeparatus Aconiti

of certain medicinals, rubbing with *Feng Gao* (Wind Paste), and moxaing the various wind points.[11]

If the *cun* pulse is slippery, there is yang repletion giving rise to congestion and fullness in the chest and counterflow vomiting. This requires taking *Qian Hu Tang* (Peucedanum Decoction)[12] and needling Greater Yang (*Tai Yang*, M-HN-9) and Great Tower Gate (*Ju Que*, CV 14) with draining.

If the *cun* pulse is bowstring, there is inflation below the heart, mild headache, and water qi below the heart. This requires taking *Gan Sui Wan* (Kansui Pills)[13] and needling Cycle Gate (*Qi Men*, Liv 14) with draining.

If the *cun* pulse is weak, there is yang qi vacuity with spontaneous perspiration and shortness of breath. This requires taking *Fu Ling Tang* (Poria Decoction)[14] and *Nei Bu San* (Internally Supplementing Powder).[15] Adjust food intake to an appropriate amount and do not tax oneself to an extreme degree. Needle Stomach Venter (*Wei Guan*, CV 12) with supplementation.

If the *cun* pulse is choppy, there is insufficiency of the stomach qi. This requires taking *Gan Di Huang Tang* (Dried Rehmannia Decoction),[16] self-nurturing, balancing drink and food, and needling Three Li (*San Li*, St 36) with supplementation [Stomach Venter (*Wei Guan*, CV 12) instead of Three Li in another version].

Carmichaeli (*Fu Zi*), Semen Pruni Armeniacae (*Xing Ren*), Herba Ephedrae (*Ma Huang*), Rhizoma Zingiberis (*Jiang*), Gypsum (*Shi Gao*), Semen Coicis Lachryma-jobi (*Yi Yi Ren*), and Cortex Cinnamomi Cassiae (*Gui Xin*).

[11] This implies, for example, Wind Mansion (*Feng Fu*, GV 16), Wind Pool (*Feng Chi*, GB 20), and Eyebrow Ascension (*Mei Chong*, Bl 3).

[12] The formula is composed of Radix Peucedani (*Qian Hu*), Radix Glycyrrhizae (*Gan Cao*), Rhizoma Pinelliae Ternatae (*Ban Xia*), Radix Paeoniae Lactiflorae (*Shao Yao*), Radix Scutellariae Baicalensis (*Huang Qin*), Radix Angelicae Sinensis (*Dang Gui*), Radix Panacis Ginseng (*Ren Shen*), Cortex Cinnamomi Cassiae (*Gui Xin*), Rhizoma Zingiberis (*Jiang*), Fructus Zizyphi Jujubae (*Hong Zao*), and Herba Lophatheri Gracilis (*Zhu Ye*).

[13] This may refer to pills prepared from Radix Euphobiae Kansui (*Gan Sui*).

[14] The ingredients of this formula are Sclerotium Poriae Cocos (*Fu Ling*), Radix Glycyrrhizae (*Gan Cao*), Radix Paeoniae Lactiflorae (*Shao Yao*), Cortex Cinnamomi Cassiae (*Gui Xin*), Radix Angelicae Sinensis (*Dang Gui*), Rhizoma Zingiberis (*Jiang*), Tuber Ophiopogonis Japonici (*Mai Dong*), and Fructus Zizyphi Jujubae (*Da Zao*).

[15] The translator has not been able to identify the ingredients in this formula.

[16] This formula is composed of dried Radix Rehmanniae (*Gan Di Huang*), Radix Paeoniae Lactiflorae (*Shao Yao*), Radix Glycyrrhizae (*Gan Cao*), Radix Salviae Miltiorrhizae (*Dan Shen*), and honey (*Feng Mi*).

If the *cun* pulse is scallion-stalk, there is blood ejection. A slightly scallion-stalk pulse reveals spontaneous external bleeding. Emptiness (of the pulse) is the result of blood loss. This requires taking *Zhu Pi Tang* (Bamboo Peel Decoction)[17] and *Huang Tu Tang* (Yellow Clay Decoction)[18] and moxaing Chest Center (*Dan Zhong*, CV 17).

If the *cun* pulse is hidden, there is qi counterflow in the chest with esophageal constriction. This is due to cold qi surging from the stomach up into the heart and chest. It requires taking *Qian Hu Tang* (Peucedanum Decoction) and *Da San Jian Wan* (Major Three Fortifying Pills),[19] needling Great Tower Gate (*Ju Que*, CV 14) and Upper Venter (*Shang Wan*, CV 13), and moxaing Chest Center (*Dan Zhong*, CV 17).

If the *cun* pulse is deep, the chest sends a dragging pain to the flanks as a result of the existence of water qi in the chest. This requires taking *Ze Qi Tang* (Helioscopia Decoction)[20] and needling Great Tower Gate (*Ju Que*, CV 14) with draining.

If the *cun* pulse is soggy, yang qi is weak, thus giving rise to spontaneous perspiration. This is an illness of vacuity taxation and requires *Gan Di Huang Tang* (Dried Rehmannia Decoction) and *Shu Yu Wan* (Dioscorea Pills),[21] *Nei Bu San* (Internally Supplementing Powder), and *Mu Li San* (Oyster

---

[17] The ingredients of this formula are Herba Asari Cum Radice (*Xi Xin*), Medulla Tetrapanacis Papyriferi (*Tong Cao*), Radix Panacis Ginseng (*Ren Shen*), Fructus Schisandrae Chinensis (*Wu Wei Zi*), Sclerotium Poriae Cocos (*Fu Ling*), Herba Ephedrae (*Ma Huang*), Cortex Cinnamomi Cassiae (*Gui Xin*), Rhizoma Zingiberis (*Jiang*), Cortex Bambusae (*Zhu Pi*), and Radix Glycyrrhizae (*Gan Cao*).

[18] This formula is composed of uncooked Radix Rehmanniae (*Sheng Di*), Radix Glycyrrhizae (*Gan Cao*), Radix Praeparatus Aconiti Carmichaeli (*Fu Zi*), Gelatinum Corii Asini (*E Jiao*), Radix Scutellariae Baicalensis (*Huang Qin*), and Terra Flava Usta (*Zao Xin Tu*).

[19] This formula is composed of Fructus Zanthoxyli Bungeani (*Chuan Jiao*), Rhizoma Zingiberis (*Jiang*), Radix Panacis Ginseng (*Ren Shen*), and malt (*Yi Tang*).

[20] The ingredients in this formula are Herba Euphobiae Helioscopiae (*Ze Qi*), Rhizoma Pinelliae Ternatae (*Ban Xia*), Radix Asteris Tatarici (*Zi Wan*), Rhizoma Zingiberis (*Jiang*), Radix Cynanchi Stauntoni (*Bai Qian*), Radix Glycyrrhizae (*Gan Cao*), Radix Scutellariae Baicalensis (*Huang Qin*), Radix Panacis Ginseng (*Ren Shen*), and Ramulus Cinnamomi Cassiae (*Gui Zhi*).

[21] This formula is composed of Radix Dioscoreae Oppositae (*Shan Yao*), Radix Angelicae Sinensis (*Dang Gui*), Ramulus Cinnamomi Cassiae (*Gui Zhi*), Massa Medica Fermentata (*Shen Qu*), Radix Rehmanniae (*Di Huang*), Fructus Germinatus Glycinis Hispidae (*Da Dou Huang Juan*), Radix Glycyrrhizae (*Gan Cao*), Radix Panacis Ginseng (*Ren Shen*), Gelatium Corii Asini (*E Jiao*), Radix Ligustici Wallichii (*Chuan Xiong*), Radix Paeoniae Lactiflorae (*Shao Yao*), Rhizoma Atractylodis Macrocephalae (*Bai Zhu*), Tuber Asparagi Cochinensis (*Tian Dong*), Radix Ledebouriellae Divaricatae (*Fang Feng*), Semen Pruni Armeniacae (*Xing Ren*), Radix Bupleuri (*Chai Hu*), Radix Platycodi Grandiflori (*Jie Geng*), Sclerotium Poriae Cocos (*Fu Ling*), Rhizoma Zingiberis (*Jiang*), Radix Ampelopsis Japonicae (*Bai Lian*), and Fructus Zizyphi Jujubae (*Da Zao*).

Shell Powder),[22] dabbing with this powder, and needling Supreme Surge (*Tai Chong*, Liv 3) with supplementation.

If the *cun* pulse is slow, there is cold in the upper burner giving rise to heart pain, acid regurgitation, and acid vomiting. This requires taking *Fu Zi Tang* (Aconite Decoction),[23] *Sheng Jiang Tang* (Uncooked Ginger Decoction),[24] and *Zhu Yu Wan* (Evodia Pills),[25] and balancing drink and food to warm (the upper burner).

If the *cun* pulse is replete, heat is generated in the spleen and lungs causing counterflow retching and qi stoppage. If the pulse is vacuous, cold is generated in the spleen and stomach causing inability to disperse and transform food. In the case of heat, it is appropriate to take *Zhu Ye Tang* (Bamboo Leaf Decoction) and *Ge Gen Tang* (Pueraria Decoction).[26] In the case of cold, it is appropriate to take *Zhu Yu Wan* (Evodia Pills) and *Sheng Jiang Tang* (Uncooked Ginger Decoction).

If the *cun* pulse is fine, there is fever with retching and vomiting. This requires taking *Huang Qin Long Dan Tang* (Scutellaria & Gentiana Decoction).[27] In case of uncheckable vomiting, it is appropriate to take *Ju Pi Jie Geng Tang* (Orange Peel & Platycodon Decoction)[28] and needle Central Treasury (*Zhong Fu*, Lu 1).

---

[22] The ingredients in this formula include calcined Concha Ostreae (*Mu Li*), Radix Astragali Membranacei (*Huang Qi*), Radix Ephedrae (*Ma Huang Gen*), and Fructus Levis Tritici Aestivi (*Fu Xiao Mai*).

[23] This formula is composed of Radix Praeparatus Aconiti Carmichaeli (*Fu Zi*), Sclerotium Poriae Cocos (*Fu Ling*), Radix Paeoniae Lactiflorae (*Shao Yao*), Radix Panacis Ginseng (*Ren Shen*), and Rhizoma Atractylodis Macrocephalae (*Bai Zhu*).

[24] This formula is composed of uncooked Rhizoma Zingiberis (*Sheng Jiang*), Radix Glycyrrhizae (*Gan Cao*), Radix Panacis Ginseng (*Ren Shen*), dried Rhizoma Zingiberis (*Gan Jiang*), Radix Scutellariae Baicalensis (*Huang Qin*), Rhizoma Pinelliae Ternatae (*Ban Xia*), Rhizoma Coptidis Chinensis (*Huang Lian*), and Fructus Zizyphi Jujubae (*Da Zao*).

[25] The ingredients of this formula consist of Fructus Evodiae Rutecarpae (*Wu Zhu Yu*), Cortex Cinnamomi Cassiae (*Gui Xin*), and Radix Angelicae Sinensis (*Dang Gui*).

[26] This formula is composed of Herba Lophatheri Gracilis (*Zhu Ye*), Radix Puerariae (*Ge Gen*), Radix Ledebouriellae Divaricatae (*Fang Feng*), Radix Platycodi Grandiflori (*Jie Geng*), Ramulus Cinnamomi Cassiae (*Gui Zhi*), Radix Panacis Ginseng (*Ren Shen*), Radix Glycyrrhizae (*Gan Cao*), Radix Praeparatus Aconiti Carmichaeli (*Fu Zi*), and Fructus Zizyphi Jujubae (*Da Zao*).

[27] The ingredients in this formula are Radix Scutellariae Baicalensis (*Huang Qin*), Radix Paeoniae Lactiflorae (*Shao Yao*), Radix Glycyrrhizae (*Gan Cao*), Fructus Zizyphi Jujubae (*Da Zao*), and Radix Gentiana Scabrae (*Long Dan Cao*).

[28] This formula is composed of Pericarpium Citri Reticulatae (*Ju Pi*), Rhizoma Zingiberis (*Jiang*), and Radix Platycodi Grandiflori (*Jie Geng*).

If the *cun* pulse is large and surging, there is fullness in the chest and flanks. This requires taking *Sheng Jiang Tang* (Uncooked Ginger Decoction) and *Bai Wei Wan* (Cynanchum Pills)[29] or *Zi Wan Tang* (Aster Decoction)[30] to precipitate and needling Upper Venter (*Shang Wan*, CV 13), Cycle Gate (*Qi Men*, Liv 14), and Camphorwood Gate (*Zhang Men*, Liv 13).

The above are seventeen conditions relating to the pulse in the *cun*.

If the *guan* pulse is floating, there is abdominal fullness with no desire for food. A floating (pulse) points to vacuity fullness. This requires taking *Ping Wei San* (Level the Stomach Powder),[31] *Fu Ling Tang* (Poria Decoction), and *Qian Hu Tang* (Peucedanum Decoction) with Rhizoma Zingiberis (*Jiang*) added and needling Stomach Venter (*Wei Guan*, CV 12) first with a draining and then with supplementation.

If the *guan* pulse is tight, there is a tormenting fullness below the heart with acute pain. A taut pulse points to repletion. This requires *Zhu Yu Dang Gui Tang* (Evodia & Dang Gui Decoction)[32] and *Da Huang Tang* (Rhubarb Decoction)[33] in addition. It is better to treat with these two (formulas combined. It also requires) needling Great Tower Gate (*Ju Que*, CV 14) and Lower Venter (*Xia*

---

[29] The ingredients in this formula include Radix Cynanchi Atrati (*Bai Wei*), uncooked Radix Rehmanniae (*Sheng Di*), Rhizoma Zingiberis (*Jiang*), Fructus Zanthoxyli Bungeani (*Chuan Jiao*), Semen Plantaginis (*Che Qian Zi*), Fluoritum (*Zi Shi Ying*), Herba Lycopi Lucidi (*Ze Lan*), Limonitum (*Yu Yu Liang*), Os Draconis (*Long Gu*), Sclerotium Poriae Cocos (*Fu Ling*), Tuber Ophiopogonis Japonici (*Mai Dong*), Radix Polygalae Tenuifoliae (*Yuan Zhi*), Radix Angelicae Sinensis (*Dang Gui*), Halloysitum Rubrum (*Chi Shi Zhi*), Radix Ligustici Wallichii (*Chuan Xiong*), Fructus Cnidii Monnieri (*She Chuang Zi*), Radix Angelicae Dahuricae (*Bai Zhi*), Radix Panacis Ginseng (*Ren Shen*), Radix Et Rhizoma Ligustici Sinensis (*Gao Ben*), Gypsum (*Shi Gao*), Fructus Artemisiae Keisceanae (*An Lu Zi*), Herba Selaginellae Tamariscinae (*Juan Bai*), Cortex Cinnamomi Cassiae (*Gui Xin*), Semen Pruni Persicae (*Tao Ren*), Pollen Typhae (*Pu Huang*), Fructus Rubi (*Fu Pen Zi*), Herba Asari Cum Radice (*Xi Xin*), and Pericarpium Citri Reticulatae (*Chen Pi*).

[30] This formula may be composed of Radix Asteris Tatarici (*Zi Wan*), Radix Stephaniae Tetrandrae (*Fang Ji*), Cortex Cinnamomi Cassiae (*Gui Xin*), Herba Asari Cum Radice (*Xi Xin*), Sclerotium Rubrum Poriae Cocos (*Chi Fu Ling*), Cortex Radicis Mori Albi (*Sang Pi*), Pericarpium Arecae (*Da Fu Pi*), Fructus Aurantii (*Zhi Qiao*), Semen Lepidii (*Ting Li*), Radix Auklandiae Lappae (*Mu Xiang*), Radix Glycyrrhizae (*Gan Cao*), and Semen Arecae Catechu (*Bing Lang*).

[31] This formula is composed of Rhizoma Atractylodis (*Cang Zhu*), Cortex Magnoliae Officinalis (*Hou Po*), Pericarpium Citri Reticulatae (*Chen Pi*), and Radix Glycyrrhizae (*Gan Cao*).

[32] The ingredients in this formula are Fructus Evodiae Rutecarpae (*Wu Zhu Yu*), Fructus Chaenomelis Lagenariae (*Mu Gua*), and Radix Angelicae Sinensis (*Dang Gui*).

[33] This formula is composed of Radix Et Rhizoma Rhei (*Da Huang*), Radix Scutellariae Baicalensis (*Huang Qin*), Fructus Gardeniae Jasminoidis (*Zhi Zi*), Rhizoma Cimicifugae (*Sheng Ma*), and Mirabilitum (*Mang Xiao*).

Wan, CV 10) with draining. [The *Qian Jin* prescribes *Zhu Yu Dang Gui Tang* (Evodia & Dang Gui Decoction) with the addition of 2 *liang* of Radix Et Rhizoma Rhei (*Da Huang*). This is better.]

If the *guan* pulse is faint, there is cold in the stomach with hypertonicity below the heart. This requires taking *Fu Zi Tang* (Aconite Decoction), *Sheng Jiang Tang* (Uncooked Ginger Decoction), and *Fu Zi Wan* (Aconite Pills)[34] and needling Great Tower Gate (*Ju Que*, CV 14) with supplementation.

If the *guan* pulse is rapid, there is guest heat in the stomach. This requires taking *Zhi Mu Wan* (Anemarrhena Pills)[35] and *Chu Re Tang* (Eliminate Heat Decoction) and needling Great Tower Gate (*Ju Que*, CV 14) and Upper Venter (*Shang Wan*, CV 13) with draining.

If the *guan* pulse is moderate, the patient will have no desire for food. This is due to unbalanced stomach qi and insufficiency of spleen qi and requires *Ping Wei San* (Level the Stomach Powder), *Bu Pi Tang* (Supplement the Spleen Decoction),[36] and needling Camphorwood Gate (*Zhang Men*, Liv 13) with supplementation.

If the *guan* pulse is slippery, there is heat in the stomach. A slippery pulse points to heat repletion, and (evil) qi fullness is the cause of no desire for food and of counterflow vomiting arising upon ingestion. This requires taking *Zi Wan Tang* (Aster Decoction) to precipitate and a large dose of *Ping Wei San* (Level the Stomach Pills) and needling Stomach Venter (*Wei Guan*, CV 12) with draining.

If the *guan* pulse is bowstring, there is cold in the stomach with counterflow inversion (qi) below the heart. This arises as a result of stomach qi vacuity. It requires taking *Zhu Yu Tang* (Evodia Decoction), taking warm and balanced food, and needling Stomach Venter (*Wei Guan*, CV 12) with supplementation.

---

[34] The ingredients in this formula include Radix Praeparatus Aconiti Carmichaeli (*Fu Zi*), Fructus Pruni Mume (*Wu Mei*), Rhizoma Zingiberis (*Jiang*), and Rhizoma Coptidis Chinensis (*Huang Lian*).

[35] This formula is composed of only one ingredient, Rhizoma Anemarrhenae Asphodeloidis (*Zhi Mu*). However, because this formula is specifically effective for difficult delivery, it is not certain whether it is indeed the formula meant by the author.

[36] This formula is composed of Radix Codonopsitis Pilosulae (*Dang Shen*), Rhizoma Atractylodis Macrocephalae (*Bai Zhu*), Sclerotium Poriae Cocos (*Fu Ling*), Radix Angelicae Sinensis (*Dang Gui*), Radix Astragali Membranacei (*Huang Qi*), Semen Dolichoris Lablabis (*Bian Dou*), Radix Albus Paeoniae Lactiflorae (*Bai Shao*), Radix Ligustici Wallichii (*Chuan Xiong*), Fructus Cardomomi (*Dou Kou*), Pericarpium Citri Reticulatae (*Chen Pi*), Radix Glycyrrhizae (*Gan Cao*), Rhizoma Zingiberis (*Jiang*), and Fructus Zizyphi Jujubae (*Da Zao*).

If the *guan* pulse is weak, there is vacuity of the stomach qi and guest (*i.e.*, vacuity) heat in the stomach. A weak pulse points to vacuity heat breeding disease. There is an instruction forbidding great attacking (*i.e.*, diaphoresis) in the presence of heat. For once heat is removed, cold will arise. This is rightly a case that requires taking *Zhu Ye Tang* (Bamboo Leaf Decoction) and needling Stomach Venter (*Wei Guan*, CV 12) with supplementation.

If the *guan* pulse is choppy, blood and qi sustain counterflow cold. A choppy pulse points to blood vacuity. Since there is a slight heat in the middle burner, this requires taking *Gan Di Huang Tang* (Dried Rehmannia Decoction) and *Nei Bu San* (Internally Supplementing Powder) and needling Supreme Surge (*Tai Chong*, Liv 3) in the foot with supplementation.

If the *guan* pulse is scallion-stalk, and several *dou* (1 *dou* = 10 liters) of blood has been discharged through the stools, this is a result of an injured diaphragm point.[37] It requires taking *Sheng Di Huang Tang* (Uncooked Rehmannia Decoction)[38] and *Sheng Zhu Pi Tang* (Uncooked Bamboo Peel Decoction), and moxaing Diaphragm Shu (*Ge Shu*, Bl 17). If discharge of blood through the stools continues, needle Origin Pass (*Guan Yuan*, CV 4). In severe cases, it is appropriate to take *Long Gu Wan* (Dragon Bone Pills)[39] which will surely effect a cure.

If the *guan* pulse is hidden, there is water qi in the middle burner with duck-stool diarrhea. This requires taking *Shui Yin Wan* (Mercury Pills)[40] and needling Origin Pass (*Guan Yuan*, CV 4). Once the urine is disinhibited, the duck-stool diarrhea will stop.

If the *guan* pulse is deep, there is cold qi below the heart with tormenting fullness and acid regurgitation. This requires taking *Bai Wei Fu Ling Wan* (Cynanchum & Poria Pills)[41] and *Fu Zi Tang* (Aconite Decoction) and needling Stomach Venter (*Wei Wan*, CV 12) with supplementation.

If the *guan* pulse is soggy, the bitterness is (due to) vacuity cold and weak spleen qi and the

---

[37] The diaphragm is the meeting place of the blood. Therefore, various problems of the blood correspond with it. As to the diaphragm point, this may refer to Diaphragm Shu (*Ge Shu*, Bl 17).

[38] This formula is the same as in note 16 above with fresh Radix Rehmanniae instead of dried Rehmannia.

[39] This formula is composed of Os Draconis (*Long Gu*), Rhizoma Coptidis Chinensis (*Huang Lian*), Cortex Phellodendri (*Huang Bai*), Radix Auklandiae Lappae (*Mu Xiang*), Pericarpium Fructi Terminaliae Chebulae (*He Zi Pi*), Acetate of Lead (*Qian Fen*), Alumen (*Fan*), Rhizoma Zingiberis (*Jiang*), and Radix Angelicae Sinensis (*Dang Gui*).

[40] The translator has not been able to identify the ingredients in these pills.

[41] This formula is the same as in note 29 above except for the addition of Sclerotium Poriae Cocos (*Fu Ling*).

disease is severe diarrhea. This requires taking *Chi Shi Zhi Tang* (Halloysitum Rubrum Decoction)[42] and *Nu Wei Wan* (Clematis Pills)[43] and needling Origin Pass (*Guan Yuan*, CV 4) with supplementation.

If the *guan* pulse is slow, there is cold in the stomach. This requires taking *Gui Zhi Wan* (Cinnamon Twig Pills)[44] and *Zhu Yu Tang* (Evodia Decoction) and needling Stomach Venter (*Wei Wan*, CV 12) with supplementation.

If the *guan* pulse is replete, there is stomachache. This requires taking *Zhi Zi Tang* (Gardenia Decoction)[45] and *Zhu Yu Wu Tou Wan* (Cornus & Wu Tou Aconite Pills)[46] and needling Stomach Venter (*Wei Wan*, CV 12) with supplementation.

If the *guan* pulse is firm, there is qi congestion in the spleen and stomach with fulminant heat and fullness and rumbling in the abdomen. This requires taking *Zi Wan Wan* (Aster Pills) and *Xie Pi Wan* (Drain the Spleen Pills)[47] and needling Stomach Venter (*Wei Wan*, CV 12) with draining.

If the *guan* pulse is fine, there is [it is suspected that the words spleen and stomach have been left out here] vacuity with fullness of the abdomen. This requires taking *Sheng Jiang Zhu Yu Shu Jiao Tang* (Uncooked Ginger, Cornus & Pepper Decoction)[48] and *Bai Wei Wan* (Cynanchum Pills) and needling the Three Venters (*San Wan, i.e.,* CV 10, 12, 13).

If the *guan* pulse is surging, there is heat in the stomach invariably accompanied by distressing fullness. This requires taking *Ping Wei Wan* (Level the Stomach Pills) and needling Stomach Venter (*Wei Wan*, CV 12), first draining and then supplementing it.

---

[42] The ingredients of this formula are Hallyositum Rubrum (*Chi Shi Zhi*) and Limonitum (*Yu Yu Liang*).

[43] These pills are prepared from Caulis Clemantis Apiifoliae (*Nu Wei*).

[44] These pills are comprised of the same ingredients as Cinnamon Twig Decoction in note 1 above.

[45] This formula is composed of Fructus Gardeniae Jasminoidis (*Zhi Zi*), Radix Paeoniae Lactiflorae (*Shao Yao*), Medulla Tetrapanacis Papyriferi (*Tong Cao*), Folium Pyrrosiae (*Shi Wei*), Gypsum (*Shi Gao*), Talcum (*Hua Shi*), Radix Scutellariae Baicalensis (*Huang Qin*), uncooked Radix Rehmanniae (*Sheng Di*), Cortex Ulmi Pumilae (*Yu Bai Pi*), and Herba Lophatheri Gracilis (*Dan Zhu Ye*).

[46] This formula is the same as in note 25 above but with the addition of Radix Aconiti (*Wu Tou*).

[47] This formula may be composed of Herba Agastachis Seu Pogostemi (*Huo Xiang*), Fructus Gardeniae Jasminoidis (*Zhi Zi*), Radix Ledebouriellae Divaricatae (*Fang Feng*), Gypsum (*Shi Gao*), and Radix Glycyrrhizae (*Gan Cao*).

[48] This formula is composed of Rhizoma Zingiberis (*Jiang*), Fructus Corni Officinalis (*Zhu Yu*), and Fructus Zanthoxyli Bungeani (*Chuan Jiao*).

The above are eighteen conditions relating to the pulse in the middle position, the *guan*.

If the *chi* pulse is floating, there is heat wind in the lower (burner) with difficult urination. This requires taking *Qu Mai Tang* (Dianthus Decoction)[49] and *Hua Shi San* (Talcum Powder)[50] and needling Horizontal Bone (*Heng Gu*, Ki 11) and Origin Pass (*Guan Yuan*, CV 4) with draining.

If the *chi* pulse is taut, there is pain below the umbilicus. This requires taking *Dang Gui Tang* (Dang Gui Decoction),[51] moxaing Celestial Pivot (*Tian Shu*, St 22), and needling Origin Pass (*Guan Yuan*, CV 4) with supplementation.

If the *chi* pulse is faint, there is counterflow inversion with hypertonicity in the lower abdomen due to the existence of cold qi (there). This requires taking *Xiao Jian Zhong Tang* (Minor Fortify the Center Decoction)[52] and needling Sea of Qi (*Qi Hai*, CV 6).

If the *chi* pulse is rapid, there is aversion to cold, heat and pain below the umbilicus, and yellow or dark-colored urine. This requires taking egg soup with powdered whitefish and needling Horizontal Bone (*Heng Gu*, Ki 11) with draining.

If the *chi* pulse is moderate, there is weakness in the feet with swollen lower (limbs) and difficult urination and dribbling after voiding. This requires taking *Hua Shi Tang* (Talcum Decoction)[53] and *Qu Mai San* (Dianthus Powder)[54] and needling Horizontal Bone (*Heng Gu*, Ki 11) with draining.

If the *chi* pulse is slippery, there is qi and blood repletion. There is inhibition of the menstrual vessels in women, and hematuria in males. This requires taking *Po Xiao Tang* (Slaked Lime

---

[49] This formula is composed of Herba Dianthi (*Qu Mai*), Semen Benincasae Hispidae (*Dong Gua Zi*), Rhizoma Imperatae Cylindricae (*Bai Mao Gen*), Semen Malvae Verticillatae (*Dong Kui Zi*), Talcum (*Hua Shi*), Caulis Akebiae Mutong (*Mu Tong*), Herba Lophatheri Gracilis (*Zhu Ye*), and Radix Scutellariae Baicalensis (*Huang Qin*).

[50] The ingredients in this formula are Talcum (*Hua Shi*), Medulla Tetrapanacis Papyriferi (*Tong Cao*), Semen Plantaginis (*Che Qian Zi*), and Semen Malvae Verticillatae (*Dong Kui Zi*).

[51] This formula is composed of Radix Angelicae Sinensis (*Dang Gui*), Rhizoma Zingiberis (*Jiang*), Radix Paeoniae Lactiflorae (*Shao Yao*), Gelatinum Corii Asini (*E Jiao*), and Radix Scutellariae Baicalensis (*Huang Qin*).

[52] The ingredients in this formula include Ramulus Cinnamomi Cassiae (*Gui Zhi*), malt (*Yi Tang*), Rhizoma Zingiberis (*Jiang*), Radix Glycyrrhizae (*Gan Cao*), and Radix Paeoniae Lactiflorae (*Shao Yao*).

[53] This formula is prepared in the form of decoction with the same ingredients as in note 49 above.

[54] This formula is the same as in note 48 above but prepared in the form of a powder.

Decoction)[55] and *Da Huang Tang* (Rhubarb Decoction) to precipitate blood (stasis) from the channels and needling Origin Pass (*Guan Yuan*, CV 4) with draining.

If the *chi* pulse is bowstring, there is pain in the lower abdomen and hypertonicity of the lower abdomen and feet. This requires taking *Jian Zhong Tang* (Fortify the Center Decoction)[56] and *Dang Gui Tang* (Dang Gui Decoction) and needling Sea of Qi (*Qi Hai*, CV 6) with draining.

If the *chi* pulse is weak, there is shortage of yang qi giving rise to fever and vexation in the bones. This requires taking *Qian Hu Tang* (Peucedanum Decoction), *Gan Di Huang Tang* (Dried Rehmannia Decoction), and *Fu Ling Tang* (Poria Decoction) and needling Origin Pass (*Guan Yuan*, CV 4) with supplementation.

If the *chi* pulse is choppy, there are counterflow frigidity of the feet and lower legs and dark colored urine. This requires taking *Fu Zi Si Ni Tang* (Aconite Four Counterflows Decoction)[57] and needling Supreme Surge (*Tai Chong*, Liv 3) in the foot with supplementation.

If the *chi* pulse is scallion-stalk, there is vacuity of the lower burner with blood in the urine. This requires taking *Sheng Di Huang Tang* (Uncooked Rehmannia Decoction) with Cortex Bambusae (*Zhu Pi*) added, moxaing Cinnabar Field (*Dan Tian*, CV 5) and Origin Pass (*Guan Yuan*, CV 4), and also needling them with supplementation.

If the *chi* pulse is hidden, there is lower abdominal pain, conglomeration *shan*, and untransformed food in the stools. This requires taking a large dose of *Ping Wei Wan* (Level the Stomach Pills) and *Jie Geng Wan* (Platycodon Pills)[58] and needling Origin Pass (*Guan Yuan*, CV 4) with supplementation.

If the *chi* pulse is deep, there is pain in the upper and lower back . This requires taking *Shen Qi*

---

[55] This formula is composed of Mirabilitum (*Mang Xiao*), Slaked Lime (*Po Xiao*), Calcareous Spar (*Han Shui Shi*), and Gypsum (*Shi Gao*).

[56] This refers to Minor Fortify the Center Decoction (*Xiao Jian Zhong Tang*). See note 51 above.

[57] The ingredients in this formula include Radix Glycyrrhizae (*Gan Cao*), Rhizoma Zingiberis (*Jiang*), and Radix Praeparatus Aconiti Carmichaeli (*Fu Zi*).

[58] This formula is composed of Radix Platycodi Grandiflori (*Jie Geng*), Rhizoma Coptidis Chinensis (*Huang Lian*), Massa Medica Fermentata (*Shen Qu*), Fructus Germinatus Hordei Vulgaris (*Mai Ya*), Fructus Pruni Mume (*Wu Mei*), Cortex Magnoliae Officinalis (*Hou Po*), Rhizoma Atractylodis Macrocephalae (*Bai Zhu*), Radix Panacis Ginseng (*Ren Shen*), Halloysitum Rubrum (*Chi Shi Zhi*), Radix Scutellariae Baicalensis (*Huang Qin*), Radix Glycyrrhizae (*Gan Cao*), Os Draconis (*Long Gu*), and Cortex Cinnamomi Cassiae (*Gui Xin*).

Wan (Kidney Qi Pills)[59] and needling Capital Gate (*Jing Men*, GB 25) with supplementation.

If the *chi* pulse is soggy, there is the bitterness of difficult urination [wind *bi* with inability to move the feet in the *Qian Jin*]. This requires taking *Qu Mai Tang* (Dianthus Decoction) with powdered whitefish and needling Origin Pass (*Guan Yuan*, CV 4) with draining.

If the *chi* pulse is slow, there is cold in the lower burner. This requires taking *Gui Zhi Wan* (Cinnamon Twig Pills) and needling Sea of Qi (*Qi Hai*, CV 6) and Origin Pass (*Guan Yuan*, CV 4) with supplementation.

If the *chi* pulse is replete, there is lower abdominal pain with urinary incontinence. This requires taking *Dang Gui Tang* (Dang Gui Decoction) with 1 liang (*i.e.*, 50g) of Radix Et Rhizoma Rhei (*Da Huang*) added in order to disinhibit defecation and needling Origin Pass (*Guan Yuan*, CV 4) with supplementation to stop urination.

If the *chi* pulse is firm, there is abdominal fullness and hypertonicity of the external genitals. This requires taking *Ting Li Zi Zhu Yu Wan* (Lepidium Seed & Evodia Pills)[60] and needling Cinnabar Field (*Dan Tian*, CV 5), Origin Pass (*Guan Yuan*, CV 4), and Central Pole (*Zhong Ji*, CV 3).

The above are sixteen conditions relating to the pulse in the lower position, the *chi*.

---

[59] This formula is composed of Radix Rehmanniae (*Di Huang*), Radix Dioscoreae Oppositae (*Shan Yao*), Fructus Corni Officinalis (*Zhu Yu*), Sclerotium Poriae Cocos (*Fu Ling*), Rhizoma Alismatis (*Ze Xie*), Cortex Radicis Moutan (*Mu Dan Pi*), Ramulus Cinnamomi Cassiae (*Gui Zhi*), and Radix Praeparatus Aconiti Carmichaeli (*Fu Zi*).

[60] This formula is composed of Semen Lepdii (*Ting Li*) and Fructus Evodiae Rutecarpae (*Wu Zhu Yu*).

Chapter Four

A Discussion of the Pulses of the Eight Extraordinary Vessels

There are eight extraordinary vessels. What are they?

The answer is as follows:

They are the yang linking and yin linking, the yang motility and yin motility, the penetrating, governing, conception, and girdling vessels. These eight vessels are all independent of the channels and, therefore, are called extraordinary vessels. There are twelve channels and fifteen vessel networks, twenty-seven altogether. The qi follows these up and down. But why are the extraordinary vessels alone independent of the channels? The sages designed and dug canals and ditches and dredged waterways against unexpected dangers. If it rained (heavily), the canals and ditches would brim and flood. Rainwater then ran wild (everywhere). At that moment, the sages were unable to bring this water back (into the ditches and canals). These (extraordinary) vessels (are vessels to collect) the flooded water that is no longer confined to the channels.

Given that the eight extraordinary vessels are independent of the channels, where do they start and to what are they linked?

The answer is as follows:

The yang linking vessel originates at the meeting point of the various yang (channels, *i.e.*, Metal Gate *Jin Men*, Bl 63), and the yin linking vessel originates at the confluence of the various yin (*i.e.*, Guest House, *Zhu Bin*, Ki 9). The yang and yin linking vessels link and connect (every part of) the body, gathering the flooded (qi and blood) that are no longer able to circulate along or irrigate the channels.

The yang motility originates in the heel, ascending via the lateral malleolus and submerging in Wind Pool (*Feng Chi*, GB 20). The yin motility also originates within the heel, ascending via the medial malleolus to the throat, where it joins and communicates with the penetrating vessel.

The penetrating vessel originates at Origin Pass (*Guan Yuan*, CV 4), going straight upward inside the abdomen and reaching the throat. [In another version it is said that the penetrating vessel originates at Surging Qi (*Chong Qi*, St 30), joins the yang ming channel, travels upward by the side of the umbilicus, and disperses in the chest when it reaches there.]

The governing vessel originates at the point of the Lowest Extremity (*Xia Ji*, CV 1), joining the inside of the spine, reaching Wind Mansion (*Feng Fu*, GV 16) through the back. While the penetrating vessel is the sea of all the yin vessels, the governing vessel is the sea of all the yang vessels.

The conception vessel originates from Uterine Gate (*Bao Men*, Ki 13, left) and Infant Door (*Zi Hu*, Ki 13, right), travels upward bilateral to the umbilicus, and reaches the chest. [It is said in another version that the conception originates from below Central Pole (*Zhong Ji*, CV 3), rises to the pubic hair region, proceeds inside the abdomen up through Origin Pass (*Guan Yuan*, CV 4), and ends in the throat.]

The girdling vessel originates in the region of the free rib [lateral costal region in the *Nan Jing*] and encircles the body.

These eight are vessels independent of the twelve channels and, therefore, are called extraordinary vessels.

What kinds of diseases are the extraordinary vessels capable of?

The answer is as follows:

The yang linking vessel links the yang (channels), while the yin linking vessel links the yin. If the yin and yang (linking vessels) fail to perform their linking functions, there will arise abstraction, loss of orientation, and lethargy. [A person abstracted is susceptible to fright. As a result of apprehension, the linking vessels become slack. Slackness makes the body feckless, thus giving rise to loss of orientation, impaired memory, and abstraction.]

The disease of the yang linking vessel is the bitterness of cold and heat (*i.e.*, fever and chills). The disease of the yin linking vessel is the bitterness of heart pain. [The yang linking is the defensive, and the defensive is capable of giving rise to cold and heat. The yin linking is the constructive, and the constructive is the blood. Blood rules the heart and, therefore, the yin linking is capable of giving rise to heart pain.]

The disease of the yin motility is slack yang and tense yin. [The yin motility is located in the medial malleolus. When it is diseased, it is tense. Thus tension occurs from the medial malleolus upward and slackness occurs from the lateral malleolus upward.]

The disease of the yang motility is slack yin and tense yang. [The yang motility is located in the lateral malleolus. When it is diseased, it is tense. Thus the (sick) person suffers from tension from the lateral malleolus upward and slackness from the medial malleolus upward.]

The disease of the penetrating vessel is qi counterflow with abdominal urgency (*i.e.,* cramping). [The penetrating vessel goes from Origin Pass (*Guan Yuan,* CV 4) to the throat. Therefore, it is capable of giving rise to qi counterflow and abdominal urgency.]

The disease of the governing vessel is rigidity of the spine and inversion. [The governing vessel is located in the back. When it is diseased, it becomes tense, causing rigidity of the spine.]

The disease of the conception vessel is the bitterness of internal binding developing into the seven *shan*[1] in males and conglomeration and gathering[2] in females. [The conception vessel originates at Uterine Gate (*Bao Men,* Ki 13, left) and Infant Door (*Zi Hu,* Ki 13, right). Therefore, its disease, binding, may develop into the seven *shan* and conglomeration and gathering.]

The disease of the girdling is the bitterness of abdominal fullness and weakness in the lower back as if sitting in water. [The girdling vessel circles around the body. When it is diseased, it is slack, thus causing the lower back to be weak.]

These are the diseases of the eight extraordinary vessels.

If the yang linking pulse[3] is found to be floating, visual dizziness will arise on attempting to rise up. This is due to exuberance and repletion of yang. There is (also) the bitterness of lifting the shoulders to facilitate breathing and shivering as if in the cold.

If the yin linking pulse is found to be large, deep, and replete, the bitterness is pain in the chest, propping fullness in the lateral costal regions, and heart pain.

If the yin linking pulse is found to be like a string of pearls, there is repletion in the lateral costal regions and pain in the lower back in males and pain in the external genitals as with sores in females.

---

[1] The seven *shan* include those of the five viscera as well as fox and *tui shan*. However, there are also other ways to categorize these conditions. In short, any enlargement in the abdomen and scrotum can be referred to as *shan*.

[2] Conglomeration and gathering is a glomus or mass that is movable. It gathers and disperses unpredictably.

[3] For the location of this pulse, see Book Ten.

If the girdling vessel pulse is perceived,[4] there is pain from around the umbilicus to the (lateral) abdomen and the lumbar spine. This pain radiates to the medial aspects of the thighs.

When the pulse on both hands displays yang at the superficial level and yin at the deep level,[5] both yin and yang[6] are replete and exuberant. This is the pulse of the governing and the penetrating vessels.[4] The penetrating and governing vessels are the thoroughfares for the twelve channels. If they overplay their power, the twelve channels will no longer meet at the *cun* opening and the (sick) person will experience the bitterness of abstraction, mania, and feeble-mindedness. If not, the person must suffer from vacillation and being of two minds.

When the yang pulses[7] at both hands are so floating, fine, and faint that they are hardly palpable and if the yin pulse,[7] though present, is also very fine, this is the (pulse of) the yang and yin motility.[4] This house has had a death from obsession by ghosts or from wind. The bitterness is abstraction, a disaster brought on by the dead person. [The last two sentences are suspected to be interpolations.]

If the yang motility (pulse) is perceived, there is a disease of hypertonicity. If the yin motility (pulse) is perceived, there is a disease of slackness.

A pulse floating in the *chi* to the *cun*, (beating) straight up and down, is a governing vessel pulse. (If it appears,) there will be stiffness and pain in and inability to bend either forward or backward the upper and lower back. In adults, there will be the disease of madness, while in children, there will be trouble of wind epilepsy.[8]

If the pulse arrives floating in the middle position, beating straight up and down, this is a pulse of the governing vessel. When (this vessel) is affected, there will be the bitterness of cold in the

---

4   For the locations of the pulses of the eight extraordinary vessels, see Book Ten as well as the following discussions in this chapter. One should note that the pulses corresponding to the eight extraordinary vessels do not mainly have to do with their location as in the case of the viscera or bowels but with their images. In other words, one should not feel these images in normal cases. If a pulse of an extraordinary vessel is present, some disorder related to that vessel already does exist.

5   Yin and yang in this context mean nearly the same, *i.e.,* an exuberant pulse image.

6   In this context, yin and yang respectively mean the deep and superficial levels. They are also simultaneously indicative of yin qi and yang qi.

7   Here, a yang pulse refers to the *cun* pulse, while a yin pulse refers to the *chi* pulse.

8   This refers to epilepsy due to wind seen in infants. The child is seen to cry with convulsive spasms and contracted fingers.

upper and lower backs and knees. In adults, there will be madness, and in children, epilepsy. (To treat this,) moxa the vertex with three cones, right in the center of the top.

If the pulse is firm from the *chi* to the *cun*, (beating) straight up and down, this is a pulse of the penetrating vessel revealing that there is cold *shan* in the chest.

If the pulse arrives hard and replete at the middle position, popping up in the *guan*, this is a pulse of the penetrating vessel. When (this vessel) is affected, there will be the bitterness of lower abdominal pain, (qi) rushing into the heart, the existence of concretion *shan*, infertility, fecal and urinary incontinence, and distressing propping fullness of the lateral costal regions.

If a pulse stays in the *cun* like rolling pellets, this is a pulse of the conception vessel. When (this vessel) is affected, there will be the bitterness of a finger-shaped qi mass in the abdomen which may surge up into the heart. There will be inability to bend (the body) either forward or backward and hypertonicity (in the abdomen).

If the pulse arrives tight, fine, replete, and long (from the *chi*) to the *guan*, this is a pulse of the conception vessel. When (this vessel) is affected, there will be the bitterness of periumbilical pain in the lower abdomen radiating down to the pubic bone and sending a lancinating pain to the external genitals. Treat the point three *cun* under the umbilicus.

BOOK THREE

Collated and edited by Honorary Minister Without Portfolio,
Curator of the Imperial Library,
Imperial Courier and Senior Army Protector,
Lin Yi *et al.*

The Section on the Liver & Gallbladder

The liver is analogous to wood and united with the bowel of the gallbladder. Its channel is the foot *jue yin* which has an interior/exterior relationship with the foot *shao yang*. Its pulse is bowstring. [Bowstring is typical of the liver pulse.] It is minister (*xiang*)[1] in the three months of winter. [In winter, water is king and wood is its minister.] It is king (*wang*)[1] in the three months of spring. It abdicates (*fei*)[1] in the three months of summer. It is confined in the last month of summer, *i.e.*, the sixth month. [In the last month of summer, earth is king but wood is confined.] It is dead (*si*)[1] in the three months of autumn. [In autumn, metal is king and wood is dead.]

Its king days are *jia* and *yi*. Its king watches are calm dawn (3-5 a.m.) and sunrise (5-7 a.m.). [All of these are ascribed to wood.] Its confined days are *wu* and *ji*. Its confined watches are breakfast (7-9 a.m.) and sun's descent (1-3 p.m.). [All of these are ascribed to earth.] Its dead days are *geng* and *xin*. Its dead watches are late afternoon (3-5 p.m.) and sundown (5-7 p.m.). [All of these are ascribed to metal.]

Its spirit is the ethereal soul (*hun*). That which it rules is color. That which it nourishes are the sinews. Its expression is the eyes. [The liver is reflected in the eyes. Therefore, in case of liver repletion, the eyes are red.] Its sound is shouting. Its color is green-blue. Its smell is of urine. [It is said in the "*Yue Ling* (Lunar Order)"[2] that it smells like a ram.] Its fluid is tears. [Tears come from the liver.] Its flavor is sour. That which becomes it is bitterness. [Bitterness is the flavor of fire.] That which it is averse to is acridity. [Acridity is the flavor of metal.]

---

[1] According to five phase theory, a viscus is king during the months, days, or hours corresponding to the same phase. Thus the liver, wood, is king during wood months, days, or hours. Continuing to take liver wood as an example, wood is child to water. During water's king time, liver wood enjoys assistance from its mother, water. This period is the ministerial time for liver wood. Fire is the child of wood and relies on wood for nourishment. In summer, fire is king and wood, the mother, is dwindling away because it has to meet the extravagant demands of its child. In this period, liver wood abdicates. In long summer or the last month of summer, earth, which should be restrained by wood, is king. During this period, earth will become too strong to be restrained by wood. Therefore, during the sixth month in the Chinese lunar calendar, liver wood remains confined. Metal restrains wood. In the metal king's months, days, or hours, wood suffers doubly and can be nothing other than defunct. Therefore, autumn, *geng* and *xin* days, or the late afternoon watch (3-5 p.m.) are perishing times for liver wood.

[2] This is a chapter in the *Li Ji* (*Record of Rituals*) which is virtually an almanac based on five phase theory.

Its transporting point is located at the ninth vertebra in the back, and its alarm point is Cycle Gate (*Qi Men*, Liv 14). The transporting point of the gallbladder is located at the tenth vertebra in the back, and its alarm point is Sun & Moon (*Ri Yue*, GB 24).

The above is newly compiled. [It is derived from the *Su Wen (Simple Questions)* and other classics. In the past, people compiled this section in such a confused and incoherent way that it was too complex to understand. Now (the present author) presents a copy of the relevant essentials divided into five parts based on the five viscera.]

On the first *jia zi* day[3] after the Winter Solstice, the *shao yang* inaugurates at midnight and the liver begins its reign. [The Winter Solstice is a term at the end of the year, and the *jia zi* day is the switching day between yin and yang. The *shao yang* is the gallbladder, and the gallbladder is wood which is generated from water. Therefore, (the *shao yang*) inaugurates at midnight. Because its qi is usually faint and meager, it is called *shao yang* (lesser yang). Midnight, the *zi* watch, is ascribed to water.] The liver is ascribed to the east and wood. (During spring) tens of thousands of things are beginning to engender and the qi comes soft and weak, loose and vacuous. [Spring sees *shao yang* qi which is warm and gentle, soft and weak. Hence everything is growing day by day.] Therefore the pulse is bowstring. [Liver qi nourishes the sinews. Therefore, its pulse is (like a) rigid bowstring. This is an analogy to the rigidity of material wood.] Softness forbids diaphoresis, while weakness forbids precipitation. Looseness means open (interstices) and openness, in turn, means disinhibition. Disinhibition is free flow. This is what is meant by the statement that (the *shao yang* qi) is loose and vacuous. [This tells that at its beginning, the *shao yang* is still soft and weak and that the constructive, the defensive and the interstices are open and free. (Therefore,) diaphoresis may induce uncheckable perspiration. Precipitation is also prohibited, since precipitation may induce uncheckable diarrhea. This is what is signified by looseness and vacuity when they are spoken of as disinhibition and free flow.] In spring, the root (of the liver) is the stomach qi which must not be violated. [The stomach is earth, while the tens of thousands of things rely on earth to grow. The stomach also nourishes the five viscera. For that reason, the liver in its king period must take the stomach qi as its root. Not to violate (the stomach qi) is to prevent it from damage.]

The above is derived from the classics on the four seasons.

The Yellow Emperor asked:

---

[3] When one combines the ten Heavenly Stems (*jia, yi, etc.*) and the twelve Earthly Branches (*zi, chou, etc.*), one gets a sixty day cycle with *jia zi* as the first day in this cycle. After the Winter Solstice is the time when the liver/gallbladder, *i.e.*, the *shao yang* qi, reigns.

The spring pulse is like a bowstring. Why is this so?

Qi Bo answered:

The spring pulse is of the liver which is ascribed to the east and wood. (In spring,) tens of thousands of things begin to engender. Therefore, the (pulse) qi comes soggy, weak, gentle, vacuous, and slippery. Because it is straight and long, it is called bowstring. (Pulses) contrary to this indicate disease.

The Yellow Emperor asked:

What are the contrary pulses like?

Qi Bo answered:

If (the pulse) qi comes not only replete but strong, this is known as excess, suggesting disease in the external. If (the pulse) qi comes not only unreplete but faint, this is known as insufficiency, suggesting disease in the center.

The Yellow Emperor asked:

What illnesses are there when the spring pulse shows excess and insufficiency?

Qi Bo answered:

Excess causes people impaired memory [irritability should take the place of impaired memory], abstraction, dizziness, oppression, and troubles involving the head. Insufficiency causes people pain in the chest and flanks radiating to the upper back and, below, fullness in the lateral costal and subaxillary regions.

The Yellow Emperor said:

Good. If the liver pulse arrives soggy and weak, undulating gently, giving a sensation of touching the end of a long pole, this is a normal pulse. [It is said in the *Chao Yuan (Chao's Origin)*[4] that when the pulse is leisurely, feeling like touching the string of a musical instrument or touching along a pole, it is known as normal.] The spring (pulse) relies on the stomach qi as its root. If the liver pulse arrives brimming, replete, and slippery, feeling like touching along a long pole, this suggests liver disease. If the liver pulse arrives not only urgent but forceful like a full-drawn bowstring, this indicates that the liver is dead.

____

[4] The *Zhu Bing Yuan Hou Lun* (*Treatise on the Origins & Symptoms of Various Diseases*) in full by Chao Yuan-fang published in 610 CE.

The true liver pulse[5] is a pulse that is urgent inside and at the sides, giving a sensation of sharpness as when one feels the edge of a knife or presses on the string of the musical instrument. If the facial complexion is whitish green-blue and lusterless with brittle hair, then death will ensue.

The spring pulse with stomach[5] is slightly bowstring. This is a normal pulse. If the pulse is very bowstring with little stomach, liver disease is suggested. If it is completely bowstring with no stomach, death is suggested. If it is hair-like with a shade of stomach,[6] disease will arise in autumn. If (the pulse) is very hair-like, imminent disease is suggested.

The liver stores blood and blood houses ethereal soul (*hun*). When sorrow and lamentation disturb the center, the *hun* is injured. When the *hun* is injured, there arise mania and frenzy, absence of essence (*i.e.*, feeble-mindedness), not daring to face people [for the last two conditions, another version gives essence insecurity and retracted testicles], retracted testicles, sinew hypertonicity, inability to lift the free ribs, brittle hair, and a perishing facial complexion. Then death will come in autumn.

In spring, liver wood is the king. If the pulse is bowstring, fine, and long, it is a normal pulse. If, on the contrary, it feels floating, choppy, and short [faint, choppy, and short in the *Qian Jin*], this shows that the lungs are overwhelming the liver. Since metal should restrain wood, the evil is murderous. It is a greatly unfavorable (condition). Ten out of ten cases will die without a remedy.

If, on the contrary, the pulse is surging, large, and dissipated [floating, large, and surging in the *Qian Jin*], this shows that the heart is overwhelming the liver. Because the child should assist its mother, the evil is repletion. Even though it causes disease, it will cure by itself.

If, on the contrary, the pulse feels deep, soggy, and slippery, this shows that the kidneys are overwhelming the liver. When the mother turns to its child, the evil is vacuity. Even though it causes disease, it is easy to treat.

---

5 In normal cases, there is a distinctive pulse image in each season. In spring, for example, if the pulse is a little bowstring, this is normal. But in normal cases, every pulse image should contain a shade of stomach or stomach qi. This is characterized by a quality of moderateness. If, in a certain season or a particular condition, the pulse expresses its seasonal features too strongly without any modification of moderateness, this is called absence of stomach qi. A pulse without stomach qi is called a true pulse of a certain viscus. For example, if in winter the pulse becomes deep and hard to an extreme degree (deepness and hardness being characteristics peculiar to the winter and, by extension, the kidneys), this is a true kidney pulse, a fatal sign.

6 A hairy pulse which is floating, soft, and a little dissipated is the pulse of autumn or the lungs. If the hairy pulse appears in a season other than autumn, disease is suggested.

If, on the contrary, the pulse feels large and moderate, this shows that the spleen is overwhelming the liver. When earth bullies wood, the evil is a mild one. Even though it causes disease, it will be overcome soon.

The liver pulse may arrive welling, giving a sensation of standing against a pole or touching a string drawn on a musical instrument. If it beats twice (in one inhalation or one exhalation), it is a normal pulse. If it beats thrice, it suggests an illness of channel aberration. If it beats four times, it suggests desertion of essence. If it beats five times, this is death (*i.e.*, death will ensue). If it beats six times, life is at an end.

The above is (a discussion of) the pulses of the foot *jue yin*.

A very urgent liver pulse points to blasphemy (*i.e.*, confused speech), while a slightly urgent liver pulse to fat qi[7] which is located under the lateral costal region like an upside down cup. A very moderate liver pulse points to frequent retching, while a slightly moderate liver pulse to water conglomeration *bi*.[8] A very large liver pulse points to internal *yong*, frequent retching, and external spontaneous bleeding, but a slightly large liver pulse to liver *bi*[9] with retracted testicles and cough provoking a discomfort in the lateral abdomen. A very small liver pulse points to massive drinking, while a slightly small liver pulse to pure heat wasting thirst. A very slippery liver pulse points to *tui shan*,[10] but a slightly slippery liver pulse to enuresis. A very choppy liver pulse points to phlegm rheum, while a slightly choppy liver pulse to tugging and slackening and sinew cramps.

When the qi of the foot *jue yin* expires, the sinews contract, making the testicles retracted and the tongue curled. The *jue yin* is the liver vessel, while the liver is associated with the sinews. The sinews gather around the external genitals and connect with the root of the tongue. Therefore, when the (liver) vessel receives no nourishment, the sinews become contracted and tense. When the sinews become contracted and tense, they withdraw the tongue and the testicles. Thus cyanic lips, curled tongue, and retracted testicles show that the sinews are already dead. (Liver disease) may become exacerbated on *geng* days and end in death on *xin* days, for metal overcomes wood.

---

7   Liver accumulation is called fat qi. It refers to a mass located under the ribs on the left side of the abdomen.

8   This is a condition due to water evils blocking. In this case, water gathers into a mass in the region below the heart. This mass gathers and disperses unpredictably and may develop into generalized edema.

9   This condition is characterized by sleep fraught with fright and terror, thirst, massive drinking, frequent urination, and abdominal distention.

10   *Tui shan* refers to scrotal swelling with pain affecting the lateral sides of the lower abdomen in males and pain and hypertonicity in the lower lateral abdomen in females.

The liver is a dead viscus if the pulse is weak at the superficial level and, when pressure is applied, becomes like a rope with no beat palpable or like a winding snake. Then this is death.

The above is derived from the *Su Wen (Simple Questions)*, the *Zhen Jing (Classic of Needling)*,[11] and Zhang Zhong-jing.

____

[11] This is another name for the *Ling Shu (Spiritual Pivot)*.

_____________Chapter Two_____________
The Section on the Heart & Small Intestine

The heart is analogous to fire and is united with the bowel of the small intestine. [The small intestine is a bowel which receives and contains.] Its channel is the hand *shao yin* which has an interior/exterior relationship with the hand *tai yang*. Its pulse is surging.

It is minister in the three months of spring. [(In spring,) wood is king and fire is its minister.] It is king in the three months of summer. It abdicates in the last summer month, the sixth month. It is confined in the three months of autumn. [(In autumn,) metal is king and fire is confined.] It is dead in the three months of winter. [(In winter,) water is king and fire is dead.]

Its king days are *bing* and *ding*, and its king watches are outlying region (9-11 a.m.) and midday (11 a.m.-1 p.m.). Its confined days are *geng* and *xin*, and its confined watches are late afternoon (3-5 p.m.) and sundown (5-7 p.m.). Its dead days are *ren* and *gui*, and its dead watches are serenity (9-11 p.m.) and midnight (11 p.m.-1 a.m.).

That which it stores is spirit. That which it rules is smell. That which it nourishes is blood. Its expression is the tongue. Its sound is speech. Its color is red. Its smell is a charred odor. Its fluid is sweat. Its flavor is bitterness. That which becomes it is sweetness. That which it is averse to is saltiness. The transporting point of the heart is located at the fifth vertebra in the back. [It also can be said to be at the seventh vertebra.] Its alarm point is Great Tower Gate (*Ju Que*, CV 14). The transporting point of the small intestine is located at the eighteenth vertebra in the back, and its alarm point is Origin Pass (*Guan Yuan*, CV 4).

The above is newly compiled.

The heart is ascribed to the south and fire. [The heart governs blood, and its color is red. For that reason, it is king in the south in summer and corresponds to the phase of fire.] (In summer,) tens of thousands of things are exuberant and extravagant. (Trees) are growing drooping twigs and heavy foliage, all of which bend, hanging down. (Therefore, the summer pulse) is called hook-like. The heart pulse is surging, large, and long. This surging is produced by replenished defensive qi. When (the defensive qi) is replenished, qi can find nowhere to escape. [A surging pulse shows replenished defensive qi. When defensive qi is replenished, the interstices are compact, and, when (the interstices) are compact, the qi cannot find anywhere to escape.] The largeness is produced by luxuriant constructive qi. Luxuriant (constructive qi) and surging (defensive qi) work together, making diaphoresis possible and producing a long (pulse). Since a long and surging (pulse) are present at the same time, one has to drink (quantities of) water to irrigate the channels and vessel networks and to moisten the skin with fluid. That the *tai yang* becoming surging and large is entirely credited to its mother's body and its lucky acquisition of *wu* and *ji* which is utilized to fasten the root of the plant. [The *tai yang* is summer fire, and its mother is spring wood. Yang does not begin to generate till spring comes, and (during spring) yang is called *shao* (lesser) yang. When summer comes, (yang) becomes surging and exuberant and is, therefore, called *tai* (great) yang. On that account, the *shao yang* is said to be the mother's body (of the *tai yang*). *Wu* and *ji* mean earth. Earth is the child of fire. When fire is king, earth is its minister. Therefore, earth should be used to help fix the root of the plant (*i.e.* the *tai yang*).]

When yang qi exits from the upper (body), perspiration appears on the head, the five internal (organs) become desiccated, and the bladder is empty. (In this situation,) if a physician misuses precipitation, this will cause double vacuity.

A floating pulse reveals the presence (*i.e.*, repletion) of the exterior with absence (*i.e.*, vacuity) of the interior and that yang acts as envoy for noone. [When yang is exuberant and (the pulse) is floating, it is appropriate to promote perspiration. If precipitation is administered instead, yin qi will be injured. Yang is the exterior, while yin is the interior. It is stated in the classic that yang is the envoy of yin, while yin is the guard of yang. They are thus interdependent on one another. (In this sense,) a floating pulse suggests the absence of the interior. If this is treated in an erroneous way, yin and yang will be separated and no longer able to act reciprocally as agents.] This not only endangers (the *tai yang*) itself, but strikes its mother. [This says that precipitation not only brings damage to the heart but also strikes the liver.]

The above is derived from the classics on the four seasons.

The Yellow Emperor asked:

The summer pulse is like a hook. Why is this so?

Qi Bo answered:

The summer pulse is of the heart which is ascribed to the south and fire. (In summer,) every living thing flourishes. Therefore, (the pulse) qi arrives exuberant but retreats in decline. Because of this, (the pulse) is called hook-like. (Pulses) contrary to this indicate disease.

The Yellow Emperor asked:

What are the contrary pulses like?

If the (pulse) qi not only arrives exuberant but retreats exuberant, this is known as excess. (It) reveals that there is disease in the external. If the (pulse) qi does not arrive exuberant but retreats exuberant, this is known as insufficiency and suggests that there is disease in the center.

The Yellow Emperor asked:

What kinds of disease are there when the summer pulse shows excess and insufficiency?

Qi Bo answered:

Excess causes people bodily heat and pain in the skin developing into a disease known as sapping (*jin yin*).[1] Insufficiency causes people vexation of the heart and coughing of foamy sputum above with qi leakage[2] below.

The Yellow Emperor said:

Good. If the heart pulse feels like a string of pearls or glossy jade, this is a normal pulse. The summer (pulse) relies on the stomach qi as its root. If the pulse arrives as if gasping,[3] beating continuously without a break, with small amplitude of modulation,[4] this suggests heart disease. If the heart pulse arrives first crooked and then straight, giving a sensation of holding a crook-

---

[1] The word sapping implies evil qi growing rampantly. In this case, the evil grows in an aggressive, threatening way causing heat to pervade the body. However, this term may also refer to the outbreak of sores due to effulgent fire or damp heat.

[2] *I.e.*, passing of gas or flatulence

[3] A pulse as if gasping is a pounding, urgent pulse. It arrives tense and exuberant, but when it retreats, it flops weakly.

[4] Concerning the description of this type of pulse, there is another interpretation which says that the pulse is one that strikes forcefully and very rapidly but occasionally pauses.

shaped girdle,[5] this indicates that the heart is dead.

The true heart pulse is a pulse that is hard and striking forcefully, feeling like a string of Job's tears. If the facial complexion is reddish black and lusterless with brittle hair, death will ensue.

The summer (pulse) with stomach is slightly hook-like. This is a normal pulse. If the pulse is very hook-like with little stomach, heart disease is suggested. If it is completely hook-like with no stomach, death is suggested. If it has stomach with a stone-like shade,[6] disease will occur in winter. If it is very stone-like, imminent disease is suggested.

The heart stores the vessels, and it is the vessels that house the spirit. Apprehension, thought, and worry damage the spirit. When the spirit is damaged, there arise susceptibility to fright, spontaneous flux,[7] shedding and cleaving of the major limb muscles, brittle hair, and a perishing facial complexion. Then death will occur in winter.

In summer, heart fire is king, and its pulse is surging, large and dissipated [floating, large, and surging in the *Qian Jin*]. This is a normal pulse. If, on the contrary, it is deep, soggy, and slippery, this shows the kidneys are overwhelming the heart. Since water should restrain fire, the evil is a murderous one. It is a greatly unfavorable condition. Ten out of ten cases will die without a remedy.

If, on the contrary, the summer pulse is large and moderate, this shows the spleen is overwhelming the heart. Since the child should assist its mother, the evil is repletion. Even though it causes disease, it will heal by itself.

If, on the contrary, the summer pulse is bowstring, fine, and long, this shows the liver is overwhelming the heart. When the mother turns to the child, the evil is vacuity. Even though it causes disease, it is easy to treat.

If, on the contrary, the summer pulse is floating [faint in the *Qian Jin*], choppy, and short, this shows the lungs are overwhelming the heart. When metal bullies fire, the evil is a mild one. Even though it causes disease, it will be overcome soon.

---

[5] This refers to a belt decorated with a hook-shaped, ornamental buckle worn in ancient times. Running one's finger over such a hook-shaped buckle, one would first feel a high part followed by flatness. This is what is being suggested here. However, there is another interpretation that the pulse is hard and shaped like a clothes hook.

[6] A stone-like pulse is a deep, hard pulse which is ascribed to the kidneys.

[7] Flux here means spermatorrhea in males and vaginal discharge in females.

The heart pulse may appear like a string of pearls, smooth and slippery. If it beats twice (for an inhalation or an exhalation), this is normal. If it beats thrice, this indicates a disease of channel aberration. If it beats four times, there is desertion of essence. If it beats five times, this is death. If it beats six times, life is at an end.

The above is (a discussion of) the pulses of the hand *shao yin.*

A very urgent heart pulse points to tugging and slackening, while a slightly urgent heart pulse to heart pain radiating to the upper back and inability to ingest. A very moderate heart pulse points to manic laughing, while a slightly moderate heart pulse to deep-lying beam[8] located below the heart which, moving up and down, may give rise to blood ejection. A very large heart pulse points to constriction of the throat, but a slightly large heart pulse to heart *bi*[9] sending a discomfort to the upper back with frequent tearing. A very small heart pulse points to frequent retching, while a slightly small heart pulse to pure heat wasting thirst. A very slippery heart pulse points to constant thirst, while a slightly slippery heart pulse to heart *shan*[10] sending discomfort to the umbilicus with rumbling in the lower abdomen. A very choppy heart pulse points to loss of voice, but a slightly choppy heart pulse to bleeding and inversion frigidity of the four limbs, ringing in the ears, and troubles involving the head.

When the qi of the hand *shao yin* expires, (the blood) vessels are blocked. This is because the *shao yin* is the heart vessel, and the heart is associated with (the blood) vessels. When the vessels are blocked, blood circulation is at a stop. When blood stops circulating, the hair and the complexion become lusterless. Therefore, a facial complexion which is as black as a lacquer faggot shows that the blood is already dead. (Heart disease) becomes exacerbated on *ren* days and ends in death on *gui* days, for water overcomes fire.

The heart is a dead viscus if the pulse is replete at the superficial level, striking against the fingers like beans or hemp seeds. If it also feels agitated and racing, this is death.

The above is derived from the *Su Wen* (*Simple Questions*), the *Zhen Jing* (*Classic of Needling*), and Zhang Zhong-jing.

---

[8] Deep-lying beam is a mass transversely lying in the upper or lower abdomen. It can be as large as an arm.

[9] This refers to inhibited blood vessels manifesting as vexation, palpitations, panting, dry throat, belching, and apprehension.

[10] *I.e.,* a painful mass in the lower abdomen due to heart and, therefore, small intestine disease.

The Section on the Spleen & Stomach

The spleen is analogous to earth and is united with the bowel of the stomach. Its channel is the foot *tai yin* which has an interior/exterior relationship with the foot *yang ming*. Its pulse is moderate. It is minister in the three months of summer. [(In summer,) fire is king and earth is its minister.] It is king in the last summer month or the sixth month. It abdicates in the three months of autumn. It is confined in the three months of winter. It is dead in the three months of spring.

Its king days are *wu* and *ji*. Its king watches are breakfast (7-9 a.m.) and sun's descent (1-3 p.m.). Its confined days are *ren* and *gui*. Its confined watches are serenity (9-11 p.m.) and midnight (11 p.m.-1 a.m.). Its dead days are *jia* and *yi*. Its dead watches are calm dawn (3-5 a.m.) and sunrise (5-7 a.m.). [Both of these are watches ascribed to wood.]

Its spirit is reflection (*yi*). That which it rules is flavor. That which it nourishes is the flesh. Its expression is the mouth. Its sound is singing. Its color is yellow. Its smell is fragrance. Its fluid is saliva. Its flavor is sweetness. That which becomes it is acridity. That which it is averse to is acidity.

The transporting point of the spleen is located at the eleventh vertebra in the back, and its alarm point is Camphorwood Gate (*Zhang Men*, Liv 13). The transporting point of the stomach is located at the twelfth vertebra in the back, and its alarm point is Supreme Granary (*Tai Cang*, CV 12).

The above is newly compiled.

The spleen is attributed to earth. (Earth) is bountiful and generous. Bountifulness is richness. (Thus to earth are credited) tens of thousands of things in diversified colors. [The spleen governs water and grain. If its qi is faint and weak, water and grain cannot be transformed. The spleen is ascribed to the earth phase and is king in the last summer month. Earth is bountiful and rich by nature. It breeds and nourishes the tens of thousands of living things. In the last summer month, all kinds of plants are seen with luxuriant branches and leaves. There are a multitude of species of them in various different colors — green, yellow, red, white, and black.] For this reason, (earth) is said to be virtuous. Generosity is vastness. [Earth produces and nourishes tens of thousands of things. Similarly, the spleen provides supplies for the various viscera. On this account, (the spleen) is boundlessly beneficent.] All living things, including plants with hanging roots or crawling vines and leaves (growing) on the top, wriggling wrigglers or moving midges, flying insects or any breathing animals, receive grace from earth. Virtue is (something) moderate, and grace is expected to be leisurely. Therefore the *tai yin* pulse is moderate and slow, and it is different between the *chi* and the *cun*. [In the *chi*, (the pulse) is slow, and in the *cun*, it is moderate.]

Sourness, saltiness, bitterness, and acridity are all products of the great sand (*i.e.*, earth). At the time (when the spleen is exuberant), they all go around (the body), but they each have their own routes. They never head for the same place. (Therefore,) one can take them all constantly. [The liver is sour; the kidneys are salty; the heart is bitter; and the lungs are acrid and astringent. These flavors are those of the four viscera. The spleen governs the balancing of the five flavors to nourish the four viscera, while the four viscera receive flavors from the spleen. When the spleen is king, its vessels reach (all) the muscles and flesh. (The five flavors) travel around the body, and then they each take a separate route, going along the four limbs, making their qi pervade the whole body to sustain the various viscera and bowels and nourish the skin and hair. They do not go to the same place in a group. For that reason it is said that one can take them all constantly.]

Earth is warm in cold (weather) but cool in hot (weather). [In winter, yang qi lies below and earth is warm. In summer, yin qi lies below and earth is cool. The case is the same with the spleen qi.]

Earth has one child known as metal. It carries metal in its bosom, never allowing it to leave its body. Metal, (however,) is afraid of fire. For fear of heat fuming (it), it may forsake its mother and flee to water. Water is the child of metal and is able to keep the fire spirit out of sight. (Inside water, metal is safely sealed, as if living) with doors and windows shut up, the inside shut up from the outside. This is likened to the winter time. [When yang qi settles in the center (*i.e.*, earth spleen) — yang is ascribed to the fire phase — because metal is afraid of fire by nature, it fears being fumed (by fire) and returns to water to escape from fire. (Thus,) the mother and the child (*i.e.*, lung metal and kidney water) mutually help each other and both become exuberant. Being shut up implies that within replenished water qi, metal is secure and fortified so that fire can find no opportunity to restrain it any more. This says that (metal) is tightly sealed.][1] Since earth has lost its child, its qi becomes diminished and debilitated. (In consequence,) water floods, inundating and causing pools. It penetrates and strikes the skin, causing puffy swelling of the face and eyes and gathers in the limbs. [This describes (the consequence of) damage and debilitation of the spleen. Earth is capable of defending against water. Now earth is weak, while water is strong. Therefore, water finds a chance to overwhelm (earth) and run wild.] When seeing (the case of)

---

[1] According to the annotation, it seems that the escape of metal from fire makes the lung metal secure. However, the present translator has a different understanding of this passage. In long summer, summerheat, or in some heat conditions, the lungs (metal) are subjected to the torment of fire. Thus, they tend to turn to water (or the kidneys) for help. In doing so, metal creates a potential danger for earth (spleen). This is because it strengthens water undesirably. Since water is ascribed to winter, when water is replenished too much, winter gains its reign in an untimely manner or, in other words, water floods.

water, an ignorant physician may recklessly administer precipitation (only) to evacuate the spleen and empty the stomach. (As a result,) water overlies (the spleen and stomach), causing the lungs to float and develop dyspnea. [When the spleen and stomach are already diseased, it is appropriate to bank up and nourish their qi and to disinhibit the waterways. Ignorant physicians do not know this but administer precipitation. This causes double injury (to the spleen qi) and water qi will bully it ever more. (Then water qi) invades the chest. Meeting with water, the lungs are upborne. Therefore, the lungs are said to float and become dyspneic.] On the other hand, the liver fears the lungs. So it sinks and submerges below. [The lungs are metal, while the liver is wood. The former restrains the latter. When the lungs are floating, they become replete and inevitably restrain the liver ever more. For fear of them, (the liver) sinks and submerges below.] (Now) there appears brambles underneath. For fear that it will injure its body, (the spleen) evades to the side, giving way to water flow. [Brambles are a kind of wood. The liver is just wood. When it is sunken below, it turns into a bramble. The word body means the spleen's body. The spleen is earth. Earth is afraid of wood. Therefore, (the spleen) evades. It is shunning wood. Water flow means the passageways of water flow. Earth restrains water originally. Now, however, it is faint, weak, and, in addition, struck by wood. It is no longer able to restrain water. Therefore, water has a chance to prevail.]

Since the heart is debilitated, the pulse is hidden. Because the liver is faint, the pulse is deep. Therefore, now the pulse is hidden and deep. [The heart is fire, while the liver is wood. Fire fears water and wood fears metal. When metal and water conspire, their qi becomes replete so as to overwhelm the liver and heart. Thus the two viscera (the liver and heart) are debilitated and faint. (Therefore,) the pulse becomes deep and hidden.] If an experienced physician comes to handle the case, he will twist (the needle) at the (right) point to disinhibit the stools and urine. In consequence, the waterways are freed and sweet fluids flow out from below. (He) will (also) balance yin and yang. Then dyspnea will be alleviated and sweat exits and flows in a normal way. The liver is able to fix its root, and, as the heart qi rises, yang moves around the four limbs. The lung qi becomes tranquil, and dyspnea is quieted down. [Twisting at the point means turning the various viscera to normal through needling their well and spring points. Sweet fluids refer to the fluids of the spleen. Balancing yin and yang aims to send them back to their normal positions. As a result, the flow of the constructive and defensive are freed, water qi is eliminated, and the liver has its root fixed again. The liver is mother to the heart child. When the liver becomes firm, the heart qi rises. Then the lung qi is leveled and balanced. This is what is meant by the word tranquil which has the sense of upright and graceful.]

The kidneys are capable of calming down sound. Their flavor is saltiness. [The lungs rule sound. The kidneys are their child and render assistance to the lungs. This is what is meant by calming down sound. Saltiness is the flavor of the kidneys.]

(In sum,) it is due to loss of reliance that the mother collapses into a filthy mess of stench. [Metal, which is mother to water, flees into water. This is mother turning to child. Thus the spleen qi (*i.e.,* the mother of metal) is made vacuous. The five viscera restrain and fell each other in turn in such a way that (one) failing to sustain (another) will cause the (whole) house to collapse into a filthy mess of stench. This is what the above implies.] If earth finds (support from) its child, it will become (as gigantic as) a mountain. If metal finds (support from) its mother, it can be said to be (as gigantic as) a hill.

The above is from the classics on the four seasons.

The Yellow Emperor asked:

(The pulses of the five viscera except for the spleen) undergo vicissitudes in order of the four seasons, but in what (season) does the spleen pulse rule by itself?

Qi Bo answered:

The spleen is earth. It is the solitary viscus that irrigates the four sides.[2]

The Yellow Emperor asked:

Are the favorable and unfavorable spleen (pulses) observable?

Qi Bo answered:

The favorable is not observable, but the unfavorable is.

The Yellow Emperor asked:

What is the unfavorable like?

Qi Bo answered:

It arrives like water running. This shows excess and that there is disease in the external. If it feels like a bird's beak, this indicates insufficiency and that there is disease in the center. Excess causes

---

[2] The pulses of the other four viscera each prevail in only one season. In spring, for example, the liver pulse is prevalent. The spleen pulse, however, should appear in every season as a modifier of the pulses of other viscera. This is because the spleen should provide supplies of nourishment for all the viscera and bowels throughout the year.

people heaviness of and inability to lift the four limbs. Insufficiency causes people congestion and block in the nine portals.[3] This is called superimposition (*chong qiang*).[4]

If the spleen pulse arrives soft and gentle and at even intervals, feeling like a cock putting down its feet on the ground,[5] this is a normal pulse. In long summer, (the pulse) relies on the stomach qi as its root.[6] If the spleen pulse arrives replete and brimming as well as rapid, feeling like a cock lifting its feet,[7] this indicates spleen disease. If the spleen pulse arrives hard and sharp, like a bird's beak or the spur of a bird or if it is like a leak in the roof[8] or water flowing, this suggests that the spleen is dead.

The true spleen pulse is a pulse that is weak, beating at long intervals at times but dissipated (rapid in another version) at others. If the facial complexion is yellowish green-blue and lusterless with brittle hair, death will ensue.

The long summer pulse with stomach is slightly soggy and weak. This is a normal pulse. If the pulse is very weak with little stomach, spleen disease is suggested. If it is completely weak with no stomach, death is suggested. If it is soggy and weak with a stone-like shade, disease will occur in winter. If the pulse is very stone-like, imminent disease is suggested.

The spleen stores the constructive, and the constructive stores reflection (*yi*). Endless worry and anxiety damage reflection. When reflection is damaged, there arise oppression, disturbance, inability to lift the limbs, brittle hair, and a perishing facial complexion. Then death will come in spring.

---

3 In the head, there are seven portals — two ears, two eyes, two nostrils, and one mouth — and below there are two — the anus and urethra in males or anus and vaginal meatus (including the urethra) in females.

4 Superimposition means the qi of the various viscera overlie and interfere with one another.

5 This describes a gentle and leisurely pulse beat.

6 This sentence implies that the stomach qi is expressed as an image of moderation and, therefore, the spleen pulse should be moderate, *i.e.*, soft and gentle.

7 This describes an abrupt and rapid pulse beat.

8 This describes and irregularly beating pulse pausing with long intervals.

The sixth or the last summer month sees the *wei* establishment[9] which falls within the position of earth that lies between *kun* and *wei*.[10] Now the spleen is king. The pulse may be large, leisurely, and moderate. This is a normal pulse. If, on the contrary, the pulse feels bowstring, fine, and long, this shows that the liver is overwhelming the spleen. Because wood should restrain earth, the evil is a murderous one. It is a greatly unfavorable condition. Ten will die out of ten cases without a remedy.

If, on the contrary, the pulse feels floating [faint in the *Qian Jin*], choppy, and short, this shows the lungs are overwhelming the spleen. Since the child should assist its mother, the evil is repletion. Even though it causes disease, it will heal by itself.

If, on the contrary, the pulse feels surging, large, and dissipated, this shows that the heart is overwhelming the spleen. When the mother turns to its child, the evil is vacuity. Even though it causes disease, it is easy to treat.

If, on the contrary, the pulse feels deep, soggy, and slippery, this shows that the kidneys are overwhelming the spleen. When water bullies earth, the evil is a mild one. Even though it causes disease, it will be overcome soon.

The spleen pulse may be long and weak, slow in coming and swift in retreating. If it beats twice (for an exhalation or an inhalation), this is a normal pulse. If it beats thrice, this shows a disease of channel aberration. If it beats four times, this shows desertion of essence. If it beats five times, this is death. If it beats six times, life is at an end.

The above is (a discussion of) the foot *tai yin* pulse.

A very urgent spleen pulse points to tugging and slackening, while a slightly urgent spleen pulse to fullness in the diaphragm giving rise to reflux of ingested food and foamy stools. A very moderate spleen pulse points to wilting inversion, while a slightly moderate spleen pulse to wind wilting with disabled limbs. (The patient) is serene as if there were no disease. A very large spleen pulse points to sudden collapse, but a slightly large spleen pulse to glomus qi and a great mass of

---

9   The Big Dipper completes a cycle of rotation of 360° in a year. This cycle is divided into twelve parts and each part is matched with one of the twelve Earthly Branches. The movement of the Big Dipper from one section to a succeeding section is called establishment. Further, the movements of the Big Dipper and the Earthly Branches correspond with the twelve months. In the sixth month, the Big Dipper points to *wei* in the cycle of the Earthly Branches.

10 *Kun* is one of the eight trigrams and is associated with earth. *Wei* is one of the twelve Earthly Branches, also ascribed to earth.

pus and (decayed) blood in the abdomen outside the intestines and stomach. A very small spleen pulse points to cold and heat, while a slightly small spleen pulse to pure heat wasting thirst. A very slippery spleen pulse points to *tui shan* and urinary block, while a slightly slippery spleen pulse to worm toxins like roundworms and rumbling and heat in the intestines. A very choppy spleen pulse points to prolapse of the rectum, but a slightly choppy spleen pulse to internal festering with much pus and blood in stools.

When the qi of the foot *tai yin* expires, the vessel will not nourish the lips. The lips are the root of the muscles and flesh. When the vessel does not nourish the muscles and flesh anymore, they will become soggy and the philtrum full. Because the philtrum is full, the lips are out-turned. When the lips are out-turned, the flesh is already dead. (Spleen disease) becomes exacerbated on *jia* days and ends in death on *yi* days, for wood overcomes earth.

The spleen is a dead viscus if the pulse is large and moderate at the superficial level and like an inverted cup, hard and rolling when pressure is applied.

The above is derived from the *Su Wen* (*Simple Questions*), the *Zhen Jing* (*Classic of Needling*), and Zhang Zhong-jing.

_____________ Chapter Four _____________
The Section on the Lungs & Large Intestine

The lungs are analogous to metal and are united with the bowel of the large intestine [which is the bowel of conveyance and transportation]. Its channel is the hand *tai yin* which has an interior/exterior relationship with the hand *yang ming*. Their pulse is floating.

They are minister in the last summer month, the sixth month. [(In this month,) earth is king and metal is its minister.] They are king in the three months of autumn. They abdicate in the three months of winter. They are confined in the three months of spring. They are dead in the three months of summer. [(In this period,) fire is king and metal is dead.]

Their king days are *geng* and *xin*, and their king watches are late afternoon (3-5 p.m.) and sundown (5-7 p.m.). Their confined days are *jia* and *yi*, and their confined watches are calm down

(3-5 a.m.) and sunrise (5-7 a.m.). Their dead days are *bing* and *ding*, and their dead watches are outlying region (9-11 a.m.) and midday (11 a.m.-1 p.m.).

Their spirit is the corporeal soul (*po*). That which they rule is sound. That which they nourish is the skin and hair. Their expression is the nose. Their sound is crying. Their color is white. Their smell is fishy. Their fluid is snivel. Their flavor is acridity. That which becomes them is saltiness. That which they are averse to is bitterness.

The transporting point of the lungs is located at the third vertebra in the back [or rather at the fifth vertebra]. Their alarm point is Central Treasury (*Zhong Fu*, Lu 1). The transporting point of the large intestine is located at the sixteenth vertebra in the back. Its alarm point is Celestial Pivot (*Tian Shu*, St 25).

The above is newly compiled.

The lungs are ascribed to the west and metal. (In autumn,) tens of thousands of (living) things come to an end. [Metal is rigid; so it reigns the west. It cuts everything; therefore every (living) thing ends in autumn.] Old leaves and fallen twigs litter everywhere, while sparse branches stand erect and lonely (on the trees). The pulse is faint and floating or hairy because the defensive qi is slow (in circulation), while the constructive qi circulates rapidly. That which is rapid goes above, while that which is slow goes below. This is why hairiness is caused. [The various yang vessels are rapid, while the various yin vessels are slow. The constructive is yin and should not circulate rapidly. On the contrary, now it is said to be rapid. This is because, in the autumn season, yin ascends to the position of yang, and, for the moment, it becomes rapid and stands high up. At the time when yin is beginning to work, yang is descending to hide itself, and (thus) its qi becomes slow. As a result, the lung pulse (*i.e.*, a yin pulse) is rapid, and scattered like hair.] If yang is not sinking when it ought to be, and yin is not upborne when it ought to be, this suggests strike by an evil. [When yin and yang do not exchange with one another on time (in position), the two qi will affect and interfere with one another. Then wind cold will strike.]

When yang is struck by evils, there is cuddling up. When yin is struck by evils, there is tension. Cuddling up is accompanied by aversion to cold, and tension by shivering. (Aversion to) cold and shivering combine to form a disease known as malaria. When the pulse becomes weak, there is fever, and when it becomes floating, (the evil qi) has exited. [Cuddling up refers to curling up of the body, while tension here refers to a tight pulse. This is spoken of when wind cold first strikes. A tight pulse reveals cold in the body. When cold (*i.e.*, chills) comes to a stop, the pulse becomes fainter and weaker. The (very) weak pulse suggests fever. When fever comes to a stop, the pulse becomes floating. A floating pulse reveals that the malaria (episode) is resolved and the king (*i.e.*, the lung) pulse shows itself.]

If stroke (by wind cold) occurs in the morning, (the episode) occurs in the morning. If (the stroke) occurs in the evening, (the episode) occurs in the evening. [This means that the malaria attacks (subsequently and repeatedly) at the same hour as the wind evils first struck (the body).] Because the viscera may be located remote or near, so their pulses may be slow or rapid. (The vessels) have certain lengths, and (the constructive and the defensive) travel a constant number of circuits (in a day). These are in agreement with the divisions of the clepsydra. [The word viscera means the five viscera of the human being — the liver, heart, spleen, lungs, and kidneys. The heart and lungs are located above the diaphragm, and, on exhalation, their qi exit. Therefore, they are said to be near. Exhalation is yang. The pulses (of the heart and the lungs) are rapid. The kidneys and liver are located below the diaphragm. With inhalation, their qi enter. Therefore, they are said to be remote. Inhalation is yin. The pulses (of the kidneys and liver) are slow. The number of circuits (etc.) tells that though the channel vessels vary in length, the constructive and the defensive (qi) travel around the body twenty-five circuits in yin and yang each to complete one round. This corresponds with the hundred divisions of the clepsydra.] If a slow pulse appears above (*i.e.,* in the *cun*), there is injury to the luster of the hair. If a rapid pulse appears below (*i.e.,* in the *chi*), there is injury to the lower burner. An unfavorable (pulse) of the middle burner is observable, but a favorable one is kept out of sight. [In autumn, yang qi is slow, while yin qi moves rapidly. (In normal cases,) a slow pulse is expected to be in the lower (*i.e.,* the *chi*), while a rapid (pulse) should be found in the upper (*i.e.,* the *cun.* The pulse qualities) change with the seasons. The hair and luster are said to be injured since the skin and hair of the human being is the place where the lung qi travels. The lower burner is below the umbilicus within the precinct of yin. Its pulse should be slow. Now, on the contrary, it is rapid. Therefore, it is said that the lower burner is injured. The middle burner is the spleen. In peaceful and favorable times, its own (typical) pulse is often unobservable. It appears only when (the spleen) is debilitated. Therefore, it is said that once it is unfavorable, it is tangible.]

When yang qi is sunken below, yin qi becomes warm. [This means (the normal state) where yang qi is sunken to warm and nurture the various viscera.] If, (in autumn,) yang lies below rather than (yin), and yin lies above, rather than (yang), then longevity and keeping fit can be said (to be possible.) [The vicissitudes of yin and yang carry on in accordance with the seasons and terms. Thus a person's blood vessels are peaceful and tranquil, and one can be said to enjoy longevity and keep fit.]

The above is derived from the classics on the four seasons.

The Yellow Emperor asked:

The autumn pulse is like (something) floating. Why is this so?

Qi Bo answered:

The autumn pulse is of the lungs which are ascribed to the west and metal. With (autumn,) tens of thousands of things are harvested. Therefore, the (autumn pulse) qi is light, vacuous, and floating, the qi [the last two words are suspected to be redundant] arriving urgent but retreating scattered. Therefore, it is called floating. Pulses contrary to this indicates disease.

The Yellow Emperor asked:

What are the contrary pulses like?

Qi Bo answered:

If the (pulse) qi arrives hair-like and hard in the center but vacuous at the sides, this is known as excess, indicating that there is disease in the external. If the (pulse) qi arrives hair-like and faint, this is known as insufficiency, suggesting that there is disease in the center.

The Yellow Emperor asked:

What kinds of disease are there when the autumn pulse shows excess and insufficiency?

Qi Bo answered:

Excess causes people qi counterflow with pain and discomfort in the back. Insufficiency causes people dyspnea, diminished qi, cough, qi ascent, blood seen (in the sputum), and a pathological sound (*i.e.,* rales) heard below.

If the lung pulse arrives flapping gently like a falling elm pod, the lungs are normal. In autumn, (the lung pulse) relies on the stomach qi as its root. [It is said in the *Nan Jing* that (a pulse) flapping gently giving the sensation of stroking an elm leaf is a normal spring pulse and that a pulse soft like the canopy of the cart and becoming larger at a deeper level is a normal autumn pulse.] If the lung pulse arrives neither rising nor falling (*i.e.,* sluggish and rough), feeling like stroking a chicken's feather, this indicates lung disease. If the lung pulse feels like flotsam or like hair being blown in wind, this indicates that the lungs are dead.

The true lung pulse is a pulse that feels large and vacuous like a feather touching the skin. If the complexion is whitish red and lusterless with brittle hair, death will ensue.

The autumn pulse with stomach is slightly hair-like. This is a normal pulse. If the pulse is very hair-like with little stomach, lung disease is suggested. If it is completely hair-like with no stomach, death is suggested. If it is hair-like with a shade of bowstring, disease will occur in the spring. If the pulse is very bowstring, imminent disease is indicated.

The lungs store qi, and it is qi that houses the corporeal soul (*po*). Excessive joy and delight brings damage to the *po*. When the *po* is injured, there arises mania. A manic person does not recognize people. If the skin becomes parched with the hair brittle and the complexion perishing, death will come in summer.

In metal autumn, the lungs are king. Their pulse is floating, choppy, and short. This is a normal pulse. If, on the contrary, it feels surging, large, and scattered [floating, large, and surging in the *Qian Jin*], this shows that the heart is overwhelming the lungs. Since fire should restrain metal, the evil is a murderous one. It is a greatly unfavorable condition. Ten out of ten cases will die without a remedy.

If, on the contrary, the pulse feels deep, soggy, and slippery, this shows that the kidneys are overwhelming the lungs. Since the child should assist its mother, the evil is repletion. Even though it causes disease, it will heal by itself.

If, on the contrary, the pulse feels large and moderate, this shows the spleen is overwhelming the lungs. When the mother turns to the child, the evil is vacuity. Even though it causes disease, it is easy to treat.

If, on the contrary, the pulse feels bowstring, thin, and long, this shows the liver is overwhelming the lungs. When wood bullies metal, the evil is a mild one. Even though it causes disease, it will be overcome soon.

The lung pulse may arrive buoyant, feeling like the down on the back of a bird being blown in the breeze. If it beats twice (for one inhalation or exhalation), this is a normal pulse. If it beats thrice, this indicates a disease of channel aberration. If it beats four times, there is desertion of essence. If it beats five times, this is death. If it beats six times, life is at an end.

(The above is a discussion of) the pulses of the hand *tai yin*.

A very urgent lung pulse points to madness, while a slightly urgent lung pulse to lung cold and heat, lethargy, coughing and spitting of blood, (cough) giving rise to pain in the upper and lower back and chest, and tormenting inhibited breathing due to nasal polyp. A very moderate lung pulse points to profuse sweating, while a slightly moderate lung pulse to fistulas and hemilateral wind [leaking wind[1] instead of fistulas and hemilateral wind in another version, and this is acceptable] with sweat exiting uncheckably from below the head. A very large lung pulse points to swelling in the lower leg, but a slightly large lung pulse to lung *bi*[2] which affects the chest and upper back yet starts in the lower back. A very small lung pulse points to swill diarrhea, while a slightly small lung pulse to pure heat wasting thirst. A very slippery lung pulse points to inverted cup surging (*xi ben*)[3] with qi ascent, while a slightly slippery lung pulse to bleeding above and below. A very choppy lung pulse points to retching of blood, but a slightly choppy lung pulse to rat's fistulas[4] in the neck and/or in the armpit, inability of the lower (limbs) to bear the upper body, and a predilection for sourness.

When the qi of the hand *tai yin* expires, the skin and hair become parched. It is the *tai yin* that moves qi to warm the skin and hair. When its qi stops providing nourishment, the skin and hair become parched. When the skin and hair are parched, fluids are gone. When fluids are gone, the nodes of the skin are injured. When the nodes of the skin are injured, the nails become desiccated and the hair becomes brittle. When the hair is brittle, qi is already dead. (Lung disease) becomes exacerbated on *bing* days and ends in death on *ding* days, for fire overcomes metal.

The lungs are dead viscera if (their pulse) is vacuous at the superficial level and feels weak like a scallion-stalk when pressure is applied. If (the pulse) is deprived of its root[5] below (*i.e.*, in the *chi*), this is death.

The above is derived from the *Su Wen* (*Simple Questions*), the *Zhen Jing* (*Classic of Needling*), and Zhang Zhong-jing.

---

[1] This refers to invasion of wind evils while intoxicated which is characterized by massive perspiration, particularly while eating, dyspnea, aversion to wind, thirst, and inability to stand any exertion.

[2] This is a condition characterized by vexation, fullness in the chest, dyspnea, and retching.

[3] This is a mass shaped like an inverted cup located in the right lateral costal region. It gives rise to rapid distressed dyspneic breathing with qi surging up.

[4] This refers to an open persistent fistula constantly discharging pus.

[5] This implies that no pulse is felt at the deep level.

Chapter Five

The Section on the Kidneys & Urinary Bladder

The kidneys are analogous to water and are united with the bowel of the urinary bladder [which is the bowel of fluids and humors]. Their channel is the foot *shao yin* which has an interior/exterior relationship with the foot *tai yang*. Their pulse is deep.

They are minister in the three months of autumn. [(In autumn,) metal is king and water is its minister.] They are king in the three months of winter. They abdicate in the three months of spring. They are confined in the three months of summer. They are dead in the last summer month, the sixth month.

Their king days are *ren* and *gui*, and their king watches are serenity (9-11 p.m.) and midnight (11 p.m.-1 a.m.). Their confined days are *bing* and *ding*, and their confined watches are outlying region (9-11 a.m.) and midday (11 a.m.-1 p.m.). Their dead days are *wu* and *ji*, and their dead watches are breakfast (7-9 a.m.) and sun's descent (1-3 p.m.).

Their spirit is the will (*zhi*). That which they rule are fluids. That which they nourish are the bones. Their expression is the ears. Their sound is groaning. Their color is black. Their smell is rancid. Their fluid is sputum. Their flavor is saltiness. That which becomes them is acidity. That which they are averse to is sweetness.

The transporting point of the kidneys is located at the fourteenth vertebra in the back, and their alarm point is Capital Gate (*Jing Men*, GB 25). The transporting point of the urinary bladder is located at the nineteenth vertebra, and its alarm point is Central Pole (*Zhong Ji*, CV 3).

The above is newly compiled.

The kidneys are ascribed to the north and water. (In winter,) tens of thousands of things are in store. [Things germinate in spring, grow in summer, harvest in autumn, and are stored in winter.] And the hundreds (of kinds) of insects and worms lie hibernating. Yang qi is sunken below, while yin qi is ascending. If yang qi emerges from confinement when yin qi is rigorous, it turns into frost. Since (the emerged yang qi) is unable to rise, it transforms into snow and frost. Wild beasts lie dormant and worms lie hidden. [When yang qi is spoken of as sunken below, it means that it has submerged into the ground. (At the same time), however, yang qi keeps emerging and rising (from the ground). Because yin qi, which lies above, is cold and exuberant, yang qi, which, though it manages to emerge and rise, cannot go anywhere but transform into snow and frost.] (Therefore,) the pulse (during winter) is deep. Deepness is yin, indicating (yang qi lying) internally and that diaphoresis is not allowed. If perspiration is promoted, (the consequence will be like that when) worms are let out and exposed to frost and snow.

When yin qi is in the exterior while yang is in the viscera, one must be careful not to administer precipitation, for precipitation will bring damage to the spleen. If spleen earth is made weak, water qi will become frenzied. Precipitation is likened to taking a fish from water or pitching a moth into boiling water. When the respectable guest stays internally, one should be careful not to fume it. Fuming will irritate the guest, giving rise to dyspnea. [The respectable guest refers to yang qi. Fuming refers to (the application of) red-hot needling, fire, or boiling water steaming, etc.] One should not keep the guest hot, for heat will cause festering sores in the mouth. (Diaphoresis) may disintegrate the yin (i.e., blood) vessels. Then blood will become dispersed or blocked, and the righteous yang will be inverted. (In consequence,) yin (and yang) no longer follow one another, and guest (i.e., exogenous) heat will invade frenziedly. This will lodge internally to develop into chest binding.[1] The spleen qi is subsequently made weak and there will develop clear urine (i.e., frequent voidings) and diarrhea.

The above is derived from the classics on the four seasons.

The Yellow Emperor asked:

The winter pulse is secretive. Why is it secretive?

Qi Bo answered:

The winter pulse is of the kidneys which are ascribed to the north and water. (In winter,) every living thing lies hidden under shelter. Therefore, (the kidney pulse) qi is deep and pounding. This is why it is called secretive. Pulses contrary to this indicate disease.

The Yellow Emperor asked:

What are the contrary pulses like?

---

[1]   This refers to fullness, tightness, and pain in the upper abdomen.

Qi Bo answered:

If the (pulse) qi arrives (hard) like striking a pellet, this is known as excess, indicating that there is disease externally. If (the pulse) is swift in retreating, this is known as insufficiency, suggesting that there is disease in the center.

The Yellow Emperor asked:

What kinds of disease are there when the winter pulse shows excess and insufficiency?

Qi Bo answered:

Excess causes people slackness and listlessness, pain in the spinal vessels, diminished qi, and no desire to speak. Insufficiency causes people (to feel) as if the heart were suspended as in the illness of hunger, chilling of the lateral abdomen, pain in the spine, fullness in the lower abdomen, and yellow or dark-colored urine.

If the kidney pulse arrives as if gasping, undulating without a break and hook-like, and becomes hard under pressure, the kidneys are normal. In winter, (the pulse) relies on the stomach qi as its root. If the kidney pulse arrives like a vine drawn straight and becomes harder with pressure, this indicates that the kidneys are diseased. If the kidney pulse arrives like a rope being hauled or a pellet striking repeatedly, this indicates that the kidneys are dead.

The true kidney pulse is a pulse pounding with interruption, giving a sensation of striking a pellet with the finger. If the complexion is blackish yellow and lusterless with the brittle hair, death will ensue.

The winter pulse with stomach is a little stone-like. This is a normal pulse. If the pulse is very stone-like with little stomach, kidney disease is suggested. If it is completely stone-like with no stomach, death is suggested. If it is stone-like with a hook-like shade, disease will occur in summer. If (the pulse) is very hook-like, imminent disease is suggested.

For everyone, water and grain are the root. Therefore, when people are deprived of water and grain, they die. If the pulse has no stomach qi, death will also come. What is meant by absence of stomach qi is the appearance of the true visceral pulse with no stomach qi. What is meant by absence of stomach qi from the pulse is absence of a bowstring (quality) in terms of the liver (pulse), absence of stone-like (quality) in terms of the kidney (pulse, etc.).[2]

---

[2] Translated freely, this sentence can be rendered as follows: Absence of stomach qi from the pulse means, for example, that the liver pulse is devoid of the *slight* bowstring quality peculiar to it. There is, however,

The kidneys store essence, and it is essence that houses the will (*zhi*). Violent and endless anger damages the will. When the will is injured, one is liable to forget what one has just said and suffers from pain in the lumbar spine with inability to bend (the body) either forward or backward. If the hair is brittle and the complexion is perishing, death will come in the last summer month.

In winter, kidney water is king. If the kidney pulse is deep, soggy, and slippery, this is a normal pulse. If, on the contrary, it feels large and moderate, this shows that the spleen is overwhelming the kidneys. Since earth should restrain water, the evil is a murderous one. It is a greatly unfavorable condition. Ten out of ten cases will die without a remedy.

If, on the contrary, the pulse feels bowstring, fine, and long, this shows that the liver is overwhelming the kidneys. Because the child should assist its mother, the evil is repletion. Even though it causes disease, it will heal by itself.

If, on the contrary, the pulse feels floating [faint in the *Qian Jin*], choppy, and short, this shows the lungs are overwhelming the kidneys. When the mother turns to its child, the evil is vacuity. Even though it causes disease, it is easy to treat.

If, on the contrary, the pulse feels surging, large, and dissipated [floating, large, and surging in the *Qian Jin*], this shows that the heart is overwhelming the kidneys. When fire bullies water, the evil is a mild one. Even though it causes disease, it will be overcome soon.

The kidney pulse may be deep, fine, and tight. It is a normal pulse if it beats twice (for one inhalation or exhalation). If it beats thrice, it indicates a disease of channel aberration. If it beats four times, there is desertion of essence. If it beats five times, this is death. If it beats six times, life is at an end.

(The above is a discussion of) the pulses of the foot *shao yin*.

---

a quite different interpretation of the true visceral pulse. According to this alternate interpretation, the true liver pulse, for example, is a completely bowstring pulse without the moderateness typical of the stomach qi. The true kidney pulse is a completely stone-like (*i.e.*, hard and deep) pulse without the moderateness typical of the stomach qi. From this point of view, the word "absence" in "absence of bowstring" and "absence of stone-like" is a redundancy, the result of garbling of the text.

A very urgent kidney pulse points to bone wilting[3] and madness, while a slightly urgent kidney pulse to running piglet,[4] heaviness and inversion frigidity of the lower limbs, disabled feet, and inability to urinate and defecate. A very moderate kidney pulse points to pain in the spine as if fit to break, while a slightly moderate kidney pulse to throughflux diarrhea. In throughflux diarrhea, there is untransformed grain in the stools and food refluxing upon ingestion. A very large kidney pulse points to impotence, but a slightly large kidney pulse to stone water.[5] (Stone water) is a swelling progressing from the infra-umbilical region to the (whole) lower abdomen which may appear sagging. If the swelling spreads to the upper abdomen, death is inevitable without a remedy. A very small kidney pulse points to throughflux diarrhea, while a slightly small kidney pulse to pure heat wasting thirst. A very slippery kidney pulse points to dribbling urinary block and *tui*, while a slightly slippery kidney pulse to bone wilting, inability to rise from a sitting position, eyes not seeing , or black flowery vision. A very choppy kidney pulse points to major *yong*, but a slightly choppy kidney pulse to amenorrhea and chronic hemorrhoids.

When the qi of the foot *shao yin* expires, the bones become dried and withered. The *shao yin* is a winter vessel. It goes hidden to moisten the bone marrow. Therefore, when the bones are deprived of moisture, the flesh cannot be fixed to it. If the bones and flesh have lost their affinity between them, then the flesh becomes floppy and dwindles away. Since the flesh is floppy and dwindled, the teeth seem to be longer and are covered with tartar [desiccated instead of "covered with tartar" in the *Nan Jing*], and the hair is lusterless. When the hair is lusterless, the bones are already dead. (Kidney disease) becomes exacerbated on *wu* days and ends in death on *ji* days, for earth overcomes water.

The kidneys are dead viscera if their pulse feels hard at the superficial level and pell-mell like a rolling pellet under pressure. If this (quality) appears down to the *chi* part, this is death.

The above is derived from the *Su Wen* (*Simple Questions*), the *Zhen Jing* (*Classic of Needling*), and Zhang Zhong-jing.

---

3   This is a condition due to heat in the kidneys which is characterized by aching and weakness of the lower back, atony of the lower limbs, desiccated teeth, and a black facial complexion.

4   Accumulation of the kidneys is called running piglet. It is characterized by qi rushing up from the lower abdomen into the chest and the throat.

5   This is a water disease whose symptoms are a deep pulse, abdominal dropsy, and fullness of the lower abdomen.

BOOK FOUR

Collated & edited by Honorary Minister Without Portfolio,
Curator of the Imperial Library,
Imperial Courier and Senior Army Protector,
Lin Yi *et al.*

Discrimination of the Three Positions &
the Nine Indicators, Their Pulses &
Their (Reflected) Patterns

The classic (*i.e.*, the *Nan Jing*) says, "What is known as the three positions is the *cun, guan,* and *chi.* The nine indicators refer to heaven, earth, and human in each of these three positions."[1] The upper position[2] mainly reflects (the area) from the chest up to the head. The middle position mainly reflects (the area) from the diaphragm down to the (qi) thoroughfare (*i.e.*, the groin). The lower position[2] mainly reflects (the area) from (qi) thoroughfare down to the feet.

There are various different (pulse) descriptions such as floating, deep, firm, bound, slow, racing, slippery, and choppy. One should have the (vessel) theory in mind when trying to discriminate these and be attentive when observing the changes (of the pulses). The purpose of discriminating the three positions and the nine indicators is to get knowledge of where a disease starts. Then, after consideration, one may be clear (about the nature of the disease). This also holds good for acupuncture. One should first feel the *cun* (*i.e.*, the whole wrist pulse). A floating pulse indicates (a disease) in the skin, and a deep and thin pulse indicates (disease) internally. If one is judicious of the heavenly path,[3] one will be able to dispense longevity.

If the (pulse) images in the upper position are firm, bound, deep, and slippery, there is accumulated qi in the urinary bladder. If they are faint, thin, and weak, there are abdominal urgency while lying down, headache, cough, and qi counterflowing up and down. If there is heat around the heart and diaphragm, there is a dry mouth and burning thirst. If the disease (pattern) is in agreement with the *cun* (pulse) and the evil has entered the upper (part of the body), one may declare resolution.

If the pulse arrives like a string drawn on a musical instrument, the bitterness is lower abdominal pain and, in females, inhibited menstruation and sores in (genital) orifices, while in males, the

---

1   Heaven means the superficial level; earth, the deep level; and the human, the medium level.

2   One should take special note that the *cun* or distal part of the wrist pulse is called the upper. The *guan* or middle position is the middle. And the *chi* or proximal position is the lower.

3   *I.e.*, studies and pays attention to classical explanations of the pulse theories

trouble of hemorrhoids and sores on the left and right lateral costal regions. If the pulse is bound in the upper position, the bitterness is lower abdominal pain and rumbling in the intestines. If the pulse is vacuous and weak in the *cun*, there is injury to and insufficiency of qi. There is a mass the size of a plum or peach seed (in the abdomen) with the bitterness of *bi*. If the *cun* pulse is straight up (and down), there is (qi) counterflow vacuity. If the pulse is floating and vacuous, there is diarrhea.

In the middle position, a bound pulse reveals gatherings and accumulations in the abdomen. If (the gatherings and accumulations) are in the urinary bladder or the lateral costal regions, this is due to heat. If the pulse is floating and large, wind has invaded via the stomach venter, giving rise to water distention,[4] dry retching, a rolling sensation below the heart, and a sensation of a peach or plum seed stuck inside. If there is cold in the stomach, the bitterness is occasional vexation, pain, eating little, heart pain arising on ingestion, distention of the stomach, propping fullness, and accumulations over the diaphragm. If there is heat in the lateral costal regions, then from time to time there arises (alternating) cold and heat with sweat exiting like dew drops. If the pulse is rampant[5] and exceeds the upper position, there is an aggressive qi in the urinary bladder. This illness is persistent. If the pulse is rampant and intrudes from the *guan* into the *cun* at the right hand, there is diaphragm block and difficulty swallowing in the throat. (To treat it,) needle Origin Pass (*Guan Yuan*, CV 4) and enlist the *shao yin*.[6]

Of the pulses in the lower position, the one that arrives floating and large indicates spleen (disease). Joining hands with wind, (this disease) may cause pain in the top of the head from time to time which radiates to the upper and lower back. If the pulse is small and slippery, there is inversion which is characterized by heat in the soles of the feet, distressed fullness, and (qi) counterflowing up into the heart and further into the throat. There seems to be malign flesh[7] (inside the throat). This is due to damage of the spleen. If the disease is located below the lower abdomen, there is cold and frigidity in and inability to bend or stretch the knees and other joints (of the legs). If the pulse is urgent like a bowstring, the sinews are tense. If the feet are afflicted with hypertonicity, the four limbs are heavy. If (wind) evils find an expression from the *chi* to the

---

[4] Water distention refers to swelling starting from the eyelids which gradually spreads to the legs and feet, finally making the belly enlarged like a water bag.

[5] A rampant pulse is a very strong and exuberant pulse.

[6] The phrase, "enlisting the *shao yin*", means to needle the *shao yin* channel.

[7] Malign flesh refers to a sudden growth of hyperplasia somewhere in the body.

yang ming,[8] there will be (alternating) cold and heat. If great wind evils appear in the *shao yin*,[9] there is white and red vaginal discharge in females and hematuria, impotence, and a pain radiating (from the penis) to the lower abdomen in males.

A human being has 360 vessels corresponding to the 360 days (of the year). The three positions are the *cun, guan,* and *chi*. The *chi* pulse is yin, and a yin pulse is usually deep and slow. The *cun* and *guan* are yang, and yang pulses are floating and rapid. Breathing out is motion, while breathing in is respite. A yang pulse beats thirteen times for six or seven respites, and a yin pulse beats fifteen times for seven or eight respites. This is a normal (state).

The twenty-eight vessels[10] are coupled with each other and circulate up and down (the body). If one vessel fails to appear, this makes known the afflictions that disease inflicts. If the *chi* prevails,[11] treat the lower (part of the body). If the *cun* prevails, treat the upper. If the *chi* and *cun* are normal, treat the center.

(The region) from the umbilicus above is yang and is analogous to heaven. (The region) from the umbilicus down is yin and is analogous to earth. The umbilicus is the central pivot. The head is heaven, while the feet are earth.

If the exterior (pulse) is present but the interior is absent, evils have settled (in the body). This is a ghost disease.[12] What is meant by presence of the exterior but absence of the interior? The *cun* and *chi* are the exterior, while the *guan* is the interior. (Therefore, the term refers to) a pulse being present at the two ends but failing to appear in the *guan*. If the pulse, (though appearing) at the *chi*, cannot reach up to the *guan*, yin is expiring. If the pulse, (though appearing) at the *cun*, cannot reach down to the *guan*, yang is expiring. Expiring yin with faint yang indicates death without a remedy. If the pulse appears in the three positions at one time but disappears at another, there is cold qi in the stomach which is responsible for the blocked pulse.

---

[8] Because the *yang ming* (stomach) is reflected in the radial aspect of the bar pulse on the right hand, this expression may refer to a pathological pulse image starting in the cubit and then progressing distally and outward.

[9] The *shao yin* is the lower position or cubit of the pulse.

[10] The 28 vessels include the twelve channels of the hand and foot bilaterally, the governing vessel, conception vessel, and the yin and yang motility vessels.

[11] Prevalence here means conspicuous abnormality.

[12] In "ghost disease", the word ghost is an epithet expressing severity. Therefore, ghost disease means nothing more than a mortal or critical condition.

If the pulse is present in the upper position but absent from the lower position, the person ought to vomit. Those who do not vomit will die. If the pulse is absent from the upper position but present in the lower position, even though there is trouble, there is no (serious) affliction. This can be explained by a simile. A person having a pulse in the *chi* is likened to a tree having its root. Even though its branches and leaves have withered, its root will engender them of itself. Just as a tree has its root, so the human being has its qi. Thus one knows that there is no dying.

Why can one die when one's pulse is normal in the *cun* opening? All the twelve channels count on the source of the life qi. What is known as the life qi is (the word not has been omitted by the tr.) the radix of the twelve channels, known as the stirring (or moving) qi between the kidneys. This is the foundation of the five viscera and six bowels, the root of the twelve channels, the gate of respiration, and the source of the triple burner. It has another name of guardian against evils. For that reason, (this stirring) qi is the root and foundation of human beings. Once the root expires, the stem withers. The reason why one dies with the pulse normal in the *cun* opening is total expiration of the life qi internally. [The stirring qi between the kidneys refers to the kidney at the left side and the life gate at the right. The life gate is the place where spirit and essence are housed, a place on which the source qi hangs.]

Qi Bo explained:

Those with an exuberant form,[13] a fine pulse, and diminished qi not enough for breath will die. Those with a thin shape, a large pulse, and abundant qi in the chest (*i.e.*, chest fullness and gasping for breath) will die. Compatibility between the form and the (pulse) qi suggests survival, while any sort of incompatibility suggests disease. If the pulses in the three positions and nine indicators are out of line, death is a certainty. If the pulses in the upper and lower positions at the left and right hand are all out of step with each other as if (several) pestles are pounding (at varied speeds), the disease is severe. If the pulses in the upper and lower positions at the left and right hand are all abnormal and impossible to count, this is death. If the (pulse) image in the middle position is harmonious but out of line with (the pulses of) all the other viscera, death is a certainty. If the (pulse) image in the middle position is (conspicuously) diminished, this is death. Sunken eyes suggest death.

The Yellow Emperor asked:

What does winter yin and summer yang mean?

Qi Bo answered:

---

[13] An exuberant form is a stout appearance. However, such conditions as a red facial complexion with rapid dyspneic breathing and some other repletion signs can be also called exuberant form.

When the pulses in all the nine indicators are deep, fine, suspended, and expiring, this is yin, which rules winter.[14] Therefore, death will come at midnight.[15] (If the pulses in all the three positions) are exuberant, agitated, as if gasping, and rapid, this is yang, which rules summer. Therefore, death will come at midday. It follows that those with (alternating) cold and heat die at the calm dawn watch, while those with heat in the center or febrile illness die at midday. Those with wind illness die in the evening. Those with water illness die at midnight. Those with the pulse rapid at one time but retarded at another, slow at one time but racing at another, die at the (earth)-prevalent watch of the four seasons of the day.[16] Those with shedding of the formal flesh will die even though their pulses in the nine indicators are in harmony.

In spite of the appearance of the seven (mortal)[17] signs, those with the nine indicators (of the pulse) favorable will not die. What is not diagnosed as mortal includes diseases of wind qi or diseases of menstruation. They look like but are not diseases of the seven (mortal) signs. Therefore, they are not diagnosed as mortal. Those (really) with the seven (mortal) signs and with collapsing pulse images in addition will die.

When there is bound to be dry retching and belching, one must inquire about the initial and the present condition and then palpate the pulse in each (position). After that, determine whether (the qi of) the channels and vessel networks is upborne or downborne by feeling them up and down. If the pulse is racing, there is no disease. If the pulse is slow, there is disease. If the pulse stops coming and going, death is a certainty. If the skin is fixed (to the bone), this is death.

The pulse will be soggy at the two hands if there is binding in its upper (position). It will be moderate if there is binding in its middle position. It will present a bean-shaped prominence if there is binding at Three Li (*San Li*, LI 10). There is a pulse which is weak in the *guan* and soggy in the top (i.e., the *cun*), faint in the upper (i.e., the *cun*) and choppy in the lower (i.e., the *chi*). In the presence of faintness, there is an insufficiency of yang qi giving rise to vacuity fever and

———————————————

[14] Winter here means exuberant yin or critical conditions of a yin nature.

[15] One should note that winter is yin and midnight is the winter season in terms of the periods of the day. See note 16 below.

[16] There are twelves watches in the day, marked by the twelve Earthly Branches: *zi, chou, yan, mou, chen,* etc. The twelve watches are each divided into four periods corresponding with the four seasons of the year. As in the four seasons, earth prevails in one watch in each of the four periods. They are *chen* (7-8 a.m.), *xu* (7-8 p.m.), *chou* (1-2 a.m.) and *wei* (1-2 p.m.).

[17] The seven mortal signs are those discussed in the immediately preceding paragraph. That is, an exuberant form with a fine pulse, diminished qi not enough for breath, etc.

sweating. In the presence of choppiness, there is absence of blood giving rise to inversion with cold (of the limbs).

The Yellow Emperor asked:

Whenever I study colors and feel the pulse, a desire occurs to me that I should try to diagnose a disease merely by examining the cubit skin. Then how can one know the internal through (studying) the external (cubit skin)?

Qi Bo answered:

By scrutinizing the slackness and tension, the largeness and smallness, the slipperiness and roughness of the cubit skin, and the hardness and fragility of the (cubit) flesh, one can determine pathological changes.

(The Yellow Emperor) asked:

Then how to determine (them this way)?

(Qi Bo) answered:

When the pulse is urgent, the cubit skin is tense. When the pulse is moderate, the cubit skin is slack. When the pulse is small, the cubit skin is reduced and thin. When the pulse is large, the cubit skin is large (*i.e.*, thick). When the pulse is slippery, the cubit skin is slippery. When the pulse is choppy, the cubit skin is rough. These six variations vary in degree. Therefore, those who are good at studying the cubit skin need not study the *cun* (pulse). Those who are good at studying the pulse need not study colors. (Yet only) those who are able to make a synthetic study of them all can be physicians of high proficiency.

If the cubit skin is slippery, moist, and lustrous, there is wind. If the inner (ulnar) aspect of the cubit skin is weak (or flabby) and if there are slackness and listlessness, liking the comfort of lying down, and shedding of flesh, then there is cold and heat. If the cubit skin is rough, there is wind *bi.*[18] If the cubit skin is coarse like the scales of a dried fish, there is water phlegm rheum. If the cubit skin is very hot and the pulse is exuberant and agitated, there is warm disease. If the pulse is exuberant and slippery, sweat is about to exit. If the cubit skin is very cold and the pulse is small [urgent in another version], there are diarrhea and diminished qi. If the cubit skin is burning hot with fever followed by chills, there is (alternating) cold and heat. If the cubit skin feels cold at first but hot after held for a long (time), there is also (alternating) cold and heat. If the cubit skin is

---

[18] This refers to migratory pain in the muscles.

burning hot and the *ren ying* (pulse)[19] is large, there has been loss of blood in the past. If the cubit skin is tense and the *ren ying* pulse is small, there is diminished qi. If the complexion is gradually becoming white, death is imminent.

If there is heat which is confined to the elbow, there is heat from the lumbus up. If there is heat which is confined to the anterior portion of the elbow, there is heat in the bosoms. If there is heat which is confined to the posterior portion of the elbow, there is heat in the shoulders and upper back. If the posterior region 3-4 *cun* below the prominence of the elbow is coarse, there are worms in the intestines. If there is heat which is confined to the hands, there is heat from the lumbus up. If there is heat which is confined to the middle part of the forearm, there is heat in the lower back and abdomen. If there is heat in the palm, there is heat in the abdomen. If there is cold in the palm, there is cold in the abdomen. If there are green-blue blood vessels in the white flesh of the fish's border, there is cold in the stomach.

Any floating, deep, slippery, choppy, bowstring, or taut pulse in the *cun* points to disease above the diaphragm. If they appear in the *guan*, there is illness below the stomach. If they appear in the *chi*, there is disease below the kidneys.

If the *cun* pulse is slippery and slow, neither deep nor floating, neither long nor short, this shows no disease. This holds true of either hand.

Of the excessive and insufficient *cun* pulses, the one that the fingers feel to be short indicates headache. The one that the fingers feel to be long indicates pain in the lower leg and foot. The one that the fingers feel to be skipping and pounding indicates pain in the shoulder and upper back.

If the *cun* pulse is floating and exuberant, there is disease externally. If the *cun* pulse is deep and hard, there is disease internally.

If the *cun* pulse is deep and weak, this indicates cold and heat [cold qi in another version, and cold in the center in yet another] and *shan* conglomeration with lower abdominal pain.

If the *cun* pulse is deep and weak, hair is bound to come off.

If the *cun* pulse is deep and tight, the bitterness is cold below the heart with occasional pain and gatherings and conglomerations.

---

[19] The *ren ying* pulse here refers to the pulse in the *cun* position.

If the *cun* pulse is deep, the chest is short of qi. If the *cun* pulse is deep and as if gasping, there is cold and heat.

If the *cun* pulse is replete all the time, there is heart taxation.[20]

If the *cun* pulse is tight or floating, there is cold around the diaphragm with water qi below the lungs.

If the pulse is tight and so long as to exceed the *cun*, there is pouring disease.[21]

If the pulse is tight and reaches the *cun*, there is wind stroke.[22] The case is the same with wind headache [cold damage with headache in the *Qian Jin*].

If the pulse is bowstring and reaches the *cun*, there is accumulated food. If it descends,[23] there is headache.

If the pulse exceeds the *cun*, reaching the fish's border, there is enuresis.

If the pulse emerges at the fish's border, there is qi counterflow dyspnea.

If the *cun* pulse is wafting like oil over the soup, yang is faint. If it undulates like a spider's web (*i.e.*, is fine and soft), yin qi is debilitated.

If the *cun* pulse is expiring on one hand, one arm is paralyzed. If the person's pulse is expiring on both hands, there is no cure. If the yang of the pulse is expiring[24] at the distal position on both hands, the bitterness is cold toxins below the heart with heat in the mouth.

____

[20] Heart taxation refers to insomnia and sleep fraught with dreams due to overwork of the brain.

[21] In the term, pouring disease, the word pouring means infectious. Thus pouring disease refers to chronic, infectious troubles, particularly TB.

[22] Wind stroke often refers to cold damage or febrile disease and not necessarily to wind stroke which may give rise to hemilateral withering.

[23] According to the ordinary definition, descent should be understood as extending up to the *chi*, but in this context, it means the reverse. Therefore, this phrase says that a bowstring image extends from the *guan* to the *cun*.

[24] A pulse which is very faint or hardly perceptible in the *cun* is called yang expiring.

If the *guan* pulse is floating and large, there is wind in the stomach with lifting the shoulders to facilitate breathing and an open mouth, a rolling sensation below the heart, and a desire to vomit arising after ingestion.

If the *guan* pulse is slightly floating, there is accumulated heat in the stomach with vomiting of roundworms and forgetfulness.

If the *guan* pulse is slippery and varying in size, [counterflow vomiting is inevitable in the *Qian Jin*] this shows that the disease is advancing. Within one or two days it will start a relapse. The person has a desire to drink quantities of water, but, upon drinking, downpour diarrhea will be induced. If the diarrhea stops, (the person) will survive. If not, death is a certainty.

If the *guan* pulse is tight and slippery, roundworms are stirring.

If the *guan* pulse is choppy and hard, large and replete, no less forceful under pressure, there is repletion in the middle burner, a hidden binding in the spleen, congestion of the lung qi,[25] and repletion heat in the stomach.

If the *guan* pulse is wobbling in a large amplitude but the *chi* and *cun* pulse are thin, the person must have accumulated cold in the cardiac and abdominal regions, concretions and conglomerations, bindings and gatherings, and desire for hot drink and food.

If the *guan* pulse appears and disappears irregularly and becomes large at one time but small at another, slow at one time but rapid at another, there is cold and heat in the stomach, marked emaciation, no desire for drink and food, and malaria-like disorder.

If the *chi* pulse is floating, there is guest yang (*i.e.*, exogenous heat) in the lower burner.

If the *chi* pulse is fine and faint, there is duck-stool diarrhea and cold dysentery.

If the pulse is weak in the *chi* but strong in the *cun*, the stomach vessel network is injured.

If the *chi* pulse is vacuous and small, there is cold in the lower legs with wilting *bi* and pain in the feet.

---

[25] Congestion of the lung qi often refers to rapid dyspneic breathing with chest fullness.

If the *chi* pulse is choppy, there is hemafecia, inhibited defecation, and profuse perspiration.

If the pulse is slippery and racing, this shows blood vacuity.

If the *chi* pulse is deep and slippery, there are tapeworms.

If the *chi* pulse is thin and urgent, there is hypertonicity of the sinews with *bi* and inability to walk.

If the *chi* pulse is thick frequently with fever, this indicates heat in the center giving rise to pain in the lower back and crotch and hot, dark-colored urine.

If the *chi* pulse is slippery and racing on one hand with a red facial complexion as if intoxicated, there is an illness due to external heat.

Chapter Two
A Discussion on the Pulses of Miscellaneous Diseases

A slippery pulse points to repletion and [debilitated yang qi] in the lower (burner). A rapid pulse points to vacuity and heat. A floating pulse points to wind and vacuity. A stirring pulse points to pain and fright.

A deep pulse points to water (problems), repletion, [and ghost pouring[1]]. A weak pulse points to vacuity and palpitations.

A slow pulse points to cold. A choppy pulse points to shortage of blood. A moderate pulse points to vacuity. A surging pulse points to qi (exuberance) [heat in another version]. A taut pulse points to cold. A bowstring and rapid pulse points to malaria-like disease.

Malaria-like disease is featured by a bowstring pulse. If the pulse is rapid as well as bowstring, there is much heat. If it is slow as well as bowstring, there is much cold. If it is (also) faint, there is vacuity. If it is regularly interrupted and dissipated, this is death.

---

[1] This refers to an infectious disease caught from a dead body.

A bowstring (pulse) points to painful *bi*. [It is said in another version that a floating pulse points to wind pouring.[2]] A bowstring pulse appearing on one hand (only) points to rheum. If the bowstring pulse appears on both sides, there is hypertonicity of and pain in the lateral costal regions and the patient is averse to cold with shivering.

A large pulse indicates that there is cold and heat in the center. A hidden pulse indicates choleraic disease. An exuberant pulse accompanied by liking the comfort of lying down suggests desertion of blood. If there is collapsing perspiration (*i.e.*, massive sweating), cold rheum in the lungs, cough due to cold water, diarrhea, or vacuity cold in the stomach, the pulse is tight. A floating and large (pulse) points to wind. A floating, large pulse points to wind stroke with top-heaviness and nasal congestion. A floating and moderate (pulse) points to insensitivity of the skin due to wind cold invading the muscles and flesh. A slippery, floating, and dissipated pulse points to paraplegic slack wind (*huan feng*).[3] A slippery pulse points to ghost pouring. A choppy and tight (pulse) points to the illness of *bi*. A floating, surging, large, and long pulse points to wind dizziness and disorders involving the head. A large, hard, and racing pulse points to epilepsy.

If (the pulse) is bowstring and hook-like with stabbing pain in the lateral costal regions which swoops down (dramatically) like a corpse (*i.e.*, a spirit), this does not cause death even though the trouble is very severe.

A tight, urgent pulse points to fleeing corpse (*dun shi*).[4]

A surging large pulse points to febrile disease of cold damage.

A floating, surging, and large pulse points to cold damage. If (cold damage) comes on in spring, it is favorable. If it develops in autumn, it will give rise to a (serious) disease.

A floating, slippery pulse points to accumulated food.

A floating, slippery, and racing pulse points to untransformed food in stools due to inability of the spleen to grind it.

A short, racing, and slippery pulse points to disease due to wine.

---

[2] This refers to migratory pain due to vacuity and wind.

[3] This is a type of foot qi. Its symptoms include insensitivity of the legs and feet, cardiac disorders, and edema. In severe cases, mental disorders may also be present.

[4] This refers to a very severe case of distention and acute pain in the chest and abdomen. In this case, the patient dares not to breathe for fear of chest pain. In addition, there is qi surging up into the chest and attacking the flanks, masses springing up suddenly, and hypertonicity of the lower back.

A floating, thin, and slippery pulse points to damage by rheum.

A slow and choppy pulse points to cold in the center and concretion binding.[5] A swift and tight pulse points to gatherings and accumulations with tenderness. A bowstring and urgent pulse points to *shan* concretions and pain in the lower abdomen or the illness of elusive masses (in the lateral costal regions) [illness of *bi* in another version]. A slow and slippery pulse points to distention. An exuberant and tight pulse suggests distention. A bowstring and small pulse points to cold elusive masses. A deep, bowstring pulse points to suspended rheum with internal pain. A bowstring, rapid pulse points to existence of cold rheum which is difficult to treat in winter or summer. A tight and slippery pulse points to counterflow vomiting. A small, weak, and choppy pulse points to stomach reflux.

If the pulse is slow and moderate, there is cold. If the pulse is faint but tight, there is cold. If the pulse is deep and slow, there is a cold disease in the viscera in the abdomen. If the pulse is faint and weak, there is cold with diminished qi. If the pulse is replete and tight, there is cold in the stomach and distressing inability to take in food. The case with frequent diarrhea is difficult to treat. [In another version it is said that, in case of frequent retching, (the condition) will linger on and is difficult to treat.] A slippery and rapid pulse points to binding below the heart and exuberant heat. If the pulse is slippery and racing, there is heat in the stomach. A moderate, slippery pulse suggests heat in the center. A deep but urgent pulse points to the disease of cold damage with sudden fulminant vacuity heat.

If the pulse is floating but expiring, there is qi urgency.[6] If the pulse is a bit large and slippery, the center is short of qi (*i.e*, there is shortness for breath). If the pulse is floating and short, the patient suffers from injured lungs with the various qi scant and diminished. Then death will come within one year. There ought to be coughing. A deep and rapid pulse points to water stroke (*zhong shui*)[7] which will heal by itself without the need to treat it if it starts in winter. A short, rapid pulse points to heart pain and vexation. A bowstring and tight pulse points to pain in the lateral costal region due to injured viscera with blood stasis [cold blood in another version]. A deep and slippery pulse indicates heaviness of the lower (limbs) and/or pain in the paravertebral muscles. If the pulse arrives fine and slippery and is capable of becoming vacuous under pressure, there will arise sudden collapse when straightening up abruptly with a weight. (This may be caused by) having fallen from a height. The disease lies internally.

---

[5] Binding here means concretions and conglomerations in the abdomen.

[6] Qi urgency refers to such conditions as gasping for breath or rapid distressed dyspneic breathing.

[7] This refers to disease due to toxins in the water in some mountainous areas.

A faint and floating pulse is favorable if it appears in autumn but suggests illness if it appears in winter.

If the pulse is faint and rapid, even though (the evil) is serious, no disease has yet developed. (However,) one should not tax oneself.

The floating, slippery, racing, or tight pulse may present itself in hundreds of diseases. The disease, if enduring, is easy to cure.

When a yang evil comes, there will appear a floating and surging pulse. When a yin evil comes, there will appear a deep and thin pulse. When water and grain (retention) comes, there will appear a hard, replete pulse.

If the pulse is large at one time but small at another, long at one time but short at another, this shows a ghostly disaster (sui).[8]

If the pulse is surging and large, beating gracefully, the Local Guardian is working the ghostly disaster.[9]

If the pulse is deep and floppy, there is insensitivity and heaviness of the four limbs. Earth is working the ghostly disaster.[9]

If the pulse is fixed within the muscles[10] but discernible after a long time of feeling, precipitation is appropriate.

If the pulse is bowstring, small, and tight, precipitation is appropriate.

If the pulse is tight and rapid with fever and chills, recovery cannot be effected except through precipitation.

If the pulse is bowstring and slow, it is appropriate to administer warm medicinals.

If the pulse is tight and rapid, diaphoresis is appropriate.

---

[8] *Sui* is a disastrous event caused by an evil spirit. However, it is also sometimes used as an epithet for something which is clandestine, evil, erratic, or unpredictable. In this sentence, it means an unpredictably transmutable disease.

[9] A Local Guardian or Earth Guardian are one and the same type of spirit. They are a type of protector of a local area. Ghostly disaster here refers to transmutable patterns of odd natures.

[10] This refers to a hidden, elusive pulse tangible only after careful palpation.

Examination of the Signs & Symptoms of Expiry of the Qi of the Five Viscera & Six Bowels

If a sick person's liver has expired, death will come in eight days. What indicates (such liver expiry)? A green-blue facial complexion, desire for nothing but to sleep lying down, looking but seeing no people, and sweat exiting uncheckably like running water.

If a sick person's gallbladder has expired, death will come in seven days. What indicates (such gallbladder expiry)? The eyebrows are slanting.

If a sick person's sinews have expired, death will come in nine days. What indicates (such sinew expiry)? Green-blue nails of the fingers and toes and no end of shouting and cursing.

If a sick person's heart has expired, death will come in one day. What indicates (such heart expiry)? Lifting the shoulders to facilitate breathing with upturned eyes suggests instant death. [Another version says, "With the eyes fixed, death comes in one day."]

If a sick person's intestines [small intestine in another version] have expired, death will come in six days. What indicates (such small intestine expiry)? The head hair stands on end like hemp and (the body) is unable to bend or stretch with ceaseless spontaneous sweating.

If a sick person's spleen has expired, death will come in twelve days. What indicates (such spleen expiry)? A cold mouth, swollen feet, heat in the abdomen, distended belly, and fecal incontinence with evacuation at no constant hours.

If a sick person's stomach has expired, death will come in five days. What indicates (such stomach expiry)? Pain in the spine, heaviness of the lower back, and inability to turn over.

If a sick person's flesh has expired, death will come in six days. What indicates (such flesh expiry)? Dry ears [eyes in another version], swelling all over the tongue, blood in the urine, and diarrhea with red-colored stools.

If a sick person's lungs have expired, death will come in three days. What indicates (such lung expiry)? The mouth is kept open to only let breath out but not in.

If a sick person's large intestine has expired, there is no way to treat. What indicates (such large intestine expiry)? No end of diarrhea. Once diarrhea comes to an end, death ensues.

If a sick person's kidneys have expired, death will come in four days. What indicates (such kidney expiry)? The teeth suddenly become desiccated, the face becomes full black with yellow eyes, the lower back is as painful as if it were broken, and sweat exits spontaneously like flowing water.

If a sick person's bones have expired and their teeth turn yellow and fall out, death will come in ten days.

The various types of floating pulse with no root[1] all portend death. In all the above (cases), the root is the five viscera and six bowels. [2]

---

[1] This is a pulse which is only palpable at the superficial level but is absolutely impalpable at the deep level.

[2] The last sentence is quite ambiguous. One plausible interpretation may be that, as regards any floating pulses, the presence of root is crucial. This is because the root is a reflection of the viscera and bowels. Another possible interpretation is that the crucial point in all the above problems discussed in this chapter is the condition of the viscera and bowels.

_____________Chapter Four_____________
Examination of the Pulse Signs
Counter to the Four Seasons

In the three months of spring, wood is king and the liver pulse is in the government. (Therefore,) the liver pulse should appear first (in the year). Then the heart pulse appears next. Following it is the lung pulse. The kidney pulse appears last. This is the order of (the pulses decided by) their king and ministerial times in the four seasons. (Following this order,) the pulses are normal ones.

When the sixth month comes, earth becomes king and the spleen pulse should be the first to appear. If the spleen pulse fails to appear but instead the kidney pulse is acquired, this shows the kidneys rebelling against the spleen. Death will come in seventy days. What indicates the kidneys rebelling against the spleen? In summer, fire is king, the heart pulse should appear first, and then the lung pulse will follow.[1] Now, the kidney pulse is acquired instead. Thus this makes known that the kidneys are rebelling against the spleen. (Disease) is expected to occur in the fifth and sixth months. *Bing* and *ding* are lethal.[2]

If the spleen rebels against the liver, death comes in thirty days. What indicates that the spleen is rebelling against the liver? In spring, the liver pulse should be the first to appear. If it fails to come but instead the spleen pulse appears first, this makes known that the spleen is rebelling against the liver. (Disease) is expected to occur in the first and second months. *Jia* and *yi* are lethal.

If the kidneys rebel against the liver, death comes in three years. What indicates that the kidneys are rebelling against the liver? In spring, the liver pulse should be the first to appear. If it fails to come but instead the kidney pulse appears first, this makes known that the kidneys are rebelling against the liver. (Disease) is expected to occur in the seventh and eighth months. *Geng* and *xin* are lethal.

If the kidneys rebel against the heart, death comes in two years. What indicates that the kidneys are rebelling against the heart? In summer, the heart pulse should be the first to appear. If it fails to come but instead the kidney pulse appears first, this makes known that the kidneys are rebelling against the heart. (Disease) is expected to occur in the sixth month. *Wu* and *ji* are lethal.

---

[1] This sentence seems to be irrelevant.

[2] The ten Heavenly Stems correspond with the five phases in the following way: *jia/yi* = wood; *bing/ding* = fire; *wu/ji* = earth; *geng/xin* = metal; *ren/gui* = water

The ten stems can be used to mark the year, the month, the day, and the watch (hour). In summer, earth is prevalent, and earth is engendered by fire. This is matched with *bing* and *ding*. If kidney water rebels against spleen earth during this period, it is easy to infer that fire is debilitated. Therefore, a watch, a day, a month, or a year that is associated with fire, *i.e.*, *bing* or *ding*, is troublesome for the spleen. This explanation is likewise applicable to all the other viscera.

Examination of the Damaged (*i.e.*, Slowed Down) & Augmented (*i.e.*, Quickened) Pulses

There are damaged pulses and augmented pulses. What are they like? The answer is as follows: As far as the augmented pulse is concerned, if the pulse beats twice in one exhalation, this is normal. If it beats three times, this indicates aberration of the channel. If it beats four times, this indicates retrenchment of essence. If it beats five times, this is known as fatal. If it beats six times, this indicates that life is at an end. These pulses are augmented ones.

What are the damaged pulses like? If the pulse beats once in one exhalation, this indicates aberration of the channel. If it beats once in two exhalations, this indicates retrenchment of essence. If it beats once in three exhalations, this is known as fatal. If it beats once in four exhalations, this indicates that life is at an end. These pulses are damaged ones.

An augmented pulse shows (that the disease tends to transmit) from the lower to the upper,[1] while a damaged pulse shows (a tendency for disease to transmit) from the upper to the lower.

What kinds of disease does the damaged pulse reflect? The first damage is done to the skin and hair, causing contraction of the skin and loss of hair. The second damage is done to the blood vessels, causing them to be vacuous and diminished so that they are unable to nourish the five viscera and six bowels. The third damage is done to the muscles and flesh, causing them to be emaciated since food and drink cannot serve the muscles and skin. The fourth damage is done to the sinews, causing them to be slack and unable to contract. The fifth damage is done to the bones, causing bone wilting and inability to rise from bed. The diseases reflected by the augmented pulses are respectively just the opposite to the above. (A condition developing) from the upper (*i.e.*, externally) to the lower (*i.e.*, internally) ends in death when bone wilting appears with inability to rise from bed. (A condition developing) from the lower to the upper ends in death when skin contraction appears with loss of hair.

What methods are there to treat these damages? The answer is as follows: When the lungs are damaged, one may boost the qi of the lungs. When the heart is damaged, one may balance the

---

[1] The upper and lower do not merely refer to the upper and lower parts of the body but also respectively the external and internal or exterior and interior.

constructive and the defensive. When the spleen is damaged, one may balance food and drink and try to adapt to cold and heat. When the liver is damaged, one may moderate the center (with sweet medicinals). When the kidneys are damaged, one may boost the essence and qi. These are the methods of treating damages.

The pulse may beat twice in one exhalation and twice in one inhalation, three times in one exhalation and three times in one inhalation, four times in one exhalation and four times in one inhalation, five times in one exhalation and five times in one inhalation, or six times in one exhalation and six times in one inhalation. The pulse may beat once in one exhalation and once in one inhalation, once in two exhalations and once in two inhalations, or twice in one exhalation and inhalation.

This is the frequency of the pulse beat. Then what kinds of diseases do these pulses reveal? The answer is as follows: If the pulse beats twice in one exhalation and twice in one inhalation and it is neither large nor small, this is normal. If the pulse beats three times in one exhalation and three times in one inhalation, the disease is just taken. If the pulse is large in the distal position and small in the proximal, there is headache with visual dizziness. If it is small in the distal position and large in the proximal, there is fullness in the chest with shortness of breath.

If the pulse beats four times in one exhalation and four times in one inhalation, the disease is just tending to become severe. If the pulse is surging and large, the bitterness (*i.e.*, the suffering) is vexation and fullness. If it is deep and thin, there is abdominal pain. If it is slippery, there is heat damage. If it is choppy, there is mist and dew stroke.

If the pulse beats five times in one exhalation and five times in one inhalation, the person must be having trouble. If the pulse is deep and thin, (the condition) becomes worse at night. If it is floating and large, (the condition) becomes worse during the day. If it is neither large nor small, it is curable even though there is trouble. If the pulse varies in size, it is difficult to treat.

If the pulse beats six times in one exhalation and six times in one inhalation, this pulse suggests ten deaths out of ten cases. If the pulse is deep and thin, death comes at night. If it is floating and large, death comes during the day.

A pulse beating once in one exhalation and once in one inhalation is known as a damaged pulse. Though the person is able to move about, they should lie in bed since the qi and blood are both insufficient.

If the pulse beats once in two exhalations and once in two inhalations, this is known as absence of *hun*.[2] Those deprived of *hun* are expected to die. Though such a person is able to move about, they can be said to be a walking corpse.

Bian Que explained:

(In terms) of the pulse, if its emerging and submerging are equal (in duration), this is a normal state. If its submerging is twice as long as its emerging, this is *shao yin*.[3] If its submerging is three times as long as its emerging, this is *tai yin*. If its submerging is four times as long as its emerging, this is *jue yin*. If its emerging is twice as long as its submerging, this is *shao yang*. If its emerging is three times as long as its submerging, this is *yang ming*. If its emerging is four times as long as its submerging, this is *tai yang*. The emerging pulse is yang, while the submerging pulse is yin.

Supposedly, while a person finishes one exhalation, the pulse beats twice and the qi moves three *cun*, and while a person finishes one inhalation, the pulse beats twice (more) and the qi moves another three *cun*. During one exhalation, one inhalation, and the interval (between them), the pulse beats five times. One exhalation and one inhalation comprise one respiration, during which time the qi moves six *cun*. When a person completes ten respirations, the pulse has beaten fifty times and the qi has covered six *chi*. During twenty respirations, the pulse beats 100 times, providing a totality of qi corresponding with the four seasons.

Heaven has 365 days (in the year) and the human being has 365 joints. There are 100 divisions on the clepsydra for one day and night. For one totality of qi, the vessel (qi) moves twelve *chi*. In one day and night, the qi travels for twelve watches and then comes to an end, having covered the whole body. This is in compliance with the heavenly path and hence is a normal (state). Normalcy is freedom from disease — one yin matching with one yang. Two beats of the pulse is called one bout. If (the pulse) beats two bouts (during one exhalation) and is tight, there is retrenchment of qi. There are 135 respirations during one division (of the clepsydra), 1,350 respirations for ten divisions, and 13,500 respirations for 100 divisions. Two divisions amount to one circuit, and one

---

[2] This term means exhausted yang qi.

[3] The submerging pulse is categorized as yin, while the emerging pulse as yang. In this case, submerging takes double the time that emerging takes. This means that yin is twice as much as yang. Therefore, this state is called (exuberance of) *shao yin* or lesser yin. If the situation is worse, we have *tai yin*. If it further deteriorates, *jue yin* appears. If the relation is reversed in terms of yin and yang, then we will see *shao yang*, etc.

circuit means that the qi has completed its traveling around the body.[4] In one day and night, (the qi) runs fifty circuits.

If the pulse beats three times (during one exhalation), there is aberration of the channel. Since the pulse beats three times during one exhalation, the qi covers four and a half *cun* (during the same duration of time. Thus,) when a person completes one respiration, the pulse has beaten seven times and qi has covered nine *cun*. During ten respirations, the pulse beats seventy times and the qi covers nine *chi*. During one totality of qi, the pulse beats 140 times and the qi covers eighteen *chi*. When qi has completed one circuit round the body, it has exceeded 180 degrees.[5] Therefore, this is called aberration of the channel. Aberration of the channel is a disease. It is one yin matching two yang.

If the pulse beats thrice (during one exhalation) and is tight, there is retrenchment of blood.

If the pulse beats four times (during one exhalation), there is retrenchment of essence. Since the pulse beats four times during one exhalation, the qi covers 6 *cun* (during the same duration of time). When a person has completed one respiration, the pulse has beaten nine times and the qi has covered one and two tenths *chi*. When a person has completed ten respirations, the pulse has beaten ninety times and the qi has covered twelve *chi*. For one totality of qi, the pulse beats 180 times and the qi moves twenty-four *chi*. When qi completes one circuit round the body, it has exceeded 360 degrees, doubling (the normal number of degrees) round the body. Thus the qi has covered the body twice in this duration of time. If the pulse is floating and choppy, the five viscera are deprived of essence. This is difficult to treat since it is one yin matching with three yang. If the pulse beats four times (during one exhalation) and is tight, the form is retrenched.

If the pulse beats five times (during one exhalation), death is a certainty. Since the pulse beats five times during one exhalation, the qi moves six and a half *cun* (for the same duration of time). [It should be seven and a half *cun*. This note is acceptable. (tr.)] When a person has completed one respiration, the pulse has beaten eleven times and the qi has covered one and three tenths *chi*. [It should be one and half *chi*. This note is acceptable. (tr.)] When a person has completed ten respirations, the pulse has beaten 110 times and the qi has covered thirteen *chi*. [It should be

---

4   The total length of the channels measures, on average, 162 *chi*. If the qi travels 81 *chi* during one division of the clepsydra, then in two divisions, the distance the qi covers is 162 *chi*. This means that the qi completes a circuit round the whole body in that duration of time.

5   One circuit around the body is divided into 360 degrees. During two divisions of the clepsydra, the qi covers 180 degrees at its normal speed. But now the pulse beat is quicker than normal. Therefore, during two divisions, the qi covers more than that number of degrees.

fifteen *chi*. This note is acceptable. (tr.)] For one totality of qi, the pulse beats 220 times and the qi covers twenty-six *chi*. [It should be thirty *chi*. This note is acceptable. (tr.)] When (the qi) has visited the 365 joints around the whole body, it has exceeded 540 degrees, exceeding 170 degrees even after it has covered the body twice. This situation is related to each of the joints in terms of the qi. Because the (pulse) qi is floating and choppy, the channels have exhausted the blood and qi circulating in them. (The essence and qi) are unable to keep to the center, and, (in consequence,) the five viscera become atrophic and wasted, while the essence spirit is dispersed and lost. (Therefore,) if the pulse beats five times (during one exhalation) and is tight, death is a certainty, for the three yin and three yang (are all exhausted). Even though the five viscera are not wilted or wasted, there is no help.

In the case of the first damage reflected by a dual pulse beat, the pulse beats once when the person completes one exhalation or beats twice when the person completes one respiration. (During this time) the qi covers three *cun*. During ten respirations, the pulse beats twenty times and the qi covers three *chi*. During one totality of qi, the pulse beats forty times and the qi covers six *chi*, leaving 180 joints of the body yet to visit. Because the qi is too short to go round the body, the bitterness is diminished qi and listlessness and slackness of the body.

In the case of the second damage, during one respiration, the pulse beats once and the qi covers one and half *cun*. When the person completes ten respirations, the pulse has beaten ten times and the qi has covered one and half *chi*. For one totality of qi, the pulse beats twenty times and the qi covers three *chi*, leaving 200 joints of the body yet to visit. Since the qi and blood are exhausted, they cannot reach the channels. Therefore, this is called aberration of the channel. Since the blood does not go where it should, there is blood in both the stools and urine.

In the case of the third damage, during one respiration plus one exhalation, the pulse beats once. During ten respirations, the pulse beats seven times and the qi covers one and half *chi*. [It should be one and five one hundredths *chi*. This note is acceptable. (tr.)] During one totality of qi, the pulse beats fourteen times and the qi covers three and one tenth *chi*. [It should be two and one tenth *chi*. This note is acceptable. (tr.)], leaving 297 joints of the body yet to visit. Therefore, this is called wrestling (*zheng*). While the qi circulates on, the blood lingers behind. They cannot coordinate and (both) become faint. If the qi is blocked and (therefore becomes) replete, there is fullness in the chest. If the viscera are withered, the qi and blood will wrestle with one another in the center. If the qi fails to come and help, blood will coagulate. Then death comes.

In the case of the fourth damage, the pulse beats once during two respirations. When a person completes ten respirations, the pulse has beaten five times and the qi has covered seven and half *cun*. For one totality of qi, the pulse beats ten times and the qi covers one and half *chi*, leaving 315 joints of the body yet to visit. Therefore, this is called blood collapse. Blood collapse means frenetic movement of the blood or blood running beyond measure. (As a result,) the body becomes emaciated and fatigued, only skin and bones. Qi and blood are both exhausted and the five viscera are deprived of their spirit. And it is clear that death is a certainty.

In the case of the fifth damage, during two respirations plus one exhalation, the pulse beats once. When the person completes ten respirations, the pulse has beaten four times and the qi has covered six *cun*. For one totality of qi, the pulse beats eight times and the qi covers one and two tenths *chi*, leaving 324 joints of the body yet to visit. Therefore, this is called expiry. Expiry means qi urgency (*i.e.*, rapid breathing), inability to rise from bed, cold breath from the mouth, and expiration of all pulses. Then death comes.

Qi Bo explained:

Incongruity of the pulse with the four seasons may be exhibited by the appearance of an (abnormal) pulse beat rate. (Such abnormal) pulse beats may be damaged or augmented pulses.

In terms of the damaged pulse, if the bones governed by the *shao yin* are heavy, this shows damaged will (*zhi*). Reduced food intake with wasted muscles and flesh shows damaged reflection (*yi*). Desire to lie down yet discomfort arising upon lying down and dim vision and hearing show a damaged ethereal soul (*hun*). Inhibited respiration and a lusterless facial complexion of (any of) the five colors show a damaged corporeal soul (*po*). The appearance of chaotic pulses on all the four limbs shows a damaged spirit (*shen*).

Major damage reduces (life) by thirty years; medium damage by twenty years; and minor damage by ten years. Each kind of damage is identified in relation to spring, summer, autumn, and winter. In regard to (the physical state of) people, if a person is tall but the pulse is short, there is a major damage subtracting thirty years. If a person is short but the pulse is long, there is a medium damage subtracting twenty years. If (the pulses on) both the hands and the feet are thin, there is a minor damage subtracting ten years. Loss of essence qi subtracts one year. If a male has a short pulse on the left hand but a long pulse on the right, his yang is damaged. This will reduce (his life) by half a year. If a female has a short pulse on the right hand but a long pulse on the left, her yin is damaged. This will reduce (her life) by half a year.

In spring, there should appear the liver pulse. If, instead, a spleen or a lung pulse appears, there is damage. In summer, there should appear the heart pulse. If, instead, a kidney or a lung pulse appears, there is damage. In autumn, there should appear the lung pulse. If, instead, a liver or a heart pulse appears, there is damage. In winter, there should appear the kidney pulse. If, instead, a heart or a spleen pulse appears, there is damage.

It is necessary to feel and examine the pulse of the *cun* opening to determine whether the pulse (qi) has expired or not. If the distal and proximal (pulses) are both gone, this is expiry (of the pulse qi).[6] If (a pulse is felt) beating in the palm and hard like a pellet, this shows that the pulse in the distal (*i.e.*, the *cun*) is vacuous and at an end. The (pulse qi) in the proximal pulse, (however,) is still present. Therefore the stomach qi still exists. If the distal pulse has come to an end but the proximal pulse is as hard as a pellet, this (also) shows the existence of the stomach qi. If both the distal and proximal pulses are at an end, death is a certainty. If neither of them have expired or disappeared, survival can be prognosed. This is (merely) damaged pulses.

In the case of the augmented pulse, if the voice sounds deep and as if coming from a distance and this is accompanied by confused vision, this shows augmented will (*zhi*). A bulky body with suddenly increased food intake shows augmented reflection (*yi*). Confused speech and confused vision with cramps of the hands and feet shows an augmented ethereal soul (*hun*). A bright green, lustrous facial complexion shows an augmented corporeal soul (*po*). If the pulses are small and out of line with spontaneously increased respiration, this shows an augmented spirit (*shen*). The above is the method (of discriminating) the augmented pulses. Death and survival depend on whether (the pulses and the disease patterns) are compatible. If the disease is helped by the qi fit to it, there is life (*i.e.*, hope of survival). Five out of ten (cases) may be carried through.

The Yellow Emperor said:

Good.

---

[6] The distal refers to the *cun* position, while the proximal refers to the *chi* position. According to the explanation given in the text, the expired pulse is a very vacuous pulse which is nearly impalpable.

______________ Chapter Six ______________
Prognosis of the Year, Month & Day of Death Through Examination of the Ratio of Beats to Interruptions of the Pulse

If one beat of the pulse is followed by one interruption, death comes in two days. If two beats are followed by one interruption, death comes in three days. If three beats are followed by one interruption, death comes in four or five days. If four beats are followed by one interruption, death comes in six days. If five beats are followed by one interruption, death comes in five or seven days. If six beats are followed by one interruption, death comes in eight days. If seven beats are followed by one interruption, death comes in nine days. If eight beats are followed by one interruption, death comes in ten days. If nine beats are followed by one interruption, death comes in nine days or in eleven days as stated in another source [in thirteen days or on the Beginning of Spring in another version]. If ten beats are followed by one interruption, death comes on the Beginning of Summer [the Beginning of Spring in another version]. If eleven beats are followed by one interruption, death comes on the Summer Solstice [Beginning of Summer in another version; Beginning of Autumn in yet another version]. If twelve or thirteen beats are followed by one interruption, death comes on the Beginning of Autumn [Beginning of Winter in another version]. If fourteen or fifteen beats are followed by one interruption, death comes on the Beginning of Winter [Beginning of Summer in another version]. If twenty beats are followed by one interruption, death comes in one year or on the Beginning of Autumn. If twenty-one beats are followed by one interruption, death comes in two years. If twenty-five beats are followed by one interruption, death comes on the Beginning of Winter [in one or two years in another version]. If thirty beats are followed by one interruption, death comes in two or three years. If thirty-five beats are followed by one interruption, death comes in three years. If forty beats are followed by one interruption, death comes in four years. If fifty beats are followed by one interruption, death comes in five years. If more than fifty beats are followed by one interruption, death comes in five years.

If the pulse beats fifty times without one interruption, all the five viscera are furnished with qi. That is to say, there is no disease. If the pulse beats forty times with one interruption, one viscus[1] is dispossessed of qi. Death comes four years later in the spring when the grass begins to grow.

---

[1] This implies the kidneys.

If the pulse beats thirty times with one interruption, two viscera are dispossessed of qi. Death comes three years later when wheat ripens. If the pulse beats twenty times with one interruption, three viscera are dispossessed of qi. Death comes two years later when the mulberry turns red. If the pulse beats ten times with one interruption, four viscera are dispossessed of qi. Death comes half a year later. If (the condition) remains stable on certain nodes of qi, death comes following Pure Brightness.[3] (If not,) it comes towards the Grain Rain[4] at the latest. If the pulse beats five times with one interruption, the five viscera are all dispossessed of qi. Death comes five days later.

If one beat of the pulse is followed by one long pause, there is a persisting disease in the heart. Treat the ruler (*i.e.*, the heart). If two beats of the pulse are followed by one long pause, the disease is in the liver. Treat the twig (*i.e.*, the liver). If three beats of the pulse are followed by one long pause, the disease is in the spleen. Treat the lower (*i.e.*, the spleen). If four beats of the pulse are followed by one long pause, the disease is in the kidneys. Treat the in-between (*i.e.*, the kidneys). If five beats of the pulse are followed by one long pause, the disease is in the lungs. Treat the branches (*i.e.*, the lungs). If the (above) five kinds of pathological pulses are found in vacuous and emaciated people, death is doomed, for no medicinals are able to treat (the evil), nor is the needle able to reach it. Exuberant people, however, are curable, for their qi is intact.

---

[2]   The year is divided into twenty-four periods or solar terms. These are called the twenty-four nodes of qi and include the Spring Rain Water, the Beginning of Summer, the Summer Solstice, etc. Here the word node refers to the first day of a certain node.

[3]   The fifth node of qi in the year.

[4]   The sixth node of qi

———————— Chapter Seven ————————
The Prognosis of Life & Death
in Hundreds of Diseases

If cold damage is found with exuberant heat, there is life if the pulse is floating and large but death if the pulse is deep and small.

If cold damage has obtained perspiration, there is life if the pulse becomes deep and small but death if the pulse remains floating and large.

If there is a warm disease with sweat refusing to exit three to four days after (contracting it), there is life if the pulse is large and racing but death without a remedy if the pulse is so thin and small that it is hardly perceptible.

If there is a warm disease with raging high fever, there is death if the pulse is thin and small.

If a warm disease is accompanied by diarrhea and acute abdominal pain, there is death without a remedy.

If sweat refuses to exit in a warm disease or fails to reach the feet, there is death. If inversion counterflow (*i.e.*, chilled limbs) is accompanied by (spontaneous) sweating, there is life if the pulse is hard, strong, and urgent but death if the pulse is vacuous and moderate.

If, on the second or third day, a warm disease manifests bodily heat (*i.e.*, generalized fever), abdominal fullness, headache, normal food intake, and a straight and racing pulse, death will come eight days later. If, on the fourth or fifth day, there is headache, abdominal pain, vomiting, and a thin but strong pulse, death will come twelve days later. If, on the eighth or ninth day, there are no headache, no pain in the body, no reddening of the eyes, and no change in the complexion, if there is contrarily diarrhea, if the pulse overlaps (*i.e.*, is very swift) but does not forcefully strike against the fingers and from time to time it becomes large, and if there is tightness below the heart, death will come seventeen days later.

On the seventh or eighth day, if febrile disease manifests a pulse which is not soft [not as if gasping in another version] or dissipated [rapid in another version], there ought to be loss of voice. Three days after, if sweat does not exit in spite of heat, this is death.

If a febrile disease manifests a faint, thin pulse and inhibited urination on the seventh or eighth day, then it may end in death if suddenly there arises a dry mouth, interruption in the pulse, and a dry, parched tongue which is black in color.

If there is a febrile disease with sweat refusing to exit and an exuberant, agitated, racing pulse, there is life if perspiration is (eventually) secured, but it will be difficult to cure if perspiration fails to be secured (in the end).

If a febrile disease has seen perspiration, there is life if the pulse is quiet and tranquil, but it is difficult to cure if the pulse is agitated.

116

If a febrile disease has seen perspiration, then it may end in death (nonetheless) if high fever persists.

If a febrile disease has seen perspiration, if the fever persists, and if the pulse remains slightly agitated, one should be careful not to treat with needling.

If a febrile disease manifests fever and the fever is high, the pulse (must) be debilitated in both the yin and the yang (*i.e.*, the *chi* and *cun*). One should be careful not to apply needling. Unless sweat exits, there is bound to be diarrhea.

If a person has been taken by wind stroke with insensitivity, wilting, and limpness, and their pulse is vacuous, there is life. But if their pulse is hard, urgent, and racing, this is death.

If there is madness and the pulse is vacuous, this can be treated. If (the pulse is) replete, this leads to death.

Epilepsy may end in survival if the pulse is replete and hard, but in death if the pulse is deep, thin, and small.

Epilepsy will heal by itself in due time if the pulse beats large and slippery but is incurable if the pulse is deep, small, urgent, and replete. It is also incurable if the pulse is small, hard, and urgent.

The prognosis of headache with pain in the eyes is death if the eyes fail to see after looking for a long (time). [At the first sight instead of after looking for long in another version. This is acceptable. (tr.)]

The prognosis of a person with gatherings and accumulations in the cardiac region and abdomen is survival if the pulse is hard, strong, and urgent, but death if the pulse is vacuous and weak. In addition, a replete and strong pulse prognoses survival, while a deep pulse, death.

A person who has a large pulse, an enlarged and distended belly, and counterflow frigidity of the four limbs will die if the pulse is long in shape. Abdominal distention and fullness with blood in the stools and a large but occasionally expiring pulse may end in death when hemafecia becomes very severe and the pulse turns to become small and racing.

Pain in the cardiac region and abdomen with inability to breathe because of the pain can be prognosed as survival if the pulse is thin, small, and slow, but as death if the pulse is hard, large, and racing.

Intestinal *pi* with blood in the stools may end in death if there is bodily heat[1] but in survival if there is cold.

Intestinal *pi* with white, foamy stools may end in survival if the pulse is deep but in death if the pulse is floating.

Intestinal *pi* with pus and blood in the stools may end in death if the pulse is suspended and expiring but in survival if the pulse is slippery and large.

Diseases categorized as intestinal *pi* with bodily heat may end in survival if the pulse is slippery and large rather than suspended and expiring, but they may end in death if the pulse is suspended and choppy. The time of death is determined by (the conditions of the involved) viscera.

Intestinal *pi* with pus and blood in the stools may end in survival if the pulse is deep, small, and fluent but in death if the pulse is rapid, racing, and large and there is fever.

Intestinal *pi* with hypertonicity of the sinews may end in survival if the pulse is small, thin, and tranquil but in death if the pulse is floating, large, and tight.

Throughflux diarrhea with untransformed food in the stools, (*i.e.*, food not kept for a moment in the stomach and intestines), and with pus and blood in the stools may end in survival if the pulse is faint, small, and slow but in death if the pulse is tight and urgent.

Outpour diarrhea may end in survival if the pulse is moderate and occasionally small and bound but in death if the pulse is floating, large, and rapid.

Worms eating the anus[2] may end in survival if the pulse is vacuous and small but in death if the pulse is tight and urgent.

Cough may end in death if the pulse is deep and tight but in survival if the pulse is floating and straight; in survival if the pulse is floating and soft but in death if the pulse is small, deep, and hidden.

Cough with emaciation may end in death if the pulse displays an image of hardness and largeness.

---

[1] Bodily heat may have either of two meanings: a) generalized fever, or b) a warm feeling in the body.

[2] This means nothing more than hemorrhoids and anal fistulas.

Cough with desertion of form (*i.e.*, cachectic emaciation) and fever may end in death if the pulse is small, hard, and urgent. If the muscles are thin but there is no desertion of form, then it may end in death, (nonetheless,) if fever persists.

Cough with retching, distention of the abdomen, and diarrhea may end in death if the pulse is bowstring and urgent, near to expiring.[3]

Blood ejection or nasal bleeding may end in survival if the pulse is slippery, small, and weak but in death if the pulse is replete and large.

Perspiration accompanied by spontaneous external bleeding may end in survival if the pulse is small and slippery but in death if the pulse is large and agitated.

Spitting of blood may end in death if the pulse is tight and strong but in survival if the pulse is slippery.

Ejection of blood with cough and qi ascent may end in death if the pulse is rapid and there is fever and inability to sleep.

Qi ascent may end in death if the pulse is rapid. This refers to (the case of) reduced form (*i.e.*, cachectic emaciation).

Qi ascent dyspnea with (the head) lowering and rising (to facilitate breathing) may end in survival if the pulse is slippery and the hands and feet are warm but in death if the pulse is choppy and the four limbs are cold.

Qi ascent with a swollen face and having to lift the shoulders to facilitate breathing is incurable if the pulse is large. If there is diarrhea in addition, death is a certainty.

Qi ascent with retained fluids may end in survival if the pulse is vacuous, quiet, and deep-hidden but in death if the pulse is hard and strong.

Cold qi assaulting upward may end in survival if the pulse is replete, fluent, and slippery but in death if the pulse is replete and choppy with counterflow. [What is known as normal flow refers to warm hands and feet. What is known as counterflow refers to cold hands and feet.]

____

[3] In terms of the pulse, the word expiry/expiring often, but not always, means expiry of the pulse qi rather than excessive vacuity as defined in a preceding part in this book. Expiry of the pulse qi can be defined as absence of the quality of moderateness associated with the stomach qi.

Pure heat wasting thirst is curable if the pulse is replete and large even though the disease is enduring. (However,) if the pulse is suspended, small, hard, and urgent and the disease is enduring, it is incurable.

Wasting thirst may end in survival if the pulse is rapid and large but in death if the pulse is thin, small, floating, and short.

Wasting thirst may end in survival if the pulse is deep and small but in death if the pulse is replete, hard, and large.

Water disease is curable if the pulse is surging and large but is incurable if the pulse is faint and thin.

Water disease with (abdominal) distention and (urinary) block may end in survival if the pulse is floating, large, and soft but in death if the pulse is deep, thin, vacuous, and small.

Water disease with enlarged belly like a drum may end in survival if the pulse is replete but in death if the pulse is vacuous.

Sudden malign stroke[4] with several liters of blood ejected may end in death if the pulse is deep, rapid, and thin but in survival if the pulse is floating, large, racing, and quick.

Sudden malign stroke with an enlarged belly and fullness (*i.e.*, a distended feeling) of the four limbs may end in survival if the pulse is large and moderate; in death if the pulse is tight, large, and floating; but in survival, nonetheless, if the pulse is tight, thin, and faint.

The disease of sores with rigidity of the lumbar spine and tugging and slackening is incurable in any case.

Cold and heat with tugging and slackening will end in death if the pulse is regularly interrupted and expiring.

An incised wound with profuse bleeding may end in survival if the pulse is vacuous and thin but in death if the pulse is rapid, replete, and large.

---

[4] This refers to sudden stabbing pain in the cardiac region and abdomen with unbearable oppression and vexation in the chest.

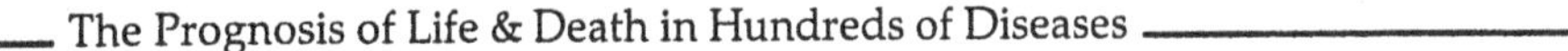

An incised bleeding wound may end in survival if the pulse is deep and small but in death if the pulse is floating and large. An axe cut with loss of one to two *dan* (1 *dan* = 100 liters) of blood will cause death in twenty days if the pulse arrives large.

Suppose an axe cut is combined with a sword cut, either of which is severe, and there is incessant bleeding with blood left scanty.[5] If the pulse arrives large, death will come seven days after the bleeding stops. If the pulse is slippery and thin, there is life.

Suppose a fall from a height has caused blood (stasis) internally giving rise to abdominal distention and fullness. If the pulse is hard and strong, there is life. If the pulse is small and weak, this is death.

A person damaged by (any of) the hundreds of medicinals may survive if the pulse is floating, choppy, and racing, die if the pulse is faint and fine, but survive if the pulse is surging, large, and slow [rapid instead of slow in the *Qian Jin*].

A person with a severe disease is difficult to cure if the pulses are out of harmony. A person with a severe disease is easy to cure if the pulse is surging.

People who are vacuous both internally and externally may die if they suffer from sweating in spite of a cold body, slight retching, vexation, restlessness, inversion counterflow frigidity of the hands and feet, and fidgeting of the body.

Suppose the pulse is replete and full with cold in the hands and feet and heat in the head. (The patient) may survive if (this happens) in the spring or autumn but die if (this happens) in the winter or summer.

Old people with a faint pulse may survive if the pulse is flaccid in the yang (*i.e.,* the *cun* and *guan*) (only) but strong in the yin (*i.e,* the *chi*). They may die if the pulse is capable of flaring up[6] in addition to being interrupted. If the pulse is weak in the yin but strong in the yang with regular interruption, they will die in a month of an odd number.

If the *chi* pulse is choppy and hard, this indicates blood repletion and qi vacuity. The diseases it causes are abdominal pain, counterflow fullness, and qi ascent. In females this is due to grave

---

[5] This phrase is also capable of being interpreted as incessant bleeding of a small amount.

[6] This describes a very weak pulse which sometimes suddenly becomes fleetingly strong but then quickly becomes flaccid again.

injury of the uterus in which exists malign blood. Over time, this develops into binding and concretions. This disease is contracted in the wintertime and ends in death when millet and glutinous millet turn red (*i.e.*, ripe).

If the *chi* pulse is thin and faint, there is insufficiency of both qi and blood. If the pulse is thin but forceful, this shows lack of grain qi. The disease tends to become active each time a node of qi begins. It ends in death when date trees grow their leaves. This disease is contracted in the autumn.

Suppose there is a *cun* pulse on the left hand which is stirring, large at one time but small at another, and arrhythmic. The pulse wobbles and varies (in quality) in the three positions from the *cun* to the *guan* and from the *guan* to the *chi*. If one falls ill in midsummer and has such a pulse, one will die when peach blossoms [leaves in another version (which is acceptable - tr.)] fall.

Suppose there is a deep and hidden *cun* pulse on the right hand which is small at one time but large at another, floating and large in the morning but deep and hidden in the evening. When there is floating and largeness, there is excess, (the pulse) appearing up on the fish's border (*i.e.*, the hypothenar eminence. However,) since the pulse is deep and hidden, it is unable to reach down to the *guan*. If this (kind of) pulse comes and goes irregularly and (this irregularity) recurs frequently, death will come when elm leaves wither and fall.

Suppose there is a *chi* pulse on the right hand which has one interruption after thirty beats at first but later has one interruption after twenty beats, stirring up at one time but slowing down at another. (This irregularity) happens continually and the pulse is out of step with the respiration. Although the person takes in grain (as usual), they cannot recuperate. Death comes when mugwort begins to grow.

Suppose there is a *chi* pulse on the right hand with one interruption after forty beats. It is capable of reappearing after interruption, but, when it comes again, it counterflows, feeling like a straight log, a full-drawn bowstring, or a taut rope as if pulled by two persons (at the ends. With such a pulse,) death will come on the Beginning of Winter [Spring in the *Qian Jin*].

The Prognosis of Life & Death in Terms of Vacuous & Replete Pulses in the Three Positions

If a pulse is harmonious in the three positions, there is life. If a pulse is collapsing in the three positions, this is death.

Suppose the pulse is vacuous in the three positions. If persons who suffer from a protracted disease have such a pulse, they will die. If the pulse is vacuous and choppy and the disease is protracted, death is also a certainty. If the pulse is vacuous and slippery, death is a certainty as well. If the pulse is vacuous and moderate, death again is a certainty. If a vacuous, bowstring, and urgent pulse appears in the disease of epilepsy, death is a certainty, nonetheless.

Suppose the pulse is replete and large in the three positions. If it appears in a protracted disease, this is death. If the pulse is replete and slippery and it appears in a protracted disease, there is life. If it appears in a sudden disease, this is death. If the pulse is replete and moderate, there is also (hope of) survival. If the pulse is replete and tight, this, too, indicates life. If a replete, tight, and urgent pulse appears in epilepsy, it is curable.

If the pulse is strong in the three positions but not congruous with the disease (pattern), the person will die.

If a flaccid pulse appears in the three positions in a person who is not flaccid, this is death.

If the pulse is thick in the three positions, a protracted disease will end in death, but a sudden disease may end in survival.

Suppose the pulse is thin and soft in the three positions. If it appears in a protracted disease, it points to survival. If the pulse is thin and rapid, this also points to survival. If the pulse is faint and tight, this points to survival as well.

If the pulse is large and rapid in the three positions, a protracted disease may end in survival, but a sudden disease will end in death.

Suppose the pulse is faint and hidden in the three positions. If it appears in a protracted disease, this is death.

Suppose the pulse is soft [soggy in another version] in the three positions. If it appears in a protracted disease, healing will ensue by itself without treatment. However, if treatment is carried out, death will ensue. If such a pulse appears in a sudden disease, there is life.

Suppose the pulse is floating and bound in the three positions. If it appears in a protracted disease, this is death. If a floating and slippery pulse appears in a protracted disease, this is also death. If the pulse is floating and rapid, a protracted disease of wind may end in survival, but a sudden disease will end in death.

If the pulse is scallion-stalk in the three positions, a protracted disease may end in survival, but a sudden disease will end in death.

If the pulse is bowstring and rapid in the three positions, a protracted disease may end in survival, but a sudden disease will end in death.

If the pulse is drumskin in the three positions, a protracted disease will end in death, but a sudden disease may end in survival.

If the pulse is hard, rapid, and (long) like a silver hairpin in the three positions, toxic drum-like distention is indicated. This will inevitably end in death. If the pulse is rapid and soft, toxic drum-like distention may end in survival.

If the pulse is wafting like oil over soup in the three positions, a protracted disease will end in death, but a sudden disease may end in survival.

If the pulse undulates like a spider's web (*i.e.*, is soft and fine) in the three positions, a protracted disease will end in death, but a sudden disease may end in survival.

If the pulse is thunderous in the three positions, a protracted disease will end in death. Death comes in thirty days.

If the pulse is like a (full-drawn) bowstring in the three positions, a protracted disease will end in death.

If the pulse beats continuously like a string of pearls, a protracted disease will end in death.

If the pulse is like sluggishly running water in the three positions, a protracted disease will heal by itself without treatment. However, it will end in death if treated. [Another version says, "If the pulse is like running water, a protracted disease will end in death in seventy days. If it is like still water, the disease will heal by itself without treatment."]

If the pulse is like a leak in the roof[1] in the three positions, a protracted disease will end in death in ten days.

If the pulse feels like a bird pecking[2] in the three positions, a protracted disease will end in death in seven days.

If the pulse feels (chaotic) like boiling water in a pot in the three positions, death will come in the evening if this pulse is obtained in the morning, at midday if it is obtained at midnight, or at midnight if it is obtained at midday.

If the pulse is urgent in the three positions and a rolling pain arises in the abdomen when pressed, needle (the points) above and below (the painful place) and then the illness will be relieved.

---

[1] This refers to an arrhythmic pulse with long pauses.

[2] This is a rapid and urgent pulse which is interrupted by pauses from time to time.

BOOK FIVE

Collated & edited by Honorary Minister Without Portfolio,
Curator of the Imperial Library,
Imperial Courier and Senior Army Protector,
Lin Yi *et al.*

_______________Chapter One_______________
Zhang Zhong-jing's Treatise on the Pulse

(The Yellow Emperor) asked:

The pulse is divided into three positions, (influenced by) the mutual overwhelming between yin and yang. In the human body, the constructive and defensive, the qi and blood follow breathing in and out, traveling up and down, and penetrate the center. By dint of breath, fluids and humors move and spread, circulating here and there. (The pulse) changes in response to the seasons. Using analogy to describe them, the spring pulse is bowstring, the autumn pulse is floating, the winter pulse is deep, and the summer pulse is surging.[1] (It is the physician's duty to) examine the colors and the pulses. (The pulses) may be different, large or small, and, in a moment, present unpredictable changes. It varies from the *chi* to the *cun*, long at one position but short at another. The (pulses in) the upper and the lower (positions) may be out of step or present here but absent there. Once the disease transmutes, (the pulse) will gain or lose (in rate), sink or mount (*i.e.*, become deep or floating). This confuses the heart and causes the reflection consternation. It often makes one lose sight of the keys and essentials (in pulse examination). I wish to have a well outlined explanation to have a clear idea (about the keys and essentials).

The master answered:

Your question touches the root and origin of the *dao* (of medicine). The pulse is divided into three positions: the *chi*, the *cun*, and the *guan*. The constructive and defensive circulate by this yardstick (*i.e.*, the pulse). The kidney pulse is deep, while the heart pulse is surging. The lung pulse is floating, while the liver pulse is bowstring. This is constant, admitting of no aberration so fine as a hundredth of *liang* (1 *liang* = approximately 31 grams). The exit and entrance (of the breath) and the ascent and descent (of yin and yang) carry on in correspondence with the divisions of the clepsydra. Each time the water falls two divisions (in the clepsydra), the pulse (qi) completes one circuit around the body, returning to the *cun* opening. Thus vacuity and repletion may manifest (in the pulse). Affected by the transmutation (of the disease), yin and yang may interfere with one another. (It follows that) wind makes the pulse floating and vacuous, while cold makes it tight and

---

[1] This line implies that the images of the seasonal pulses are based on a comparison with phenomena in the external world. For instance, in summer, plants are growing exuberantly and water floods. Therefore, the summer pulse is described as surging.

bowstring. A deep and hidden pulse reveals accumulated water. Propping rheum is made known by an urgent and bowstring pulse. A stirring and bowstring pulse points to pain, and a rapid and surging pulse indicates heat and vexation. Suppose there is no agreement (between the pulse image and the disease pattern), one should try to identify the cause of this disagreement. The pulse may be different in the three positions and, (accordingly,) different diseases are revealed. Excessive (pulse qi) challenges wondering as does insufficient (pulse qi). Evils do not come into being from nothingness. They are invariably wrought by some sinner. One should make a close study of the exterior and interior and carefully examine the three burners one by one. After having located where the evil settles, one should (further) inspect whether (the disease) is in progress or in retreat to measure (the conditions of) the viscera and bowels. Thus one will have a deep insight like a god. (I) have illustrated (the above) one by one specially for you to impart to worthy people.

———————————Chapter Two———————————
Bian Que's Method of the Yin &Yang of the Pulse

In terms of the pulse, dawn is referred to as *tai yang*, midday as *yang ming*, late afternoon as *shao yang*, twilight as *shao yin*, midnight as *tai yin*, and cockcrow as *jue yin*. These are the three yin and three yang in connection with time.

The pulse of the *shao yang*[1] is a pulse that is small at one time but large at another, long at one time but short at another, undulating in a six tenths full amplitude. It reigns at midnight of the *jia zi* day[2] of the eleventh month and reigns from the first month to the *jia zi* day of the second month.

———————————————————————

[1] In the preceding paragraph, the three yin and three yang pulses are defined in terms of the periods of the day, but in this paragraph, they are defined in terms of the month. This suggests that the pulse varies not only in different hours of the day but also in different months of the year.

[2] As mentioned above, the ten heavenly stems (*jia, yi, bing, ding,* etc.) and the twelve earthly branches (*zi, chou, yan, mou,* etc.) can be matched to form a cycle of sixty steps or divisions with *jia zi* as the first step in this cycle. The Chinese have used this sixty step cycle in order to tell dates. Because there are sixty days in such a cycle, one *jia zi* cycle covers roughly two months.

130

The pulse of the *tai yang* is a pulse that is surging and large as well as long. It floats over the sinews, undulating in a nine tenths full amplitude. It reigns from the third month to the *jia zi* day of the fourth month.

The pulse of the *yang ming* is a pulse that is floating and large as well as short, undulating in a three tenths full amplitude. It is large in the distal position but small in the proximal like a tadpole. When it arrives, (it gives a sensation of) leaping. It reigns from the fifth month to the *jia zi* day of the sixth month.

The pulse of the *shao yin* is a pulse that is tight and thin [there may be the word faint left out here], undulating in a six tenths full amplitude. It reigns at the midday of the *jia zi* day of the fifth month and reigns from the seventh month to the *jia zi* day of the eighth month.

The pulse of the *tai yin* is a pulse that is tight and thin as well as long, overriding above the sinews, undulating in a nine tenths full amplitude. It reigns from the ninth month to the *jia zi* day of the tenth month.

The pulse of the *jue yin* is a pulse that is deep and short as well as tight, undulating in a three tenths full amplitude. It reigns from the eleventh month to the *jia zi* day of the twelfth month.

If the *jue yin* pulse is urgent and bowstring, undulating in a more than six tenths full amplitude, there is a cold disease (there are two words, "low pulse", in the original text which are apparently redundant [tr.]) with lower abdominal pain radiating to the lower back. If there is dyspnea that shakes the form (*i.e.,* the body), death is a certainty. If the pulse is moderate, (the condition) is curable. Needle (the points of) the foot *jue yin* to the depth of five *fen*.

If the *shao yang* pulse is short at one time but long at another, large at one time but small at another, undulating in a more than six tenths full amplitude, there is an illness of headache and fullness in the lateral costal regions. If there is vomiting, (the condition) is curable. If there is agitation, death will ensue. Needle the foot *shao yang* (points) at the ends of the last ribs to the depth of seven *fen*.

The *yang ming* pulse is surging and large as well as floating and, when it arrives, it is slippery (and gives a sensation of) leaping. It is large in the distal position but thin in the proximal like a tadpole. If it undulates in a more than three tenths full amplitude, there is an illness of dizziness, headache, and fullness and pain in the abdomen. If there is vomiting, (the condition) is curable. If there is agitation, death will ensue. (To treat this,) needle (the points) four *cun* above the umbilicus and three *cun* below the umbilicus, each to the depth of six *fen*.

From the second to the eighth month, the yang vessel is in the exterior. From the eighth to the first month, the yang vessel is in the interior. When yang is waxing, the pulse is strong. When yin is waxing, the pulse is weak. (Either yin or yang) becoming extreme results in susceptibility to fright, while repletion (of yin and yang) results in tugging and slackening. If the pulse is thin and deep, there is diarrhea instead of tugging and slackening. Diarrhea will be followed by vexation which, in turn is followed by thirst. Then thirst will be followed by abdominal fullness which, in turn, is followed by agitation. Agitation will be followed by intestinal *pi* which presents a regularly interrupted pulse. This pulse is a pulse that arrives at one time but fails to arrive at another. If the pulse is large and deep, there is cough. Cough will cause qi ascent. When qi ascent becomes severe, the (sick person) has to lift their shoulders to facilitate breathing. If the shoulders are lifted violently, the mouth and tongue will bleed. If the bleeding is severe, there will be bleeding from the nose.

(Pathological) changes betray themselves in the *cun* opening. So does the reciprocal overwhelming between yin and yang and between the exterior and interior. Wind, for example, has its *dao* (*i.e.*, follows a certain law, expressing itself by) a yin pulse prevailing in the yang.[3] If the *cun* opening pulse is flush in both the distal and proximal positions, there is migratory wind. If the *cun* opening pulse is replete at the exterior (*i.e.*, superficial level) but empty at the interior (*i.e.*, deep level), there are three parts wind and four parts warmth. The *cun* opening pulse is able to reveal taxation wind[4] which is begun by major disease or by sweating during fast walking. The indication of soft wind is a faint pulse which is fixed to the bone in either the upper (*i.e.*, the *cun*) or the lower (*i.e.*, the *chi*). Soft wind manifests as a slack exterior with abdominal urgency. A pulse suddenly becoming thunderous and replete at the sides suggests hovering wind (*piao feng*).[5] A pulse turning from yin towards yang[6] indicates wind evils. A pulse harmonious at one time but rapid at another suggests ghost evils (*i.e.*, obsession by ghosts). If the pulse is relaxed in the yin (*i.e.*, deep level) but urgent in the yang (*i.e.*, superficial level), wind is penetrating the viscera via the exterior. If the pulse is urgent in the yin, wind has left the yang (*i.e.*, the exterior) and entered the abdomen.

---

[3] This refers to a pulse of yin nature, for instance deep and retarded, appearing in the yang positions, *i.e.*, the *cun* and *guan*.

[4] This refers to a disease caused by sweating while working in a draft. The syndrome consists of stiffness of the neck, impaired vision, copious sputum, and aversion to wind.

[5] This is a rash due to wind settling in the exterior.

[6] This implies that the pulse is deep at first but becomes, little by little, floating.

If the pulse is listless in the upper and deeply hidden in the lower, unable to reach the yang (*i.e.,* the superficial level), there is flowing rheum.[7] If there is shortage of blood in both the upper and the lower but yin is strong,[8] there is leaking glomus. If yang is strong,[9] there is wine glomus. If the pulse is neither over-cringing nor over-piratical[10] but faint contrarily in the yang (*i.e.,* the *cun* and *guan*), there is phlegm rheum. If the pulse in the yin (*i.e.,* the *chi*) is expiring, sticking to the bone, but in the yang (*i.e.,* the *cun* and *guan*) it feels swift (and strong) at first touch, there is perspiration water. If the pulse is harmonious (but dissipated like water) spreading in all directions, water disease is about to arise.

If the pulse is not piratic in the yin (*i.e.,* the *chi*) but suggests damage in the yang (*i.e.,* the *cun* and *guan*), there is additional lack of fluids. If the *cun* opening pulse is small in the distal position but large in the proximal, feeling replete in the yang (*i.e.,* the superficial level), there is food glomus. A pathological small pulse appearing in the yang (*i.e.,* the *cun* or *guan*) indicates that there is a seven-day old glomus if (the amplitude) is nine tenths (of normal). There is a ten-day old glomus if the (amplitude) is eight tenths (of normal), a fifteen-day old glomus if (the amplitude) is seven tenths (of normal), a twenty-day old glomus if (the amplitude) is six tenths (of normal), and a half year old glomus if (the amplitude) is six tenths (of normal) and the pulse is not excessively hidden.

If the pulse is impeded, not reaching one tenth full amplitude at the stomach yin,[11] there is glomus due to beverages and sweets. If the pulse is hook-like in the exterior, there is enduring glomus. If the pulse is full of drive in the interior, (the glomus) is near to ten days old. If the pulse is strong in the exterior but weak in the interior, there is glomus wrapping a big core. If the pulse is floating and bowstring on both hands, there is glomus with sap and a core. If the pulse is floating, tight, and rapid or deep on both hands, there is a disease (of glomus) due to summerheat and taking gruel. If the pulse is tight and hidden in the interior, there is (glomus due to) wheat, rice, and pancakes. If the *cun* opening pulse is confined to the yang (*i.e.,* the *cun* and *guan*), feeling tight, thin, and faint, there is (glomus due to) taking peels of melons and fruit. If the pulse is confined to the yang (*i.e.,* the *chi*) and feels tight, there is (glomus due to) taking long-stored shepherd's purse. If the pulse is deep and subtle and it is impossible to count (the beats), there is glomus due

---

[7] This refers to water spilling in the stomach and intestines giving rise to a gurgling sound.

[8] This phrase means that the pulse is very thin in the superficial level because of shortage of blood but forceful in the deep level.

[9] This phrase means that the pulse is forceful in the superficial level.

[10] Over-cringing is very weak and faint, while over-piratical describes a picture of a very hard and strong pulse image.

[11] The stomach here means the *guan* position on the right hand, and yin refers to the deep level.

to underdone meat. If the pulse is hidden but possessed of yang, there is glomus due to roasted meat. If the pulse feels somewhat small at the beginning but floating and large later, there is glomus due to underdone wheat and beans.

---

[12] Yang here refers to the qualities of rapidity and slipperiness, for example.

——————————Chapter Three——————————
Bian Que's Pulse Method

Bian Que explained:

During the time that it takes for a person to complete one inhalation or exhalation, if the pulse beats twice, this is known as a normal pulse and the bodily form is free from any affliction. During the time that it takes for a person to complete one inhalation or exhalation, if the pulse beats three times, this is known as a pathological pulse. During one inhalation or exhalation, if the pulse beats four times, this indicates *bi* due to desertion of the pulse qi.[1] If the eyes are green-blue, this portends death. During the time that it takes for a person to complete one inhalation or exhalation, if the pulse beats five times (or) above, the person will die without a remedy. In the illness of prodigious dyspnea, (however,) the pulse beats very fast, possibly as fast as five times for one inhalation or exhalation, and in some cases even six or seven times. (This will not cause death.[tr.])

Bian Que explained:

Tranquil (pulse) qi is neither slack nor urgent, neither slippery nor choppy, neither salient nor obscure, neither long nor short, neither sinking nor mounting,[2] neither subservient nor rampant.[3] This is a normal pulse. [The following words are redundant.] If the kidneys have such a pulse, the body is free from afflictions.

---

[1]   This means that the pulse is intangible and, at the same time, that there is extreme exhaustion of essence and qi.

[2]   Sinking is deep, while mounting is floating.

[3]   Subservient means weak and faint, while rampant means violent.

134

Bian Que explained:

If the pulse qi is bowstring and urgent, there is disease in the liver (manifesting possibly as) reduced food intake with constantly being fed up, abdominal urgency, talkativeness, dizziness, sore eyes, abdominal fullness, hypertonicity of the sinews, troubles in the head, qi ascent, hard accumulations in the lower abdomen, occasional spitting of blood, and dry throat.

The methods of examining disease include studying the color and sound (and voice. Since they are intended to) locate disease, how can the essentials of examining the pulse not be subtle? If the pulse is floating and rapid and if there is no heat, there is wind. If the pulse is floating and rapid and there is heat, there is qi (disease). If the pulse is surging and large, if the two breasts are twitching, and if, in addition, the pulse is rapid accompanied by fever and chills, this is a cold damage disease.

In an enduring, emaciating disease, if the pulse is floating, overreaching the *cun* opening, and there is also a slight fever, this is pouring qi disease.[4] Additionally, if there is cough with high fever and (the condition) becomes exacerbated at one time and ameliorates at another, this is difficult to treat. However, if no exacerbation happens during treatment, (the condition) is easy to cure. The case with no cough is easy to treat.

____

[4]   This is a chronic infectious disease like pulmonary tuberculosis.

_______________Chapter Four_______________
The Essentials of Bian Que's & Hua Tuo's Examination of Voice & Complexion

A sick person[1] with retrenchment of the five viscera, spirit brightness not keeping (to its abode), and a hoarse voice will die.

A sick person who has carphologia and delirious speech is beyond cure.

A sick person who suffers from expiry of both yin and yang, pulling at their clothes and catching at nothing, and raving will die.

____

[1]   Nigel Wiseman translates *bing ren* as patient. However, this implies someone who suffers in English, while the Chinese says simply a diseased or sick person.

A sick person who is raving and whose speech is confused or who is unable to speak is incurable. In heat disease such a patient (however) is curable.

A sick person who suffers from expiry of both yin and yang and loss of voice will die in three and half days.

If a sick person has a yellow color appearing at their canthi, the disease is just on the mend.

A sick person with a yellow face and green-blue eyes will not die. (However,) if the green-blue color is like that of a reed mat,[2] (the patient) will die.

A sick person with a yellow face and red eyes will not die. (However,) if the red color is like that of clogged blood, (the patient) will die.

A sick person with a yellow face and white eyes will not die. (However,) if the white color is like that of dried up bone, (the patient) will die.

A sick person with a yellow face and black eyes will not die. (However,) if the black color is like that of soot, (the patient) will die.

A sick person whose face and eyes are the same color will not die.

A sick person with a black face and green-blue eyes will not die.

A sick person with a green-blue face and white eyes will die.

A sick person with a black face and white eyes will not die.

A sick person with a red face and green-blue eyes will die in six days.

A sick person with a yellow face and green-blue eyes will die in nine days. (This disease) is known as chaotic channel. Drinking wine in a draft provides a chance for evils to enter the stomach channel. Because the gallbladder qi is drained frenetically, the eyes become green-blue. Even if heaven rendered its assistance, resurgence would be impossible.

A sick person with a red face and white eyes will die in ten days. Anxiety, indignation, thought, and worry have exhausted the heart qi internally. Even if the facial complexion improves, it is urgently necessary to prepare a coffin.

---

[2] This refers to a whitish green color.

A sick person with a white face and black eyes will die since efflorescence is already gone and the blood vessels are empty and exhausted.

A sick person with a black face and white eyes will die in eight days since the kidney qi is injured internally. The cause of this disease is retention and accumulation (of evils in the kidneys).

A sick person with a green-blue face and yellow eyes will die in five days.

A sick person who, confined to bed, suffers from heart pain, shortness of breath, and an exhausted, injured spleen internally may be relieved (a little) in a hundred days. Though able to rise from bed (at that point, this patient) can only falter (a few steps), just sit on the ground, or stand against the bed. It is a divinely excellent physician who is able to treat such a case.

A sick person whose face is devoid of the efflorescence of essence, a face whose complexion is like earth, and who suffers from inability to eat and drink will die in four days.

A sick person whose eyes are devoid of the efflorescence of essence and whose teeth are black is incurable.

A sick person with a black color starting from the ears, eyes, nose, and mouth and entering into the mouth is bound to die.

A sick person whose ears, eyes, cheekbones, and cheeks are all red will die within five days.

A sick person with a black color starting from the forehead which spreads up to the hairline and then down to the bridge of the nose and cheekbones will also die within five days.

A sick person with black qi starting in their heaven[3] and spreading down to the region between their eyebrows and cheekbones will die.

An ill or healthy person with a black or white color entering into their eyes, nose, and mouth will die within three days.

An ill or a healthy person with a facial complexion the color of horse liver, looking cyanic at a distance but black close up, will die.

A sick person with a black facial complexion with eyes staring straight and aversion to wind will die.

A sick person with a black facial complexion and green-blue lips will die.

---

[3] This refers to the region directly above the nose and beneath the hairline.

A sick person with a green-blue facial complexion and black lips will die.

A sick person with a black facial complexion with fullness in the lateral costal regions and inability to turn over by himself will die.

A sick person with blurred vision, eyes staring straight, and shoulders lifted to facilitate breathing will die in one day.

A sick person with an enduring pain in the head and eyes and sudden loss of sight will die.

A sick person who suffers from yin binding,[4] expiry of yang, desertion of the essence of the eyes, and abstraction will die.

A sick person who suffers from expiry and exhaustion of yin and yang with sunken eye sockets will die.

A sick person with a slanting eye ligation will die in seven days.

A sick person whose mouth is unable to shut like a (dead) fish's and who breathes out but scarcely in will die.

A sick person whose mouth is kept open will die in three days.

A sick person whose lips are green-blue and whose philtrum is turned out will die in three days.

A sick person whose lips are turned out and whose philtrum is full (*i.e.*, swollen) will die.

A sick person whose lips and mouth suddenly become dry is incurable.

A sick person with swollen lips and parched teeth will die.

A sick person with both yin and yang exhausted, teeth like cooked beans,[5] and a rapid pulse will die.

A sick person whose teeth suddenly become black will die in thirteen days.

A sick person with a curled tongue and retracted testicles is bound to die.

---

[4] This refers to bound stools or constipation due to yin cold.

[5] This is a description of a dull whitish color.

A sick person with sweat exiting but (too sticky to) flow and whose tongue is black and curled will die.

A sick person whose (head) hair stands on end will die in fifteen days.

A sick person whose (head) hair is like dry hemp and who is irritable will die.

A sick person whose (head) hair and eyebrows are erect will die.

A sick person with green-blue nails will die.

A sick person with white nails is incurable.

A sick person whose under the nails flesh is black will die in eight days.

A sick person whose constructive and defensive are exhausted and expired and whose face is puffy and swollen will die.

A sick person with sudden swelling and a somber black facial complexion will die.

A sick person whose palms are so swollen that the creases become invisible will die.

A sick person whose umbilicus is swollen and protruding will die.

A sick person whose testes and penis are both swollen will die.

A sick person whose pulse is expiring, whose mouth is kept open, and whose feet are swollen will die in five days.

A sick person whose insteps of the feet are swollen accompanied by vomiting and heavy-headedeness will die.

A sick person whose insteps of the feet are swollen and whose knees are as large as a *dou*[6] will die in ten days.

A sick person confined to bed with urinary incontinence will die.

A sick person who smells like a decayed corpse is incurable.

---

[6] This is a container and measuring instrument the size of a bucket with a capacity of 100 liters.

A liver disease with white skin will end in death on the *geng* or *xin* days of the lung (phase).[7]

A heart disease with black eyes will end in death on the *ren* or *gui* days of the kidney (phase).

A spleen disease with green-blue lips will end in death on the *jia* or *yi* days of the liver (phase).

A lung disease with red cheeks and swollen eyes will end in death on the *bing* or *ding* days of the heart (phase).

A kidney disease with a swollen face and yellow lips will end in death on the *wu* or *ji* days of the spleen (phase).

A green-blue (facial complexion) like lustrous green jade is desirable rather than one like indigo.

A red (facial complexion) like cinnabar wrapped in silk gauze is desirable rather than one like ochre.

A white (facial complexion) like goose feathers is desirable rather than one like salt.

A black (facial complexion) like thick lacquer is desirable rather than one like charcoal.

A yellow (facial complexion) like realgar wrapped in silk gauze is desirable rather than one like yellow clay.

If the eyes are red, the disease is in the heart. If they are white, the disease is in the lungs. If they are black, the disease is in the kidneys. If they are yellow, the disease is in the spleen. If they are green-blue, the disease is in the liver. If they are a yellow color of nondescript shade, the disease is in the chest.

When examining eye diseases, if a red vein goes from the upper towards the lower (in the eye), this is a *tai yang* disease. If it goes from the lower towards the upper, this is a *yang ming* disease. If it goes from the outer towards the center, this is a *shao yang* disease.

When examining small and large scrofulous lumps with cold and heat, red veins may be found in the eye going from the top towards the lower and ending in the pupil. If there is one such vein, death comes in one year. If there are one and a half such veins, death comes in one and a half

---

[7] The five viscera correspond with the ten heavenly stems as follows: *jia/yi* = wood/liver; *bing/ding* = fire/heart; *wu/ji* = earth/spleen; *geng/xin* = metal/lungs; *ren/gui* = water/kidneys. Based on these correspondences, the date of death is figured in terms of the restraining interrelationship among the five phases.

140

years. If there are two such veins, death comes in two years. If there are two and a half such veins, death comes in two and a half years. If there are three such veins, death comes in three years.

When examining tooth decay with pain, feel along the vessel of the *yang ming* and localized heat will be found somewhere on its route. If (the tooth decay) is on the left or right side, there will be heat on the left or right (corresponding channel route). If (the tooth decay) is in the upper or lower (teeth), there will be heat (correspondingly) in the upper or lower (part of the channel).

When examining the blood vessels, red ones usually suggest heat; green-blue ones, pain; black ones, enduring *bi*. If red, black, and green-blue vessels are seen all at once, there is (alternating) cold and heat with generalized pain. If the facial complexion is slightly yellow with yellow tooth tartar and yellow nails, there is jaundice accompanied by a desire to lie down and yellow or dark-colored urine. If the pulse is small and choppy, there is (also) no desire for food.

_______________Chapter Five_______________
The Essentials of Bian Que's Approach to the Various Incongruous, Inconsistent & Death Pulses

Bian Que explained:

On examination, death pulse qi may feel like a flock of birds gathering,[1] a tied horse galloping to and fro by the side of water,[2] or a rock falling from a precipice.[3] The pulse may appear over the sinews or hide itself under the sinews as if inside an invulnerable fortress.[4] It may flow outside the constructive and defensive. In spite of observation and cross-reference, (the pulse) may not yield its secrets.

On examination of the pulse, the sick person may complain of no disease. However, if the pulse feels like a leak in the roof or a bird pecking, this portends death. Moreover, it is said in the classic

____

[1] This is a description of a tremendously scattered pulse image.

[2] This is a terribly swift and agitated pulse.

[3] This describes a pulse rising with momentum but falling abruptly.

[4] This refers to a very deep and hardly perceptible pulse.

(*i.e.*, the *Nei Jing*) that, seven to eight days after contraction of a disease, if the pulse feels like a leak in the roof or a bird pecking, this portends death. If the pulse arrives (hard) like a pellet or a mess of entangled rope [a mess of entangled rope implies that the pulse beats rapidly and in a chaotic way, completely out of order], this portends death.

If the pulse of the sick person feels like a shrimp swimming or a fish hovering, this portends death. [A swimming shrimp pulse is a pulse which rises slowly and leisurely but, in a flash, retreats and disappears, nowhere to be found. It rises again only a long time after. (In other words,) it is a pulse that rises in a retarded way but retreats swiftly. A hovering fish (pulse) is likened to a fish staying (in one place) which only moves its tail and waves its head and trunk, staying where it is a long time.]

If the pulse feels like a rope drawing up a curtain, this portends death. If the pulse feels like rolling beans, this is death. If the pulse feels like the edge of a knife, this portends death. If the pulse feels as if it gurgles continuously without intervals, this portends death. If the pulse comes and goes suddenly, returning after a (long) pause, this portends death. If the pulse is very large in the center, this is death. If the pulse is separated, this portends death.[5]

If the pulse is present in the exterior but absent in the interior, this portends death. The pulse which is called the bound (pulse) in the classic indicates imminent death. What does the bound pulse feel like? It is a pulse floundering like a rolling hemp seed under the fingers. This pulse is ascribed to the kidneys and is named a bound pulse to indicate that death is close by. If the pulse beats five times followed by one interruption, neither increasing nor decreasing (*i.e.*, the ratio of pulse beats to interruptions remaining constant), this is death. The classic calls it a regularly interrupted pulse. What pulse is called a regularly interrupted pulse? A pulse which beats five times with one interruption. A pulse with seven beats (with one interruption) amounting to one respiration, (this rate) being observed to stay constant over half a watch, is also called a regularly interrupted pulse. It portends death without doubt.

It is said in the classic that some diseases may end in death, some diseases may heal by themselves without treatment, and some diseases may persist for months or years. Can death and survival, presence and absence of a disease be diagnosed through palpating the pulse?

The answer is that all can be diagnosed. Suppose a sick person has their eyes shut, not desiring to see people. The pulse should be the liver pulse, bowstring, long, and urgent. If, on the contrary, the lung pulse is perceived, which is floating, short, and choppy, then death is a certainty.

---

[5] This refers to a pulse which is quite out of line in the three positions.

Suppose the sick person keeps their eyes open with thirst and tightness below the heart, the pulse should be tight, replete, and rapid. If, on the contrary, the pulse feels deep, slippery, and faint, death is a certainty. Suppose the sick person suffers from blood ejection followed by runny snivel nosebleed, the pulse should be deep and thin. If, on the contrary, the pulse feels floating, large, and firm, death is a certainty. Suppose there is an illness of delirious speech and ravings, there should be fever and a surging, large pulse. If, on the contrary, there is counterflow frigidity of the hands and feet with a pulse deep, thin, and faint, death is a certainty. Suppose the sick person has an enlarged belly and diarrhea, the pulse should be thin, faint, and choppy. If, on the contrary, the pulse is tight, large, and slippery, death is a certainty. These are illustrations (of how to diagnose from pulse examination).

It is said in the classic that if the pulse shapes and the disease (patterns) are mutually contrary, this portends death. What does this mean? The answer is as follows: If the disease is headache with sore eyes but the pulse is contrarily short and choppy, this portends death. If the disease is abdominal pain but the pulse is contrarily floating, large, and long, this portends death. If the disease is abdominal fullness with dyspnea but the pulse is contrarily slippery, smooth, and deep, this portends death. If the disease is inversion counterflow frigidity of the four limbs but the pulse is contrarily floating, large, and short, this portends death. If the disease is deafness but the pulse is contrarily floating, large, and choppy, this portends death. If the disease is blurred vision but the pulse is contrarily large and moderate, this portends death.

If there is disease on the left side but pain on the right, if there is disease on the right but pain on the left, if there is disease below but pain above, or if there is disease above but there is pain below, this is known as inconsistency and there is death with no possibility of treatment. If the pulse comes expiring and soggy at the deep level but pounds endlessly against the fingers at the superficial level, death will come in half a month. If the pulse comes faint, thin, and expiring, the sick person will die of disease.

If the person is diseased but the pulse is not diseased, this is life (*i.e.*, the person will survive). If the pulse is diseased but the person is not diseased, this portends death.

If a person suffers from deathlike inversion, not responding to calls, and the pulse has expired, this is death. If the pulse is expected to be large, but, on the contrary, it is small, this portends death.

If a fat person has a pulse which is thin and small like a silk fiber, bordering on expiry, this portends death.

If a thin person has an agitated pulse, this portends death.

If the body is rough (*i.e.*, the skin is rough or, literally, choppy) but the pulse comes and goes slippery, this portends death.

If the body is slippery (*i.e.*, the skin is smooth) but the pulse comes and goes choppy, this portends death.

If the body is small (*i.e.*, slim or thin) but the pulse comes and goes large, this portends death.

If the body is short but the pulse comes and goes long, this portends death.

If the body is tall but the pulse comes and goes short, this portends death.

If the body is large (*i.e.*, bulky) but the pulse comes and goes small, this portends death.

If the *chi* pulse does not access the *cun* but, at times, is like (a horse) galloping, death will come in half a day.

If both the liver and spleen arrive (*i.e.*, show themselves in the pulse),[6] then there is an inability to transform grain. If there is more liver (than spleen),[6] death is imminent.

If both the lungs and liver arrive, then there are *yong* or *ju*[7] and heaviness of the four limbs. If there is more lungs (than liver), death is imminent.

If both the heart and lungs arrive, then there is *bi*, wasting thirst, and slackness and listlessness. If there is more heart (than lungs), death is imminent.

If both the kidneys and heart arrive, then there is difficult speech, blockage of the nine portals, and inability to lift the four limbs. If there is more kidneys (than heart), death is imminent.

If both the spleen and kidneys arrive, then the five viscera have broken down. If there is more spleen (than kidneys), death is imminent.

If both the liver and heart arrive, then there is high fever, tugging and slackening, sweat refusing to exit, and the illusion of evils (*i.e.*, ghosts and spirits).

---

[6] The liver and spleen respectively imply the pulse qualities peculiar to the liver and spleen. While more liver than spleen means that the pulse quality typical of the liver, *i.e.*, bowstring, is more conspicuous than that typical of the spleen, which is moderateness. However, this further implies that now liver wood is overwhelming spleen earth. When the restraining phase overwhelms the restrained, there is dual damage. Therefore, it is very critical.

[7] This refers to carbuncles and cellulitis.

If both the liver and kidneys arrive, then there is *shan* concretion with lower abdominal pain and, in females, absence of menstruation.

Fullness (of evil qi) in the liver, kidneys, or lungs is repletion which gives rise to swelling. Congestion[8] of the lungs results in dyspnea and fullness in the subaxillary regions. Congestion of the liver results in fullness in the subaxillary regions, susceptibility to fright while lying down, and inability to urinate. Congestion of the kidneys results in fullness from the subaxillary regions (the feet in the original text [tr.]) to the lower abdomen, legs of different sizes, severe lameness of the thighs and lower legs, and liability to hemilateral withering.

If the heart pulse is full and large, there is epilepsy with cramps and hypertonicity of the sinews. If the liver pulse is small and urgent, there is epilepsy with cramps and hypertonicity of the sinews. If the liver pulse is galloping violently, there is an experience of fright and scare. In such a case, the pulse may become imperceptible or there may be loss of voice, but (the condition) will heal by itself without treatment. If the kidney pulse is small and urgent, the liver pulse is small and urgent, or the heart pulse is small and urgent, (even though) they are not pounding (forcefully), there are concretions.

If the liver and kidney pulse are both deep, there is stone water. If they are both floating, there is wind water.[9] If they are both vacuous, this is death. If they are both small and bowstring, there is liability to fright (disease). If the kidney pulse or the liver pulse is large, urgent, and deep, there is *shan*. If the heart pulse pounds slippery and urgent, there is heart *shan*.[10] If the lung pulse is deep and pounding, there is lung *shan*.[11]

If the spleen pulse was pounding in the exterior (*i.e.*, superficial level) but now is deep, there is intestinal *pi* which will stop by itself in due time. If the liver pulse is small and moderate, there is intestinal *pi* which is easy to treat. If the kidney pulse is small, pounding, and deep, there is intestinal *pi* with blood in the stools which will end in death if the blood is warm and there is fever. Heart and liver (intestinal) *pi* is also characterized by blood in the stools. If the two viscera (*i.e.*, the heart and the liver) are both diseased, this *pi* is curable. A small, deep, and choppy (heart

---

[8]   Congestion here implies abundant evil qi.

[9]   Wind water is a species of water swelling accompanied by fever and aversion to wind. The swelling usually starts in the head and face and then gradually develops into generalized swelling.

[10]   Heart *shan* is characterized by abdominal pain, inhibited urination, rumbling in the intestines, masses in the lower abdomen, and, occasionally, difficult defecation.

[11]   Lung *shan* is characterized by swelling and pain in the lower abdomen and testicles with urinary block.

and liver) pulse is an indication of intestinal *pi*. If there is fever, this is death. Death will come seven days after the appearance of the fever.

If the stomach pulse is deep, pounding, and choppy, if it is pounding and large in the exterior, or if the heart pulse is small, tight, and urgent, there is hemilateral withering due to block (of qi and blood). If the left side is affected in males or the right side is affected in females and if there is no loss of voice and the tongue is able to move, (the condition) is curable. Recovery will ensue in thirty days. Those with loss of voice, though (otherwise) favorable (*i.e.*, progressing normally), will not recover till three years later. (Such a patient,) if under twenty years of age, will die in three years.

If the pulse arrives pounding, external spontaneous bleeding accompanied by fever will end in death. If the pulse is like a suspended hook and is floating, there is fever. If the pulse is as if gasping, there is (a disease) named qi inversion. Qi inversion is (inversion with) inability to speak to people. If the pulse is rapid, this is caused by violent fright. It will recover in three or four days.

If the pulse is floating and overlapping and, besides, is rapid, beating ten times or more in one respiration, this is due to insufficient supplies of channel qi. Death comes ninety days after the first appearance (of this pulse). If the pulse is like a newly started fire,[12] this is due to retrenchment of the supplies of heart essence. Death will come when the grass becomes dry. If the pulse is like scattered (*i.e.*, falling) leaves, this is due to inadequate supplies of liver qi. Death will come when the leaves begin to fall from the trees. If the pulse comes like a visiting guest — visiting guest implying that the pulse is blocked (at times) but pounds (at others), this is due to insufficient supplies of kidney qi. Death will come during the period from the opening to falling of the blossoms of the date trees. If the pulse is (hard) like a clay pellet, this is due to insufficient supplies of stomach essence. Death will come when elm pods begin to fall. If the pulse is like a wooden bar,[13] this is due to insufficient supplies of gallbladder qi. Death will come when crops ripen. If the pulse is like a length of (fully drawn) bowstring, this is due to insufficient supplies of bladder essence. If the disease is characterized by talkativeness, death will come when there is frost. If there is no talkativeness, (the condition) is curable. If the pulse is like filtering lacquer (sap)[14]— a

---

[12] This is an epithet for a pulse which is exuberant at first but then dies away abruptly.

[13] This is a wide and rigid pulse.

[14] Lacquer sap is very sticky. Therefore, the pulse so described is a very sluggish, indistinct pulse. However, this interpretation somewhat disagrees with the insertion of the text proper, suggesting that there might be a typographical error. According to some scholars, the term, "filtering lacquer", might be mistaken for "bramble." In that case, the impression is one of pricking here and there, *i.e.*, beating this way or that.

filtering lacquer-like pulse is one that beats to this side or that — death will come forty days after this pulse first appears. If the pulse is like a gushing spring, floating and pounding within the muscles, this is due to insufficient supplies of *tai yang* qi. If there is diminished qi, death will come when (one) tastes chives flowers (*i.e.,* chive flowers are begun to be served at table).[15] If the pulse is like a collapsed mess of earth[16] and impalpable when pressure is applied, this is due to insufficient supplies of the muscle (*i.e.,* spleen) qi. If, (on the face,) there appear the five colors with black showing itself first, death will come when Pueraria flowers begin to open. If the pulse is like the uvula — (in other words,) the less depth it is felt at, the larger it is — this is due to insufficient supplies of the twelve transporting points. Death will come when water condenses. If the pulse is like the edge of a knife — a knife-edge like pulse is one that is small and urgent at the superficial level and hard, large, and urgent at the deep — there is depressed heat in the five viscera with cold and heat joining exclusively in the kidneys. In such a case, the person is unable to sit up and will die on the Beginning of Spring. If the pulse is like a ball, so slippery as to elude the fingers, that is, untouchable to the fingers when pressure is applied, this is due to insufficient supplies of large intestine qi. Death will come when the date trees grow leaves. If the pulse is like a pestle,[17] there will be susceptibility to fear, hating either to sit or to lie down, and constantly all ears while standing or walking (*i.e.,* paranoia). This is due to insufficient supplies of small intestine qi. Death will come in late autumn or the last autumn month.

(The Yellow Emperor) said:

One spring in the second month, (we) examined the pulse of a sick person. The pulse was incompatibly deep (for the season. I) set down your prognosis that the sick person might die in autumn. If, on the contrary, the disease was relieved, a relapse would occur in the seventh month. (In autumn, we) went to examine the pulse (of the sick person again). The pulse was still deep. Then your words were set down again that (the sick person) might die in winter.

(The Yellow Emperor) asked:

When the pulse was felt deep in the second month, why did you prognose death in autumn?

The master answered:

---

[15] In China, Chinese chive flowers are eaten as a spice or a dish of their own.

[16] This pulse is wide but extremely feeble and becomes simply intangible under pressure.

[17] This is an arrhythmic pulse with varying force.

In the second month, the pulse ought to have been soggy, weak, and bowstring, but it was deep. (Therefore,) when autumn came, this pulse might remain deep. (However,) it might also become floating instead. Then death would come instantly.[18] For that reason, (I) decided that death might come in autumn.

(The Yellow Emperor continued to ask:)

In the seventh month, the pulse continued to be deep. Then why did you determine that death might come in winter?

The master answered:

A deep pulse is the kidney pulse, a true visceral pulse (of the kidneys), but it willfully appeared untimely. According to the categorization in the classic of the king, ministerial, confined, and perishing (pulses), in winter, the (deep) pulse is the king pulse. (Since it appeared earlier,) it would not appear (in winter again). Therefore, (I) knew that death would occur on the Winter Solstice. (It turned out) that in winter there was a relapse of the disease and death did come on the Winter Solstice. (From this example, we) know (the categorization of the king, ministerial, etc., pulses) to be true. It was this principle that Hua Tuo emulated.

---

[18] This sentence suggests that the autumn pulse should be floating and that, if the pulse of the sick person does become floating in the autumn, the condition will become fatal.

BOOK SIX

**Collated & edited by Honorary Minister Without Portfolio,
Curator of the Imperial Library,
Imperial Courier and Senior Army Protector,
Lin Yi *et al.***

Chapter One

Disease Patterns of the Liver
& Foot *Jue Yin* Channel

Liver qi vacuity gives rise to fear, while repletion to anger. If the liver qi is vacuous, there will be dreams of parks with grass growing. When (the liver qi) has its day,[1] one may have dreams of lying under a tree and not daring to rise. If the liver qi is exuberant, there will be dreams of being angered. If counterflow qi settles in the liver, there will be dreams of mountains with forests.

Disease in the liver is characterized by serenity at the calm dawn watch, exacerbation at the later afternoon watch, and tranquility at the midnight watch.

If disease starts first in the liver, there will be dizziness and pain and propping fullness in the lateral costal regions. In one day, (the disease) comes to the spleen, giving rise to block and congestion as well as generalized pain and heaviness. In two days, it comes to the stomach, giving rise to abdominal distention. In three days, it comes to the kidneys, giving rise to pain in the lower lateral abdomen and lumbar spine and aching in the lower legs. If it does not come to an end in ten days, death will ensue — at the sunset watch in winter, but at the breakfast watch in summer.

If the liver pulse pounds hard and long and the facial complexion is other than green-blue, there should be a disease caused by fall or impact injury. Because there is blood (stasis) in the lateral costal regions, the person suffers from counterflow dyspnea. If (the liver pulse) is soft and scattered and the complexion is lustrous, there should be the disease of spillage rheum. Spillage rheum results from massive drinking in burning thirst so that water spills into the muscles and flesh outside the intestines and stomach.

If the liver pulse is urgent in the deep level and in the superficial level as well, there is the bitterness of pain in the lateral costal regions with qi propping fullness. This pain radiates to the lateral lower abdomen. There is (also) occasional difficult urination. (In addition,) there is the bitterness of visual dizziness, headache, pain in the upper and lower back, counterflow frigidity

---

[1] Each of the five viscera is exuberant in a corresponding season. In summer, for example, the heart qi is exuberant and, therefore, it is said to have its day in this season. As to the liver, its qi is exuberant in the spring and it has its day in this season. Hence, having its day, practically speaking, means the same as a viscus's king time.

of the feet, and occasional dribbling urinary block. In females, there is absence of menstruation or the menses coming or stopping irregularly. This is a result of (injury) due to falls (in the past) at a young age.

With a green-blue complexion, if the pulse arrives long and pounding on both hands, the diagnosis is existence of accumulated qi below the heart with propping (fullness in) the subaxillary regions. The name (of this trouble) is liver *bi*. It is caused by cold dampness as in the case of *shan*. (In addition,) there is pain in the lower back, frigidity of the feet, and headache.

Wind stroke of the liver manifests as shaking head and twitching eyes, pain in the lateral costal regions, and walking with a hunched back. It may cause the person to have a predilection for sweets just as a pregnant woman does.

If taken with cold stroke of the liver, the person may suffer from aversion to cold as after a soaking, continuous mild fever, a bright red facial complexion, slight sweating, and vexation and heat in the chest.

If taken with cold stroke of the liver, the person may suffer from inability to lift their arms, a dry tongue root, frequent great sighing breaths, pain in the chest, inability to turn over, occasional thief (*i.e.*, night) sweating, cough, and vomiting of fluids upon ingestion.

The liver governs dyspnea of the chest and angry cursing. If the pulse is deep, there will inevitably be stifling in the chest with a desire for (other) people to press the chest. (In addition,) there is heat and nasal congestion.

In the case of falls, malign blood will lodge internally. In violent fury, qi will keep ascending, no longer able to descend. (Then the malign blood or qi) will accumulate in the lateral costal region on the left, thus causing damage to the liver. When the liver is damaged, the person will suffer from flesh shedding, a predilection to keep the mouth open when lying down, occasionally green-blue hands and feet, heavy eyes, and pain in the pupils of the eyes. All this is produced by a damaged liver.

Liver distention manifests as fullness and pain in the lateral costal regions affecting the lower lateral abdomen.

Liver water is characterized by an enlarged belly, inability to turn over by oneself, and pain in the lateral costal regions and abdomen. At times, fluids are generated a little (in the mouth) and (then) free urination may be resumed.

When the lungs overwhelm the liver, there is pain (*yong* in another version [tr.]) and swelling. When the heart overwhelms the liver, there will inevitably arise vomiting and diarrhea.

Liver fixation (*gan zhu*) is (a condition where) the sick person often desires to have someone tread on his or her chest (in an attack). Before attacks, the person has a desire to drink hot water.

Liver accumulation is called fat qi. It is located in the left lateral costal region and is shaped like an inverted cup. With a head and feet, it looks like a tortoise. It may persist very long, giving rise to counterflow cough and malarial disease which can last for years. It is contracted on the *wu* and *ji* days in the last summer month. Why is this? Lung disease should be transmitted to the liver and from there to the spleen. The spleen, (however,) happens to be king in the last summer month. As king, it is immune to evils. (Therefore,) the liver intends to return the disease to the lungs, but the lungs refuse to accept it (again). Thus, (the evils) have to lodge and be bound (in the liver), developing into accumulations. Because of this, one can know that fat qi develops in the last summer month.

Liver disease may manifest as a green-blue facial complexion, hypertonicity of the hands and feet, tormenting fullness in the lateral costal regions or occasional dizziness, and a bowstring, long pulse. This is curable, requiring administration of *Fang Feng Zhu Li Tang* (Siler & Bamboo Juice Decoction)[2] and *Qin Jiao San* (Gentiana Macrophylla Powder).[3] It is proper to needle Large Pile (*Da Dun*, Liv 1) in spring, Moving Between (*Xing Jian*, Liv 2) in summer, and Spring at the Bend (*Qu Quan*, Liv 8) in winter, supplementing all of them, and Supreme Surge (*Tai Chong*, Liv 3) in late summer and Central Cleft (*Zhong Xi*, Liv 6) in autumn, draining both of them. In addition, it is proper to moxa Cycle Gate (*Qi Men*, Liv 14) with 100 cones and the ninth vertebra in the back with 50 cones.

Liver disease is invariably characterized by pain in the lateral costal regions radiating to the lateral lower abdomen and irritability. In case of vacuity, there will be blurred vision, deafness, and susceptibility to fear as if fearing arrest. If one intends to treat it, one should handle the channel of the liver.

If there is qi counterflow in the foot *jue yin* and *shao yang*, there will be headache, pain in the eyes,

---

2   The translator has not been able to identify this formula.

3   This formula consists of Radix Gentianae Macrophyllae (*Qin Jiao*), Radix Rubrus Paeoniae Lactiflorae (*Chi Shao*), Cornu Rhinocerotis (*Xi Jiao*), Radix Scutellariae Baicalensis (*Huang Qin*), Radix Bupleuri (*Chai Hu*), Herba Artemisiae Capillaris (*Yin Chen Hao*), Tuber Ophiopogonis Japinici (*Mai Dong*), and Radix Et Rhizoma Rhei (*Da Huang*).

deafness or impaired hearing, and swelling of the cheeks. (To treat it,) take blood.[4]

If there are evils in the liver, there will be pain in the lateral costal regions, cold in the center, malign blood internally, frequent cramps of the lower legs, and swelling of the joints (of the lower legs. To treat this,) choose Moving Between (*Xing Jian*, Liv 2) to lead (the evil) out of the lateral costal regions, supplement Three Li (*San Li*, St 36) to warm the stomach, bleed the blood vessels (along the liver channel) to disperse the malign blood, and bleed the green-blue vessels around the auricles to resolve cramps.

The liver vessel of the foot *jue yin* originates at the border of the three hairs region of the big toe and travels upward along the surface of the instep, through the point one *cun* anterior to the medial malleolus up to a point eight *cun* above the medial malleolus. From there, it crosses behind the (foot) *tai yin* channel, ascending along the medial side of the popliteal fossa and then along the thigh, entering the region of the pubic hair and encircling the genitals. It then enters the lateral abdominal region, bypassing the stomach, and homes to the liver. It connects with the gallbladder, ascends to penetrate the diaphragm, and spreads over the lateral costal region. From there it passes behind the throat and, entering the nasopharynx, it links with the ligation of the eye and ascends to emerge at the forehead and join the governing vessel at the vertex.

A branch follows the ligation of the eye, descends inside the cheek, and encircles the inside of the lips.

Another branch starts from the liver, penetrates the diaphragm, and ascends to pour into the lungs.

If (this channel) is affected, then there will be the disease of lumbar pain and inability to bend either forward or backward. In males, there will be *tui shan*, and, in females, lower abdominal swelling. In severe cases, there will be a dry throat and a dusty facial complexion or a ghastly complexion. If the governing (viscus), the liver, becomes diseased, then there will be thoracic fullness, counterflow retching, throughflux diarrhea, fox-like *shan*, enuresis, and dribbling urinary block. Exuberance (of liver qi) is determined by a *cun* opening pulse which is twice as large as the *ren ying*.[5] Vacuity, on the contrary, is characterized by a *cun* opening pulse which is smaller than the *ren ying*.

---

[4] This refers to bleeding a superficial blood vessel.

[5] Here, as in the majority of times this term is used in this book, the *ren ying* pulse refers to the pulse in the neck by the Adam's apple.

The connecting branch of the foot *jue yin* is called Woodworm Canal (*Li Gou*, Liv 5). At a point five *cun* above the medial malleolus, it diverges into the (foot) *shao yang*. Its ramification follows the channel (of the foot *jue yin*) up to the testicles, binding with the penis. If the disease is one of qi counterflow, there will be swelling of the testicles and sudden *shan*. In the case of repletion, there will be persistent erection and heat in the penis. In the case of vacuity, there will be fulminant itching (of the genitals. To treat it,) select the branch (*i.e.*, Woodworm Canal, Liv 5).

There is a liver disease which manifests as fullness of the chest, distention of the lateral costal regions, irritability, shouting, fever followed by aversion to cold, inability to lift the four limbs, a white facial complexion, and slippery (*i.e.*, well lubricated) body (skin). If the pulse, which should be bowstring, long, and urgent (in this case), is now, on the contrary, short and choppy and if the facial complexion, which should be green-blue, is now, on the contrary, white, this shows metal overwhelming wood, a greatly unfavorable condition. Ten out of ten cases will die without a remedy.

_______Chapter Two_______
Disease Patterns of the Gallbladder
& Foot *Shao Yang* Channel

Gallbladder disease is characterized by frequent great sighing breaths, a bitter taste in the mouth, retching of old juice, a rolling sensation in the heart, apprehensiveness as if fearing arrest, a sensation of something stuck in the throat, and frequent spitting. (To treat this,) one should focus their examination on the foot *shao yang* (channel) from its beginning to its end, and then moxa the points on the vessel that are found to be depressed. If there is cold and heat, needle Yang Mount Spring (*Yang Ling Quan*, GB 34). If there is frequent retching, often of bitter juice, frequent great sighing breaths, a rolling sensation in the heart, and frequent sorrow and apprehensiveness as if fearing arrest, there are evils in the gallbladder and counterflow of the stomach. When gall spills over, a bitter taste appears in the mouth. When the stomach qi counterflows, there is retching of bitter juice. Therefore, this condition is called gall retching. (To treat this,) needle Three Li (*San Li*, St 36) to downbear stomach qi counterflow and prick the blood vessels of the foot *shao yang* to shut up the gallbladder. Then balance vacuity and repletion to eliminate the evils.

Gallbladder distention is characterized by pain and distention in the lateral costal regions, a bitter taste in the mouth, and great sighing breaths.

When inversion qi settles in the gallbladder, there are dreams of involvement in suing in court.

The vessel of the foot *shao yang* originates at the outer canthus and travels upward to the corner of the head. It then descends behind the auricle, moving along the neck and passing in front of the hand *shao yang* to arrive at the shoulder. From there, it crosses behind the hand *shao yang* to enter the supraclavicular fossa.

A branch diverges from behind the auricle, entering the ear and emerging in front of the ear to terminate in the region lateral to the outer canthus.

Another branch diverges from the outer canthus descending past Great Reception (*Da Ying*, St 5) to unite with the hand *shao yang* in the suborbital region. From there, it descends through Jawbone (*Jia Che*, St 6) and down the neck to join the preceding branch in the supraclavicular fossa. It then descends into the chest, penetrating the diaphragm, connecting with the liver, and homing to the gallbladder. From there, it travels inside the lateral costal region, emerging at the qi thoroughfare (*i.e.*, the groin), circling the region of the pubic hair to transversely enter the hip joint. Its straight branch diverges at the supraclavicular fossa, traveling down to the axilla, penetrating the chest, and passing the region of the free ribs to join the preceding branch at the hip joint. From there, it descends along the yang (lateral) aspect of the thigh, emerging at the lateral side of the knee, and descends anterior to the outer assisting bone (*i.e.*, the fibula), traveling straight down to the tip of the severed bone (*i.e.*, the lower portion of the tibia). From there, it passes in front of the lateral malleolus, traveling along the instep to emerge at the tip of the toe next to the small one.

Another branch diverges at the instep and enters the big toe. It passes between the first and second metatarsal bones to come out at the tip of the big toe in the aspect proximal to the second toe. From there, it turns back into the nail to emerge at the three hairs region.

If (this channel) is affected, there is the disease of bitter taste in the mouth, frequent great sighing breaths, pain in the heart and the lateral costal regions, and inability to turn over. In severe cases, there will be a slightly dusty complexion, sheenless and lusterless skin, and heat in the lateral side of the foot. This is yang inversion.

If the bones governed (by the channel) become diseased, there will be pain in the corner of the head, pain in the submandibular region, pain of the outer canthus, pain and swelling in the supraclavicular fossa, swelling of the axilla, saber and pearl string lumps (*i.e.*, scrofula), shivering with cold after sweating, and malaria-like disease. There will be pain all along the chest, including the lateral costal and free rib regions, the lateral aspect of the thigh and knee, the lower leg, the severed bone, and the region in front of the lateral malleolus as well as all the joints on the way. There will also be loss of the use of the toe next to the small one.

Exuberance (of the channel qi) is determined by a *ren ying* pulse which is twice as large as the *cun* opening. Conversely, vacuity is determined by a *ren ying* pulse which is smaller than the *cun* opening.

Chapter Three
Disease Patterns of the Heart
& Hand Heart-governor Channel[1]

Vacuity of the heart qi gives rise to endless sorrow, while repletion to incessant laughing. If the heart qi is vacuous, there are dreams of putting out fire and yang substances.[2] When (the heart) has its day,[3] there will be dreams of fire and burning. If the heart qi is exuberant, there are dreams of joy, laughing, fear, and apprehensiveness. When inversion qi settles in the heart, there are dreams of mounts and hills, smoke and fire.

Heart disease is characterized by serenity at the midday watch, exacerbation at the midnight watch, and tranquility at the calm dawn watch.

If disease starts first in the heart, there is heart pain. In one day, it comes to the lungs, giving rise to dyspnea and cough. In three days, it comes to the liver, giving rise to flank pain with propping fullness. In five days, it comes to the spleen, giving rise to block and congestion (of qi and blood) and generalized pain and heaviness. If the disease does not come to an end in three days, this is death. Death will come at the midnight watch in winter and at the midday watch in summer.

---

[1] One should note that, although this chapter is titled after the heart, as far as the channel is concerned, it deals with the hand *jue yin* rather than the hand *shao yin*. This is explained by the theory that the heart is immune to evils and it is the pericardium that suffers for the benefit of the heart, its governor.

[2] Yang substances are too generalized a concept even for Chinese. A different version gives instead "causing damage to articles." This seems understandable.

[3] This phrase implies summer when the heart is exuberant or days which correspond to the heart, *i.e.*, *bing* and *ding* days.

If the heart pulse pounds hard and long, there should be a disease of curled tongue with inability to speak. If the pulse is soft and scattered, there should be a disease of wasting thirst, which will heal by itself.

If the heart pulse is small and tight in the deep level and is not as if gasping in the superficial level, the bitterness is gathered qi and pain below the heart, failure of food to descend, frequently swallowing down saliva, occasional heat in the hands and feet, distressing fullness, impaired memory, melancholy, and frequent great sighing breaths. All this is produced by anxiety and thought.

If the pulse is as if gasping and hard with a red (facial complexion), the diagnosis is accumulated qi in the center which affects food intake. This is called heart *bi* which develops from an exogenous illness. Because there has been thought and preoccupation, which has caused heart vacuity, the evils find a chance to invade.

If the heart pulse is urgent, (the disease) is known as heart *shan*. There should be something tangible in the lower abdomen. The heart is regarded as a masculine viscus, and the small intestine acts as its envoy. Therefore, the lower abdomen should present something tangible[4] (in this case).

Unaccountable crying that disturbs the ethereal and corporeal souls (*i.e.*, the *hun* and *po*) is due to diminished blood and qi. Diminished blood and qi is ascribed to the heart. When the heart qi becomes vacuous, the person stands apprehensive with eyes kept shut, (always) drowsy, and has dreams of traveling far. The spirit and the essence are separated and dispersed, and the ethereal and corporeal souls are moving frenetically. If the yin qi is debilitated, there is withdrawal. If the yang qi is debilitated, there is mania. The five viscera are the dwelling places of the ethereal and corporeal souls and the support for the spirit and essence. When the ethereal and corporeal souls are soaring (*i.e.*, restless), the five viscera are empty and vacuous. Then they will be occupied by an evil spirit, (displaying the symptoms of) obsession by a goblin or being under the spell of a ghost. When the pulse is short and faint and there is insufficiency of the visceral (qi), the ethereal and corporeal souls will become restless. The ethereal soul is attributed to the liver and the corporeal soul to the lungs. The lungs govern fluids and humors which may turn into snivel and tears. (Therefore,) when the lung qi is debilitated, tears run out. When the liver qi is debilitated, the ethereal soul becomes restless. The liver governs irritability and its sound is shouting.

---

[4] This implies that, since the heart is associated with the small intestine which is located in the lower abdomen, heart troubles may manifest in the lower abdomen.

Wind stroke of the heart is characterized by continuous mild fever, inability to rise, hungering in the heart with a desire to eat, and retching upon ingestion.

If taken with cold stroke of the heart, the person will have a (burning) sensation of the heart as after eating garlic. In severe cases, there is heart pain that penetrates the back and a back pain that penetrates the heart as if in pouring *gu*.[5] If the pulse is floating, a cure will follow spontaneous vomiting.

Worry, anxiety, thought, and preoccupation injure the heart. When the heart is damaged, the bitterness will be susceptibility to fright, poor memory, and irascibility. If the heart is damaged, once taxed or fatigued, the sick person will suffer from a red face, heaviness of the lower limbs, heart pain penetrating the back, vexation, and heat. The hand can feel palpitating under the umbilicus. The pulse is bowstring. All this is produced by a damaged heart.

Heart distention is characterized by heart vexation, shortness of breath, and troubled sleep.

If taken with heart water, the person suffers from generalized heaviness, diminished qi, insomnia, vexation and agitation, and severe swelling of the genitals.

If the kidneys overwhelm the heart, there will inevitably be dribbling urinary block.

True heart pain is characterized by frigidity reaching up to the joints above the hands and feet (*i.e.*, below the elbows and knees) and severe cardiac pain. If this starts in the morning, death comes in the evening. If this starts in the evening, death comes the next morning.

(The syndrome of) pain in the heart and abdomen, a burning sensation (in the heart), swelling and gathering occurring in attacks which may move up and down, intermittent pain, heat in the heart and abdomen, tormenting thirst and drooling is produced by worms eating. (To treat it,) press the gathering with a hand, keeping up the pressure and not allowing (the worm) to move. Insert a large needle and retain it long till the worm stops moving. Then extract the needle. When there are eating worms in the intestines, one should not use a small needle (to kill them).

Heart accumulation is called deep-lying beam. It starts from above the umbilicus to the heart and (may be) as large as an arm. It may persist long, giving rise to the disease of heart vexation and

---

[5] The word pouring means infectious. *Gu* is an illness characterized by fatigue, emaciation, and heaviness of the bones. During episodes, the patient feels vexed and oppressed in the chest and a tormenting discomfort in the abdomen.

heart pain. This is contracted on the *geng* and *xin* days in autumn. Why is this? Kidney disease should be transmitted to the heart and, from there, to the lungs. The lungs, however, happen to be king in autumn. As king, they are immune to evils. (Therefore,) the heart intends to return the disease to the kidneys, but the kidneys refuse to accept it (again). Thus, (the evils) have to lodge and be bound (in the heart), developing into accumulations. Because of this, one can know that deep-lying beam develops in autumn.

Heart disease may manifest as a red facial complexion, heart pain, shortness of breath, and distressed heat in the palms possibly with crying, laughing, and insulting speech (*i.e.*, erratic change in moods), and subjection to sorrow, thought, worry, and preoccupation. If there is a red facial complexion and fever and the pulse is replete, large, and rapid, the disease is curable. (To treat this,) it is necessary to needle Central Hub (*Zhong Chong*, Per 9) in the spring, Palace of Toil (*Lao Gong*, Per 8) in the summer, and Great Mount (*Da Ling*, Per 7) in late summer, supplementing all of these, and Intermediary Courier (*Jian Shi*, Per 5) in autumn and Marsh at the Bend (*Qu Ze*, Per 3) in winter, draining both of these. In addition, it is necessary to moxa Great Tower Gate (*Ju Que*, CV 14) with 50 cones and the fifth vertebra on the back with 100 cones.

Heart disease may manifest as pain inside the chest, propping fullness of the lateral costal regions with pain below them, breast, upper back, and scapular pain, and pain in the anterior aspects of the arms. In the case of vacuity, there will be an enlarged chest and abdomen and a contracting pain between the lateral costal regions and the upper and lower back. (To treat this,) choose the channels of the hand *shao yin* and *tai yang* and (prick) the blood vessels under the tongue. For its transmuted patterns, bleed Cleft Center (*Xi Zhong*, Bl 40).

If there are evils in the heart, there will be the disease of heart pain, frequent sorrow, and occasionally dizziness and collapse. In accordance with surplus and insufficiency, administer a balancing (therapy) through these points.

The Yellow Emperor asked:

Why does the vessel of the hand *shao yin* alone not have transporting points?[6]

Qi Bo answered:

The *shao yin* is the vessel of the heart. The heart is the great governor of the five viscera and six bowels. Since the heart is the monarch, it is the abode of the spirit and essence. This viscus is

---

[6] This refers to the five transporting points below the elbow or knee, *i.e.*, the well, spring, stream, river, and sea points.

strong and impregnable. (Therefore,) it is hardly possible for evils to settle there. If they do settle there, they will damage the heart. When the heart is damaged, the spirit is gone. When the spirit is gone, the body is dead. For that reason, when various evils (are said to) be in the heart, they are actually in the enveloping network (*i.e.*, the pericardium. The channel of) the enveloping network is the vessel of the heart-governor. Therefore, the *shao yin* has no transporting points. If the *shao yin* has no transporting points, is the heart never diseased? The answer is that its external channel and the bowel (associated with it) can be diseased, but the viscus proper is immune to disease. It follows that, (in treating heart disease,) only the end of the styloid process of the ulna (*i.e.*, Spirit Gate, *Shen Men*, Ht 7) of its channel can be selected.

The vessel of the hand heart-governor (*i.e.*, the hand *jue yin*) originates in the chest and homes to the pericardium. It then travels downward through the diaphragm, connecting sequentially with the three burners.

A branch follows the chest and emerges in the lateral costal region at a point three *cun* below the axilla. From there, it ascends to the axilla and then travels along the anterior aspect of the arm, moving between the (hand) *tai yin* and *shao yin* to enter the elbow. Then it proceeds along the forearm, traveling between the two sinews (the tendons of the muscular palmaris and muscular flexor carpi radialis) to enter the palm. From there, it moves along the middle finger and finally emerges from the tip of the finger. [7]

Another branch diverges in the palm, traveling along the finger next to the small one to emerge from its tip.

If (this channel) is affected, there will be the disease of heat in the palm, hypertonicity of the elbow and the upper arm, and swelling of the axilla. In severe cases, there will be fullness of the chest and lateral costal region, a violent stirring of the heart with a rolling sensation, a red facial complexion, yellow eyes, and incessant laughing.

If the (blood) vessel governed (by the channel) becomes diseased, there will be heart vexation, heart pain, and heat in the palm.

Exuberance (of the channel qi) is determined by a *cun* opening pulse which is twice as large as the *ren ying*. On the contrary, vacuity is characterized by a *cun* opening pulse which is smaller than the *ren ying*.

The connecting branch of the hand heart-governor is called Inner Pass (*Nei Guan*, Per 6). It

---

[7] This refers to the five transporting points below the elbow or knee, *i.e.*, the well, spring, stream, river, and sea points.

emerges from between the two sinews at a point two *cun* proximal to the wrist and then follows the channel (of the hand *jue yin*) upward to link with the pericardium and connect with the heart ligation. In the case of qi repletion, there will be heart pain. In the case of vacuity, there will be heart vexation. (To treat this,) select the point between the two sinews (*i.e.,* Inner Pass).

Suppose a heart disease is characterized by vexation and oppression, diminished qi, great heat, heat going up to disturb the heart, retching and vomiting, counterflow cough, manic speech, sweat exiting (in drops) like pearls, and inversion frigidity of the body. If the pulse, which should be floating, is now, on the contrary, deep, soggy, and slippery and if the facial complexion, which should be red, is now, on the contrary, black, this shows water overwhelming fire, a greatly unfavorable condition. Ten out of ten cases will die without a remedy.

_________Chapter Four_________
Disease Patterns of the Small Intestine
& Hand *Tai Yang* Channel

Small intestine disease is characterized by lower abdominal pain, pain in the lumbar spine sending a dragging pain to the testicles, and occasional abdominal urgency in addition to heat or severe cold in the area anterior to the ears, heat confined to the shoulders, and heat in the small finger and the one next to it. The sign of small intestine disease is that the vessel (of the hand *tai yang* is) depressed somewhere.

If a dragging discomfort is sent from the lower abdomen to the testicles, affecting the lumbar spine and causing (qi) to surge up into the heart, there is an evil in the small intestine. (The small intestine) links with the ligation of the testicles, homes to the spine, penetrates the liver and the lungs, and connects with the heart ligation. If there is exuberance of qi, there will be counterflow inversion. (The counterflow qi) surges up into the intestines and stomach, disturbs the liver and the lungs, disperses over the membranes, and gathers at the epiglottis. Therefore, (to treat this,) one should select Source of the Membrane (*Huang Yuan*, CV 6) to disperse (the counterflow qi), needle the (hand) *tai yin* to replenish (the lungs), choose the (foot) *jue yin* to precipitate (liver repletion), choose Lower Ridge of the Great Hollow (*Ju Xu Xia Lian*, St 39) to remove (evil qi from the small intestine), and balance the channels involved.

If there is cold in the small intestine, the person will invariably suffer from pressure in the rectum and pus and blood in the stools. If there is heat, there must be hemorrhoids. If there is retained food in the small intestine, there is often fever in the evening which is relieved the next morning. Small intestine distention is fullness and distention of the lower abdomen causing a contracting pain in the (whole) abdomen. If inversion qi settles in the small intestine, there will be dreams of villages and townships with streets and roads.

The hand *tai yang* vessel originates from the tip of the small finger traveling along the outside of the hand up to the wrist to emerge at the styloid process of the ulna. It travels straight upward along the ulnar border of the forearm to emerge at the inside of the elbow between two bones. From there, it proceeds further upward along the posterolateral aspect of the upper arm to emerge at the shoulder joint, wrapping the scapula. (Its right and left routes) cross above the shoulder, and it submerges at the supraclavicular fossa, descending to connect with the heart. Following the esophagus, it penetrates the diaphragm to reach the stomach and homes to the small intestine.

A branch deviates at the supraclavicular fossa following the neck to the cheek, where it goes to the outer canthus and then enters the ear. A ramification deviates at the cheek, ascending to the suborbital region, then turning to the nose to reach the inner canthus, obliquely connecting with the cheekbone.

If (this channel) is affected, the disease of sore throat, swelling of the submandibular region, inability to turn the head, pain in the shoulder which feels as if it had ruptured, and pain in the upper arm which feels as if it had broken will arise.

If the humor governed (by the small intestine) becomes diseased, there will be deafness, yellowing of the eyes, swelling of the cheek and submandibular region, and pain in the lateral posterior side of the neck, submandibular region, shoulder, upper arm, elbow and the forearm.

Exuberance (of the channel qi) is determined by a *ren ying* pulse which is three times as great as the *cun* opening. Vacuity, on the contrary, is characterized by a *ren ying* pulse which is smaller than the *cun* opening.

Chapter Five

Disease Patterns of the Spleen & Foot *Tai Yin* Channel

Spleen qi vacuity gives rise to loss of use of the four limbs and unrest of the five viscera, while repletion gives rise to abdominal distention and inhibited defecation and urination.

When spleen qi becomes vacuous, there are dreams of insufficient drink and food. When the spleen qi has its day, there are dreams of building walls and houses. With the spleen qi exuberant, there are dreams of singing and (other) entertainments, generalized heaviness, and inability to lift the four limbs. If inversion qi settles in the spleen, there will be dreams of mounds and great marshes and collapsed houses in storms.

Spleen disease is characterized by serenity in the sun's descent watch, exacerbation at the calm dawn watch, keeping up at the midday watch [the above four words are suspected to be a redundant insertion], and tranquility in the late afternoon watch.

If disease starts first in the spleen, there will be block and congestion with generalized aching and heaviness. In one day, the disease comes to the stomach, giving rise to abdominal distention. In two days, it comes to the kidneys, giving rise to pain in the lower abdomen and lumbar spine and aching in the lower legs. In three days, it comes to the urinary bladder, giving rise to pain in the paravertebral sinews and urinary block. If it does not come to an end in ten days, this is death. Death will come at the serenity watch (9-11 p.m.) in winter or the breakfast watch (7-9 a.m.) in summer.

If the spleen pulse pounds hard and long and the facial complexion is yellow, there should be a disease of diminished qi. If the pulse is soft and dissipated and the facial complexion is sheenless, there should be a disease of swelling of the lower legs like water (swelling).

If the spleen pulse is soggy in the deep level and vacuous in the superficial, the bitterness is abdominal distention, distressing fullness, heat in the stomach, no desire for food, inability to transform food, difficult defecation, tormenting *bi* of the four limbs, and occasional insensitivity.

All of this is produced in the chamber.[1] (Therefore, there is also) absence of menstruation or profuse menstrual flow at short intervals. If the pulse arrives large yet vacuous with a yellow (facial complexion), there is accumulated qi in the abdomen; (that is to say) there is inversion qi which is called inversion *shan*.[2] The case is the same with females (as with males). This is caused by strenuous exertion of the four limbs and sweating in a draft.

Suppose the *cun* opening pulse is bowstring and slippery. In the presence of a bowstring (pulse), there is pain, and, in the presence of a slippery (pulse), there is repletion. Pain results in tension (of the sinews) and repletion in twitching (of the flesh). Pain and twitching [repletion is suspected instead of twitching] combine to cause (qi) to rush into and hypertonicity of the chest and lateral costal regions.

Suppose the instep pulse is floating and choppy. In the presence of a floating pulse, there is faint stomach qi, and, in the presence of a choppy (pulse), there is debilitated spleen qi. The faint (stomach qi) and the debilitated (spleen qi) combine to result in inability to breathe. This is (due to) the spleen losing its balance.

If the *cun* opening pulse is tight on both (hands), this shows that the qi has entered (deeply) and will not come out. Since (the qi) is absent from the exterior but present in the interior, there is glomus and tightness below the heart.

Suppose the instep pulse is faint and choppy. In the presence of a faint (pulse), there is absence of stomach qi, and, in presence of a choppy (pulse), there is spleen damage. When cold qi is around the diaphragm but treated by precipitation, accumulated cold will not be dispersed. (On the contrary,) the stomach will be made faint and the spleen will be damaged. Then grain qi stops moving and there arises belching upon eating. Because cold is around the diaphragm in the chest, there is vacuity above and repletion below. The grain qi is blocked, thus giving rise to the illness of constipation.

Suppose the *cun* opening pulse is moderate and slow. In the presence of a moderate (pulse), which is (an expression of) yang, the defensive qi is replenished, and, in the presence of a slow (pulse), which is of yin, there is flourishing constructive qi. Since both the constructive and

---

[1] In Chinese medicine, expressions composed of the word chamber usually mean too frequent or unhealthy sexual intercourse.

[2] Inversion *shan* is a syndrome characterized by upsurging counterflow qi in the abdomen, pain in the venter, retching and vomiting, inability to take in food, frigidity of the feet, and a discomfort radiating from the lower abdomen to the testicles.

defensive are in harmony, the unyielding and the pliant coordinate and the triple burner is consistent. Thus the (righteous) qi must be strong.

Suppose the instep pulse is slippery and tight. In the presence of a slippery (pulse), there is repletion of stomach qi, and, in the presence of a tight (pulse), there is spleen qi damage. If there is failure to disperse food after receiving it, this is due to failure of the spleen to exercise its government. Ability to eat with no abdominal fullness shows a surplus of stomach qi. Abdominal fullness with inability to take in food and a hunger-like sensation below the heart shows stagnation of the stomach qi and vacuity of the heart qi. If there is fullness arising upon eating, this is due to failure of the spleen to exercise its government.

Wind stroke of the spleen is characterized by continuous mild fever, acting like a drunk person, distressing heaviness inside the abdomen, twitching of the skin and flesh, and shortness of breath.

Impact injury or fall, entering the chamber (*i.e.*, having sex) when intoxicated or surfeit, or sweating in a draft will damage the spleen. When the spleen is damaged, the qi will be affected. Then yin and yang are separated, yang not following yin. It follows that one has to examine the three divisions (of the *cun* opening pulse) to determine death and survival.

When the spleen qi is weak, there will be disease such as diarrhea. White filthy substances in the stools, hard stools, inability to change clothes (*i.e.*, constipation), and incessant sweating are (indications of) weak spleen qi. (Weak spleen qi) may also manifest as downpour diarrhea of fluids of the five colors, green-blue, yellow, red, white, and black.

Leveling (of the area) below the nose of the sick person indicates stomach disease. If (the area) is slightly red, there is the disease of *yong*. If it is slightly black, there is heat. If it is green-blue, there is cold. If it is white, (the condition) is incurable. If the lips are black, the stomach is already diseased. If there is slight dryness (of the lips) with thirst, (the condition) is curable. If there is no thirst, it is incurable. If the umbilicus is protruding, this shows that the spleen is already fallen [dead in another version].

Spleen distention is characterized by frequent belching, hypertonicity of the four limbs, and generalized heaviness with an inability (even) to dress oneself.

If taken with spleen water, the person suffers from enlarged abdomen, tormenting heaviness of the four limbs, failure to generate fluids, tormenting diminished qi all the time, and difficult urination.

Suppose the instep pulse is floating and choppy. In the presence of a floating (pulse), the stomach qi is strong, and, in the presence of a choppy (pulse), there is frequent voiding of urine. The floating and the choppiness combine to point to hard stools due to a constricted spleen. A constricted spleen manifests as hard stools and uninhibited urination yet accompanied by no thirst.

After a person is relieved of disease and the (pathological) pulse, the person may (still) suffer from slight vexation in the evening. When people see a sick person has recovered, they (often erroneously) force food upon him. Because the spleen and stomach qi, which is still weak, are unable to disperse grain, slight vexation arises. Reduce the food intake and (full) recovery will ensue.

Spleen accumulation is called glomus qi. It is located in the venter, as large as and shaped like an inverted plate. It may persist long, giving rise to the diseases of inability to contract the four limbs, jaundice, and failure of food and drink to serve the muscles and skin. It is contracted on the *ren* or *gui* days in winter. Why is this? Liver disease should be transmitted to the spleen and from there to the kidneys. The kidneys, however, happen to be king in winter. As king, they are immune to evils. So the spleen intends to return (the evil) to the liver, but the liver refuses to receive it (again). Thus (the evils) have to lodge and be bound (in the spleen), developing into accumulations. Therefore, one can know that glomus qi develops in winter.

Spleen disease is characterized by a yellow facial complexion, untransformed grain in the stools, tormenting abdominal distention and fullness, generalized heaviness with pain in the joints, and inhibited defecation. If the pulse is slightly moderate and long, this is curable. It is appropriate to administer *Ping Wei Wan* (Level the Stomach Pills),[3] *Xie Pi Wan* (Drain the Spleen Pills),[4] *Zhu Yu Wan* (Evodia Pills),[5] and *Fu Zi Tang* (Aconite Decoction).[6] It is necessary to needle Hidden White

---

[3] This formula is suspected to be *Ping Wei San* (Level the Stomach Powder) which is composed of Rhizoma Atractylodis (*Cang Zhu*), Cortex Magnoliae Officinalis (*Hou Po*), Pericarpium Citri Reticulatae (*Chen Pi*), and Radix Glycyrrhizae (*Gan Cao*).

[4] This formula is suspected to be *Xie Pi San* (Drain the Spleen Powder) which is composed of Folium Agastachis Seu Pogostemi (*Huo Xiang Ye*), Fructus Gardeniae Jasminoidis (*Zhi Zi*), Gypsum (*Shi Gao*), Radix Glycyrrhizae (*Gan Cao*), and Radix Ledebouriellae Divaricatae (*Fang Feng*).

[5] The ingredients in this formula include Fructus Evodiae Rutecarpae (*Zhu Yu*), Cortex Cinnamomi Cassiae (*Gui Xin*), and Radix Angelicae Sinensis (*Dang Gui*).

[6] The ingredients in this formula are Radix Praeparatus Aconiti Carmichaeli (*Fu Zi*), Sclerotium Poriae Cocos (*Fu Ling*), Radix Paeoniae Lactiflorae (*Shao Yao*), Radix Panacis Ginseng (*Ren Shen*), and Rhizoma Atractylodis Macrocephalae (*Bai Zhu*).

(*Yin Bai*, Sp 1) in spring and Yin Mound Spring (*Yin Ling Quan*, Sp 9) in winter, draining both, and Great Metropolis (*Da Du*, Sp 2) in summer, Grandson of the Noble (*Gong Sun*, Sp 4) in late summer, and Shang Hill (*Shang Qiu*, Sp 5) in autumn, supplementing all of them. Moreover, it is also necessary to moxa Camphorwood Gate (*Zhang Men*, Liv 13) with 50 cones and the eleventh vertebra[7] in the back with 100 cones.

If the spleen is diseased, there will invariably be generalized heaviness, tormenting (constant) hungering, wilting feet with inability to contract, tugging frequently arising in walking, and pain in the underside of the feet. In the case of vacuity, there is abdominal distention, rumbling in the intestines, thin-stool diarrhea, and untransformed food in stools. (To treat these conditions,) choose the channels, the foot *tai yin*, *yang ming*, and *shao yin* by means of bleeding them.

If there are evils in the spleen and stomach, there is pain in the muscles. If there is a surplus of yang qi but an insufficiency of yin qi, there is heat in the center and constant hungering. If there is an insufficiency of yang qi but a surplus of yin qi, there is cold in the center with rumbling in the intestines and abdominal pain. If there is a surplus or an insufficiency of both yin and yang, there will be cold as well as heat. For any case, apply balancing through Three Li (*San Li*, St 36).

The vessel of the foot *tai yin* originates at the tip of the great toe and travels upward along the white flesh of the medial aspect of the toe, past the posterior border of the kernel bone (the head of the first metatarsal) to the front border of the medial malleolus. From there, it proceeds upwards, entering the calf, traveling along the posterior border of the tibia where it crosses the (foot) *jue yin* and then goes in front of it. It ascends further along the anterior border of the medial aspect of the knee and thigh. It enters the abdomen, homing to the spleen and connecting with the stomach. It then ascends through the diaphragm by the side of the throat to link with the root of the tongue, spreading over the underside of the tongue. A branch diverges from the stomach and, ascending through the diaphragm, pours into the heart.

If (this channel) is affected, there will be disease such as stiffness of the root of the tongue and retching upon intake of food. There will be pain in the venter, abdominal distention, and frequent belching. These can be temporarily relieved by defecation or passing flatus. There is (also) generalized heaviness.

If the governing (viscus), the spleen, becomes diseased, there will be pain in the root of the tongue, inability to turn over, failure of food to descend, heart vexation, urgency below the heart,

---

[7] As a matter of fact, this point should be located 1.5 *cun* bilateral to the vertebra or, in other words, Spleen Shu (*Pi Shu*, BL 20).

cold malaria-like disease, thin stool diarrhea, conglomeration, swill diarrhea, water blockage, jaundice, somnolence, inability to eat meat, green-blue lips, pain in the thigh and knee which occurs on attempting to stand, inversion, and loss of the use of the great toe.

Exuberance (of the channel qi) is determined by a *cun* opening pulse which is four times as large as the *ren ying*. Vacuity, on the contrary, is characterized by a *cun* opening pulse which is smaller than the *ren ying*.

The connecting branch of the foot *tai yin* is called Grandson of the Noble (*Gong Sun*, Sp 4). At one *cun* from the base joint (*i.e.*, the tubercle of the metatarsophalangeal joint of the big toe), it diverges to the (foot) *yang ming*. A ramification enters the inside to connect with the stomach and the intestines. If there is counterflow ascent of inversion qi, there will be choleraic disease. In the case of repletion, there will be lancinating pain in the intestines. In the case of vacuity, there will be inflating distention. (To treat this,) select the branch (*i.e.*, Grandson of the Noble).

Spleen disease may manifest as a yellow facial complexion, green-blue complexion of the trunk, urinary incontinence, staring straight ahead, out-turned lips, green-blue nails, counterflow vomiting upon ingestion of food and drink, generalized heaviness with pain in the joints, and inability to lift the four limbs. If the pulse, which should be floating, large, and moderate, is now, on the contrary, bowstring and urgent and if the facial complexion, which should be yellow, is now, on the contrary, green-blue, this shows wood overwhelming earth, a greatly unfavorable condition. Ten out of ten cases will die without a remedy.

_________Chapter Six_________
Disease Patterns of the Stomach & Foot *Yang Ming* Channel

Stomach disease is characterized by abdominal distention, pain right in the cardiac region of the venter, (qi) propping up against the flanks, block in the diaphragm and throat, and failure of food and drink to descend. (To treat this,) select Three Li (*San Li*, St 36).

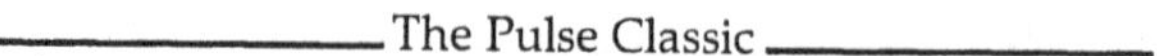

Failure of food and drink to descend due to block and congestion of the diaphragm suggests that evils are located in the venter. If they are in the upper venter, one should needle to suppress them. If they are in the lower venter, one should remove them by dispersing.[1]

If the stomach pulse pounds hard and long and the facial complexion is red, there must be a disease of (pain in) the thigh which feels as if it had broken. If the pulse is soft and scattered, there must be the diseases of food *bi*[2] and pain in the thigh.

If there is glomus in the stomach, pain will arise when eating cold substances. The pain makes eating impossible to continue. (However,) when something hot is had, eating can continue.

Stomach distention is characterized by abdominal fullness, pain in the venter, a parched smell in the nose which affects food intake, and difficult defecation.

When a (pathologic) stomach pulse is felt, what kind of disease is suggested? The answer is that a replete stomach (pulse) points to distention and a vacuous one to diarrhea.

If disease starts first in the stomach, there will be distention and fullness. In five days, the disease comes to the kidneys, giving rise to pain in the lower abdomen and the lumbar spine and aching in the lower legs. In three days, it comes to the urinary bladder, giving rise to pain in the paravertebral sinews and urinary block. In five days, it comes up to the spleen, giving rise to block and congestion and generalized heaviness and pain. If it does not come to an end in six days, this is death. Death will come at after [the preceding word is suspected to be a redundancy] midnight in winter or the sun's descent watch (1-3 p.m.) in summer.

Suppose the pulse is floating and scallion-stalk. The floating is (an expression of) yang, and the scallion-stalk, of yin. The floating and scallion-stalk combine to show that the stomach qi is generating heat and that the yang (qi) is secluded (internally).

A floating instep pulse indicates vacuity of the stomach qi. A floating and large instep pulse shows faint stomach, which gives rise to vacuity vexation and necessarily two bowel movements a day.

There is a scallion-stalk pulse which is possessed of stomach qi. It is a pulse which is large and soft in the superficial level and feels (somewhat) scallion-stalk only when slight pressure is applied. Such a pulse, though scallion-stalk, is known as possessed of stomach qi.

---

[1] This implies needling Upper Venter (*Shang Wan*, CV 13) and Lower Venter (*Xia Wan*, CV 10) respectively.

[2] This is an illness due to food retention with oppression and pain in the venter.

A rapid instep pulse indicates that there is heat in the stomach. The heat results in swift digestion with large food intake. A choppy instep pulse indicates that there is cold in the stomach giving rise to inability to transform water and grain. If the instep pulse is very thick and floating, the disease is difficult to treat. A floating and slow instep pulse indicates an enduring disease. A vacuous instep pulse indicates enuresis, and a replete one indicates flatus.

Headache and top heaviness arising on movement and tidal heat qi (*i.e.*, fever) are ascribed to the stomach. When inversion qi settles in the stomach, there are dreams of food and drink.

The vessel of the foot *yang ming* originates from the nose, (its right and left routes) crossing at the root of the nose. It travels across and then beside the (foot) *tai yang* channel and runs by the side of the nose to enter the upper teeth. It emerges again to wrap the lips, with its right and left routes crossing at Nectar Receptacle (*Cheng Jiang*, CV 24). Then it travels below and behind the jowl and emerges at Great Reception (*Da Ying*, St 5). From there, it proceeds along the mandibular border, up the region anterior to the ear, past Guest Host Person (*Ke Zhu Ren*, St 6), and then along the hairline to the corner of the forehead.

A branch diverges in front of Great Reception (*Da Ying*) and goes down to the throat via Man's Prognosis (*Ren Ying*, St 9) to submerge at the supraclavicular fossa. From there, it proceeds down through the diaphragm, homing to the stomach and connecting with the spleen.

The straight branch deviates at the supraclavicular fossa, traveling down along the medial border of the breast and then alongside of the umbilicus, and finally entering the Qi Thoroughfare (*Qi Chong*, St 30).

Another branch originates at the lower opening of the stomach, traveling down the interior of the abdomen and arriving at the qi thoroughfare to join the preceding branch. From there, it continues downward, passing through the Thigh Pass (*Bi Guang*, St 31), arriving at the Crouching Rabbit (*i.e.*, the prominent flesh above the knee) and then enters the knee cap. It continues down along the lateral aspect of the lower leg and, by way of the instep, arrives at the medial aspect of the middle toe.

Another branch descends from a point three *cun* below the knee running downward to submerge on the lateral aspect of the middle toe.

Another branch diverges from the instep, enters the big toe and finally emerges at the tip of the toe.

If (this channel) is affected, there will be illnesses such as quivering with cold, frequent stretching and yawning, and a black complexion on the forehead. In attacks of the disease, there will be aversion to the sight of people and fire, alarm and fright at hearing noise made by wood, palpitations, and a preference for privacy with doors and windows shut. In severe cases, there will be a desire to climb to heights while singing loudly and moving about naked and abdominal distention with thunderous rumbling (in the intestines). This is (called) lower leg inversion.

If the blood governed (by the channel) becomes diseased, there will be mania, malaria-like disease, rampant thermic heat with spontaneous sweating, runny snivel nosebleeding, deviated mouth, labial papules, swelling of the neck, throat *bi*, enlarged abdomen with water swelling, pain and swelling in the knee cap, and pain in the bosom, breast, qi thoroughfare, upper thigh, Crouching Rabbit, and the lateral aspect of the lower leg down to the dorsum of the foot. There will also be loss of use of the middle toe.

If there is exuberance of qi (in the channel), there will be heat all over the front of the body. If there is a surplus of qi within the stomach, there will be swift digestion with constant hungering and yellow urine. If there is an insufficiency of qi, there will be cold shudders all over the front of the body. If there is cold in the stomach, there will be distention and fullness.

Exuberance (of the channel qi) is determined by a *ren ying* pulse which is four times as large as the *cun* opening. Vacuity, on the contrary, is characterized by a *ren ying* pulse which is smaller than the *cun* opening.

_______________ Chapter Seven _______________
Disease Patterns of the Lungs
& Hand *Tai Yin* Channel

Vacuity of the lung qi gives rise to uninhibited (*i.e.*, smooth) breathing with diminished qi, and repletion gives rise to dyspneic rales and oppression in the chest with having to lie supine to facilitate breathing. If the lung qi is vacuous, there are dreams of white articles and seeing people killing each other with blood splashed everywhere. When (the lung qi) has its day, there are dreams of battles. If the lung qi is exuberant, there will be dreams of fear and dread and crying.

When inversion qi settles in the lungs, there are dreams of *hun* and *po* soaring out and seeing metal articles and rarities.

Lung disease is characterized by serenity in the late afternoon watch, exacerbation at the midday watch, and tranquility at the midnight watch.

If disease starts first in the lungs, there will be dyspnea and cough. In three days, the disease comes to the liver, giving rise to pain and propping fullness of the flanks. In one day, it will come to the spleen, giving rise to block and congestion with generalized pain and heaviness. In five days, it comes to the stomach, giving rise to abdominal distention. If it does not come to an end in ten days, this is death. Death will come at the sunset watch (5-7 p.m.) in winter or at the sunrise watch (5-7 a.m.) in summer.

If the lung pulse pounds hard and long, there must be a disease of spitting of blood. If the pulse is soggy and dissipated, there must be a disease of leaking sweat which no longer allows the use of dispersion and effusion.

If the lung pulse is rapid in the deep level but as if gasping in the superficial, the bitterness is shivering with cold, fever, abdominal fullness, heat in the intestines, dark-colored urine, pain in the shoulder and upper back, and perspiration from the lower back upward. This is produced in the chamber (*i.e.*, is due to sexual intercourse) or by sweating in a draft.

If the pulse is as if gasping, floating, and large with a white (facial complexion), there is vacuity above and repletion below with (susceptibility to) fright and accumulated qi in the chest. If the pulse is as if gasping and vacuous, (the illness) is called lung *bi* which is accompanied by cold and heat. It is caused by exertion of the internal force (*i.e.*, sexual intercourse) when intoxicated.

Wind stroke of the lungs manifests as a dry mouth, dyspnea, dizziness, generalized heaviness, oppression, and swelling and distention. Cold stroke of the lungs manifests as turbid spittle.

Cold form[1] and cold drink may injure the lungs. Because these two colds act upon one another, the interior and the exterior are both damaged. As a result, qi counterflows upward. When the lungs are damaged, the person will cough and spit blood whenever taxed and fatigued. A thin, tight, floating, or rapid pulse points to blood ejection. This is a result of damaged lungs with congested qi due to agitation, restlessness, indignation, and anger.

____

[1]   This means affection of the body by environmental cold.

Lung distention is vacuity fullness with dyspnea, counterflow cough, having to lean against something to facilitate breathing, and eyes looking as if they were coming out of their sockets. The pulse is floating.

Lung water manifests as generalized heaviness, difficult urination, and frequent duck-stool diarrhea.

Liver overwhelming the lungs will invariably give rise to vacuity fullness.

Suppose the pulse is limp and weak, weak contrarily in the *guan* and limp contrarily in the top (*i.e.*, the *cun*) or floating contrarily in the upper (*i.e.*, the *cun*) and weak contrarily in the lower (*i.e.*, the *chi*). The floating is an expression of yang, and the weakness, of insufficiency of blood. The weakness invariably points to vacuity. (However,) floating and weakness are different. Floating is spontaneous exiting (of yang qi), while weakness implies submerging (*i.e.*, yin qi lying deep). Floating means (yang qi) exiting without entering. This results in the presence (of yang qi) in the exterior and absence (of it) from the interior. Weakness means (yin qi) submerging without exiting. This results in absence (of yin qi) from the exterior and presence (of it) in the interior. When yang exits, there will be excessive sweating which is confined to the part above the lower back. This is due to the presence (of yang qi) in the exterior with absence (of it) from the interior. It is, therefore, called inversion yang (*jue yang*).[2] (This is produced by) failure to promote perspiration when diaphoresis should be carried out.

Suppose the instep pulse is floating and moderate and the *shao yang* (pulse)[3] is faint and tight. In the presence of a faint (pulse), there is blood vacuity, and, in the presence of a tight (pulse), there is slight cold. This is (an illness of) rat's breast (*shu ru*).[4] It is ascribed to the lungs.

Lung accumulation is called inverted cup surging (*xi ben*). It is located in the right lateral costal region, as large as and shaped like an inverted cup. It may persist very long, giving rise to the diseases of shivering with cold, fever, and qi counterflow cough and dyspnea. It may start lung *yong*. This is contracted on the *jia* and *yi* days in spring. Why is this? Heart disease should be transmitted to the lungs and, from there, to the liver. The liver, (however,) happens to be king in spring. As king, it is immune to evils. Then the lungs intend to return (the evil) to the heart, but

---

[2]   Inversion (*jue*) is often an equivalent of counterflow. Inversion yang, therefore, means counterflow yang in no company of yin.

[3]   This refers to the pulse around the auricle.

[4]   Rat's breast is a wart usually seen on the skin of the neck, chest, or upper back. It has a depression in the center. If pinched, it will discharge a whitish, semi-fluid substance from this depression.

174

the heart refuses to accept it (again). Therefore, (the evil) has to lodge and be bound (in the lungs), developing into accumulations. Therefore, one can know that inverted cup surging develops in spring.

Lung disease is characterized by a white facial complexion, solely cold with no heat in the body, and oft-occurring cough. If the pulse is faint and slow, this is curable. It is appropriate to administer *Wu Wei Zi Da Bu Fei Tang* (Schisandra Greatly Supplement the Lungs Decoction)[5] and *Xie Fei San* (Drain the Lungs Powder).[6] It is necessary to needle Lesser Shang (*Shao Shang*, Lu 11) in the spring and Fish Border (*Yu Ji*, Lu 10) in the summer, draining both, and Great Abyss (*Tai Yuan*, Lu 9) in the late summer, Channel Ditch (*Jing Qu*, Lu 8) in the autumn, and Cubit Marsh (*Chi Ze*, Lu 5) in the winter, supplementing all of them. Moreover, it is also necessary to moxa Chest Center (*Dan Zhong*, CV 17) with 100 cones and the third vertebra[7] on the back with twenty-five cones.

When the lungs are diseased, there must be dyspnea, cough, counterflow qi, lifting the shoulders to facilitate breathing, pain in the back, (spontaneous) sweating, and pain all the way along the sacrococcygeal region, medial aspect of the thigh, the knee which is hypertonic, gluteus, calf, lower leg, and foot. In the case of vacuity, there will be diminished qi which is not enough for breath, deafness, and a dry throat. (To treat this,) choose the hand *tai yin* channel, (the channel) lateral to the foot *tai yang*, and the foot *shao yin* channel anterior to the foot *jue yin*, bleeding them.

If there are evils in the lungs, there will arise pain in the skin, fever and chills, qi ascent, qi dyspnea, (spontaneous) sweating, and coughing shaking the shoulders and the back. (To treat this,) choose the points lateral to the breast and the point lateral to the third vertebra in the back. Needle only those of them which give relief when heavy pressure is applied. Moreover, select the point in the supraclavicular fossa[8] to evict (the evils).

The vessel of the hand *tai yin* originates in the middle burner, ascending to connect with the large intestine. It comes back up along the orifices of the stomach, ascends through the diaphragm, and

---

[5] This formula might be one composed of Fructus Schisandrae Chinensis (*Wu Wei Zi*), Radix Platycodi Grandiflori (*Jie Geng*), Radix Asteris Tatarici (*Zi Wan*), Radix Glycyrrhizae (*Gan Cao*), Radix Dypsaci (*Xu Duan*), Radix Rehmanniae (*Di Huang*), Cortex Radicis Mori Albi (*San Pi*), Caulis Bambusae In Taeniis (*Zhu Ru*), and Semen Phaseoli Calcarati (*Chi Xiao Dou*).

[6] The ingredients in this formula include Cortex Radicis Lycii (*Di Gu Pi*), Radix Et Rhizoma Rhei (*Da Huang*), Mirabilitum (*Mang Xiao*), Radix Platycodi Grandiflori (*Jie Geng*), and Radix Glycyrrhizae (*Gan Cao*).

[7] This refers to the point Lung Shu (*Fei Shu*, Bl 13).

[8] Practically speaking, this means the point Celestial Chimney (*Tian Tu*, CV 22).

homes to the lungs. From there, it proceeds along the pulmonary ligation and moves transversely towards the axilla. It emerges from there, circulating downwards in front of the (hand) *shao yin* channel and the heart-governor channel on the anterior aspect of the upper arm to enter the elbow. It then continues along the anterior aspect of the forearm, passing by the medial border of the styloid process of the radius to submerge at the *cun* opening. It then ascends at the fish margin (*i.e.*, the thenar prominence) and, moving along the fish margin, emerges from the tip of the thumb.

A branch diverges from the region distal to the wrist, moving along the radial border of the forefinger and emerging from its tip.

If (this channel) is affected, there will be illnesses such as distention and fullness of the lungs, inflating distention with dyspnea and cough, and pain in the supraclavicular fossa. In severe cases, the arms will fold across the chest and there will be visual distortion. This is called arm inversion.

If the governing (viscus), the lungs, become diseased, there will be cough, qi ascent, dyspneic rale, heart vexation, fullness of the chest, pain in the radial border of the anterior aspect of the upper arm and forearm, and heat in the palms. An exuberance or surplus of qi results in painful wind in the shoulder and upper back, spontaneous sweating, and frequent voiding of scanty urine. A vacuity of qi results in pain and cold in the shoulder and the upper back, diminished qi not enough for breath, a change in the color of urine, and sudden incessant diarrhea.

Exuberance (of the channel qi) is determined by a *cun* opening pulse which is four times as large as the *ren ying*. Vacuity, on the contrary, is characterized by a *cun* opening pulse which is smaller than the *ren ying*.

The connecting branch of the hand *tai yin* is called Broken Sequence (*Lie Que*, Lu 7). It originates at the parting of the muscles in the wrist and diverges to the (hand) *yang ming*. Together with the *tai yin* channel, its ramification goes straight to enter the palm and disperse in the fish margin. In the case of repletion, there will be heat in the palm and styloid process of the radius. If there is vacuity, there will be yawning, coughing, and enuresis or frequent voidings. (To treat this,) select the point one and a half *cun* proximal to the wrist (*i.e.*, Broken Sequence).

When the lungs are diseased, there should be generalized heat, cough, shortness of breath, and coughing of pus and blood. If the pulse which should be short and choppy, is now, on the contrary, floating and large and, if the facial complexion which should be white, is now, on the contrary, red, this shows fire overwhelming metal, a greatly unfavorable condition. Ten out of ten cases will die without a remedy.

_______________Chapter Eight_______________
Disease Patterns of the Large Intestine & Hand *Yang Ming* Channel

Large intestine disease is characterized by a lancinating pain and a gurgling sound in the intestines. In the case of dual affection by cold in winter, there will be diarrhea, pain right around the umbilicus, and inability to stand for long. (In that case,) the same reaction can be taken as in stomach (disease, *i.e.,*) to select Upper Ridge of the Great Hollow (*Ju Xu Shang Lian*, St 37).

If there is thunderous rumbling in the intestines with qi surging up into the chest, dyspnea, and inability to stand for long, there are evils in the large intestine. Needle Source of the Membrane (*Huang Yuan*, CV 6), Upper Ridge of the Great Hollow (*Ju Xu Shang Lian*, St 37), and Three Li (*San Li*, St 36).

Cold in the large intestine gives rise to duck-stool diarrhea, while heat gives rise to rotten flesh in the stools. If there is food retention in the large intestine, there will be quivering with cold, fever, and, sometimes, malarial disease.

Large intestine distention manifests as rumbling and pain in the intestines. In case of cold, there is diarrhea with untransformed food in the stools.

When inversion qi settles in the large intestine, there will be dreams of fields and wilderness.

The vessel of the hand *yang ming* originates at the tip of the radial aspect of the finger next to the thumb. It goes along the radial side of the finger to emerge between the two bones of Valley Union (*He Gu*, LI 4) and then moves upward to submerge between the two sinews. It continues upwards along the radial border of the posterior surface of the forearm to enter the outer side of the elbow. It moves further up the radial side of the posterior surface of the upper arm to arrive at the shoulder (joint) where, ascending, it emerges from the anterior aspect of the shoulder bone (*Jian Yu*, LI 15) to rendezvous (with other yang channels) at the spinal column (*Da Zhui*, GV 14).

From there, it proceeds downward, submerging at the supraclavicular fossa to connect with the lung, penetrating the diaphragm and homing to the large intestine.

A branch diverges from the supraclavicular fossa, ascending straight to the cheek via the neck and then descending to enter the spaces between the teeth. It emerges again to encircle the mouth. Crossing at the philtrum, the left (route) goes to the right and the right to the left. It then ascends past the nostril.

If (this channel) is affected, there will be diseases such as toothache and swelling in the suborbital region. If the fluid governed (by the channel) becomes diseased, there will be yellowing of the eyes, dryness of the mouth, runny snivel nosebleeding, throat *bi*, pain in the anterior aspect of the shoulder and the anterior aspect of the upper arm, and pain and loss of use of the finger next to the thumb.

An exuberance or surplus of qi (in the channel) is characterized by heat and swelling along the route of the channel. If there is vacuity, there will be cold shuddering which is difficult to get over.

Exuberance (of the channel qi) is determined by a *ren ying* pulse which is four times as large as the *cun* opening. Vacuity, on the contrary, is characterized by a *ren ying* pulse which is smaller than the *cun* opening.

_______________Chapter Nine_______________
Disease Patterns of the Kidneys
& Foot *Shao Yin* Channel

Vacuity of the kidney qi gives rise to inversion counterflow (*i.e.*, frigidity of the extremities), while repletion gives rise to distention and fullness and a full black complexion of the four limbs. If there is vacuity of the kidney qi, then there are dreams of seeing people being drowned while rowing boats. When (the liver qi) has its day, there are dreams of being hidden in water with fear and terror. If the kidney qi is exuberant, there are dreams of the spine being totally separated at the lumbus. When inversion qi settles in the kidneys, there will be dreams of standing in front of an abyss or being under water.

Kidney disease is characterized by serenity at the midnight watch, exacerbation at the four seasons of the day,[1] and tranquility in the late afternoon watch.

If disease starts first in the kidneys, there will be pain in the lower abdomen and the lumbar spine and aching in the lower leg. In three days, the disease comes to the urinary bladder, giving rise to pain in the paravertebral sinews and urinary block. In two days, it comes up to the heart, giving rise to heart pain. In three days, it comes to the small intestine, giving rise to distention. If it does not come to an end in four days, this is death. Death will come at the daybreak watch in winter or at the late afternoon watch in summer.

If the kidney pulse pounds hard and long and the facial complexion is yellowish red, there must be a disease of (painful) lumbus which feels as if it had broken. If the pulse is limp and dissipated, there should be an illness of lack of blood.

If the kidney pulse is large and hard in the deep level and large and tight in the superficial, the bitterness is swelling of the bones of the hand and foot, inversion, impotence, pain in the lumbar spine, swelling of the lower abdomen, water qi below the heart, occasional (abdominal) distention with (urinary) block, and occasional diarrhea. This is produced by entering the chamber with a wet body immediately after a bath and it is started by taxation fatigue.

If the pulse is hard and large in the upper [the preceding three words are suspected to be interpolations] with a black (facial complexion), there is accumulated qi in the lower abdomen and the genitals. This is called kidney *bi*. It is contracted as a result of falling asleep after a cold bath.

Exerting oneself to lift weights, entering the chamber too frequently (*i.e.,* having sex too frequently), or perspiring as massively as in a shower will damage the kidneys.

Kidney distention is abdominal fullness affecting the back. This is quite distressing. (In addition,) there is pain in the lower back and thigh.

If taken with kidney water, the person suffers from an enlarged abdomen, swollen umbilicus, heaviness and pain of the lower back, inability to urinate, wet genitals like the sweating of a cow's nose, and counterflow frigidity of the feet. There is contrarily hard stool.

---

[1] This refers to the four watches: *chen, xu, chou,* and *wei.*

Kidney fixation (*shen zhuo*) is an illness of cold from the lower back downward which feels as heavy as if (carrying) 5,000 coins.[2] If taken with kidney fixation, the patient suffers from generalized heaviness and ice-cold of the lower back. Contrarily, there is no thirst, the urination is uninhibited, and the food intake is normal. These are the symptoms of kidney fixation. The illness is ascribed to the lower burner. Body taxation and sweating with clammy clothes on are the causes. In due time, this illness arises.

Kidney accumulation is called running piglet (*ben tun*). It starts in the lower abdomen, surging up to the infra-cardiac region. It goes up and down irregularly like a running piglet. It may persist very long, giving rise to illnesses of counterflow dyspnea, bone wilting, and diminished qi. It is contracted on *bing* and *ding* days in summer. Why is this? Spleen disease should be transmitted to the kidneys and, from there, to the heart. The heart, however, happens to be king in summer. As king, it is immune to evils. Therefore, the kidneys intend to return (the evil) to the spleen, but the spleen refuses to accept it (again). Thus, it has to lodge and be bound up (in the kidneys), developing into accumulations. Hence, one can know that running piglet develops in summer.

Water flows more swiftly at night. Why is this? The master explained, (at night,) earth is at a stop.[3] Therefore, water flows more swiftly and with a (rippling) sound. Human beings are analogous (to this). While sleeping at night, peoples' spleens are still and, (therefore,) their pulse races more rapidly (than at day).

Kidney disease is characterized by a black facial complexion, vacuous and weak kidney qi, sucking in air laboriously with qi diminished, distressed deafness, lumbago, seminal emission from time to time, reduced food intake, and frigidity from the knees down. If the pulse is deep, slippery, and slow, this is curable. It is appropriate to administer *Nei Bu San* (Supplement the Internal Powder), *Jian Zhong Tang* (Fortify the Center Decoction), *Shen Qi Wan* (Kidney Qi Pills), and *Di Huang Jian* (Rehmannia Infusion).[4] It is necessary to needle Gushing Spring (*Yong Quan*, Ki 1) in spring,

---

[2] In old times, copper coins were the prevalent form of currency, and people carried these strung on cords around their waists. Therefore, 5,000 coins were a great weight to the lumbar region.

[3] At night, kidney water is king, while its child, liver wood, is minister. The restrained phase of liver wood, *i.e.*, spleen earth, is now in confinement. This is what is meant by earth being at a stop. Since earth is at a stop, its restrained phase, water is brisk.

[4] The ingredients in this formula are Succus Radicis Rehmanniae (*Di Huang Zhi*), Succus Rhizomatis Zingiberis (*Jiang Zhi*), Succus Radicis Lycii Chinensis (*Gou Qi Gen Zhi*), butter (*Su*), Succus Viticis Negundi (*Jing Li*), Succus Bambusae (*Zhu Li*), Radix Panacis Ginseng (*Ren Shen*), Tuber Asparagi Cochinensis (*Tian Dong*), Sclerotium Poriae Cocos (*Fu Ling*), Fructus Gardeniae Jasminoidis (*Zhi Zi*), and Radix Et Rhizoma Rhei (*Da Huang*).

Recover Flow (*Fu Liu*, Ki 7) in autumn, and Yin Valley (*Yin Gu*, Ki 10) in winter, supplementing all of them, and Blazing Valley (*Ran Gu*, Ki 2) in summer and Great Ravine (*Tai Xi*, Ki 3) in late summer, draining both of them. Moreover, it is also necessary to moxa Capital Gate (*Jing Men*, GB 25) with 50 cones and the fourteenth vertebra[5] on the back with 100 cones.

If the kidneys are diseased, there must be an enlarged abdomen, swelling and pain in the lower leg, dyspnea and cough, generalized heaviness, sweat exiting in sleep, and abhorrence of wind. In the case of vacuity, there will be pain inside the chest, pain in the upper and lower abdomen, inversion frigidity (of the limbs), and melancholy. (To treat this,) choose the channels, the foot *shao yin* and the foot *tai yang*, bleeding them.

When there are evils in the kidneys, there will be yin *bi*[6] of pain in the bone. Yin *bi* is (a pain) that baffles location through palpation. There may be abdominal distention, lumbago, difficult defecation, stiffness and pain of the shoulder, upper back, and the nape of the neck, and occasional dizziness. (To treat this,) select Gushing Spring (*Yong Quan*, Ki 1) and Kunlun Mountain (*Kun Lun*, Bl 60), pricking the blood vessels found around them.

The vessel of the foot *shao yin* originates on the underside of the small toe and travels transversely towards the center of the sole. It then emerges from under the navicular bone (*Ran Gu*, Ki 2) and, passing behind the medial malleolus, it enters the heel. From there, it ascends through the calf, moving out from the medial side of the popliteal fossa and ascending along the posterior border of the medial aspect of the thigh. It then penetrates the spine to home to the kidneys and connect with the urinary bladder.

Its straight branch diverges from the kidneys, ascending through the liver and diaphragm to enter the lungs. It moves along the throat, bypassing the root of the tongue.

Another branch emerges from the lungs to connect with the heart and pour into the chest.

If (this channel) is affected, there will be diseases such as hunger with no desire to eat, a soot-black facial complexion, coughing and spitting of blood, dyspneic rales, hazy vision on attempting to rise from a sitting position, a sensation of the heart being suspended as in hunger, susceptibility to fright due to insufficiency of qi, and being apprehensive as if fearing arrest. This is called bone inversion.

---

[5]   This refers to the point Kidney Shu (*Shen Shu*, Bl 23).

[6]   Pain, insensitivity, and swelling of the joints are characteristics of *bi*. Yin *bi* refers to *bi* of a cold, damp nature.

If the governing (viscus), the kidneys, are diseased, there will be heat in the mouth, a dry tongue, swelling of the throat, qi ascent, a dry and painful throat, heart vexation, heart pain, jaundice, intestinal *pi*, pain in the spine and the posterior border of the medial aspect of the thigh, wilting inversion, somnolence, and heat and pain in the underside of the foot.

If moxibustion is applied, (the sick person) is advised to force down underdone meat, to loosen his belt and hair, to carry a large staff, and to walk in shoes with weights.

Exuberance (of the channel qi) is determined by a *cun* opening pulse which is three times as large as the *ren ying*. Vacuity, on the contrary, is characterized by a *cun* opening pulse which is smaller than the *ren ying*.

The connecting branch of the foot *shao yin* is called Large Goblet (*Da Zhong*, Ki 4). Starting from behind the (medial) malleolus, it diverges into the (foot) *tai yang*, wrapping the heel. A ramification follows the channel (of the foot *shao yin*) up to the pericardium and then descends penetrating the lumbar spine. If the illness is one of qi counterflow, there will be vexation and oppression. In the case of repletion, there will be dribbling urinary block. In the case of vacuity, there will be lumbago. (To treat this,) select the branch (*i.e.*, Large Goblet).

Kidney disease may manifest as counterflow frigidity of the hands and feet, a red face and yellow eyes, urinary incontinence, distressed pain in the bone joints, binding and pain in the lower abdomen, and qi surging into the heart. If the pulse, which should be deep, thin, and slippery, is now, on the contrary, floating and large and if the facial complexion, which should be black, is now, on the contrary, yellow, this shows earth overwhelming water, a greatly unfavorable condition. Ten out of ten cases will die without a remedy.

Chapter Ten
Disease Patterns of the Urinary Bladder & Foot *Tai Yang* Channel

Urinary bladder disease is characterized by unilateral swelling and pain in the lower abdomen which, if pressed, gives rise to a desire but inability to urinate. There is heat in the shoulder and depressions somewhere along the vessel (of the foot *tai yang*). There is heat along the lateral aspect of the small toe, in the lower leg, and in the area posterior to the lateral malleolus. If there is a depression somewhere in the vessel, select Bend Middle (*Wei Zhong*, Bl 40).

Urinary bladder distention is fullness of the lower abdomen with dribbling urinary qi block.

If disease starts first in the urinary bladder, there will be pain in the paravertebral sinews and urinary block. In five days, the disease comes to the kidneys, giving rise to pain in the lower abdomen and lumbar spine and aching in the lower leg. In one day, it comes to the small intestine, giving rise to distention. In one day, it comes to the spleen, giving rise to block and congestion with generalized pain and heaviness. If it does not come to an end in two days, this is death. Death will come at the cockcrow watch (3-5 a.m.) in winter or at the late afternoon watch (3-5 p.m.) in summer.

When inversion qi settles in the urinary bladder, there are dreams of meandering.

The vessel of the foot *tai yang* originates in the inner canthus of the eye and ascends to the forehead where its right and left routes cross at the vertex. A branch diverges from the vertex towards the tip of the auricle.

Its straight branch diverges at the vertex, submerging to connect with the brain and again emerging to descend to the nape. From there, it proceeds along the medial side of the scapula, running parallel to the spinal column into the lumbar region. It then submerges, moving along the backbone, connecting with the kidneys and homing to the urinary bladder.

Another branch diverges at the lumbar region, descending to join (other channels) at the posterior yin (*i.e.*, the anus) and then entering the popliteal fossa via the gluteus.

Another branch diverges from around the medial aspect of the scapula, traveling downward along the linking sinew (*i.e.*, the paravertebral muscles). It passes through the hip joint, traveling down the lateral posterior border of the thigh to join into the popliteal fossa. From there, it descends through the calf, emerging from behind the lateral malleolus along the base of the fifth metatarsal bone and arriving finally at the lateral aspect of the small toe.

If (this channel) is affected, there will be diseases such as (qi) surging headache, (pain in) the eyes as if they were about to burst (from their sockets, pain in) the neck as if it were being pulled up, spinal pain, (pain in) the lumbus as if it had broken, an inability to bend the thigh (*i.e.*, the hip joint), the popliteal fossa as if it were bound up, and (pain) in the calf as if it were split open. This is called malleolar inversion.

If the sinews governed (by this channel) are diseased, there will be hemorrhoids, malarial disease, mania, withdrawal, pain in the brain and the vertex, yellowing of the eyes, lacrimation, runny snivel nosebleeding, pain all the way along the nape, upper and lower back, sacrococcygeal region, popliteal fossa, calf, and foot, and loss of use of the small toe.

Exuberance (of the channel qi) is determined by a *ren ying* pulse which is three times as great as the *cun* opening. Vacuity, on the contrary, is characterized by a *ren ying* pulse which is smaller than the *cun* opening.

Chapter Eleven
Disease Patterns of the Triple Burner & Hand *Shao Yang* Channel

Triple burner disease is characterized by abdominal distention and qi fullness, tightness particularly in the lower abdomen, inability to urinate, and pressure and urgency (in the bladder). When (water) spills over, water (swelling) develops. When (water) is retained, distention develops. The reflection (of the condition) is found along the major vessel network lateral to the foot *tai yang* between the (foot) *tai yang* and the (foot) *shao yang*, where a red vessel may appear. (To treat this,) select Bend Yang (*Wei Yang*, Bl 39).

If there is a lower abdomen disease of swelling and inability to urinate, the pathogen is constriction of the triple burner. Choose the major connecting vessel of the (foot) *tai yang*, bleeding the blood binds in this vessel and the minute vessel network of the (foot) *jue yin*. If the swelling has spread up to the venter, select Three Li (*San Li*, St 36).

Triple burner distention is qi filling up the skin which, though inflated, is not tight or painful.

Heat in the upper burner may produce cough, and subsequently, lung wilting. Heat in the middle burner may produce abdominal tightness. Heat in the lower burner may produce hematuria.

The vessel of the hand *shao yang* originates from the tip of the finger next to the small one. It emerges between the two fingers, traveling across the back of the wrist, emerging between the two bones on the posterior aspect of the forearm, ascending to penetrate the elbow. It travels along the posterior aspect of the arm upward to arrive at the shoulder. From there, it crosses and moves behind the foot *shao yang* channel, submerging at the supraclavicular fossa to spread over the center of the chest. It then disperses to connect with the pericardium, descending through the diaphragm and homing to the three burners consecutively.

A branch diverges from the center of the chest, ascending to emerge at the supraclavicular fossa. It then ascends along the nape, curving behind the auricle, and moves straight upward to emerge from the upper aspect of the auricle. From there, it turns down and then crosses the cheek to reach the suborbital region.

Another branch diverges from behind the auricle, entering the ear and emerging anterior to the auricle. It then passes Guest Host Person (*Ke Zhu Ren*, GB 3) to join the preceding branch at the cheek and ultimately reaches the outer canthus.

If (this channel) is affected, there will be diseases such as deafness, muddle-headedness, swelling of the throat, and throat *bi*.

If the qi governed (by the channel) becomes diseased, there will be (spontaneous) sweating, pain in the outer canthus, swelling of the cheek, pain radiating down along the back of the auricle and the posterior aspect of the shoulder, upper arm, elbow, and forearm, and loss of use of the finger next to the small one.

Exuberance (of the channel qi) is determined by a *ren ying* pulse which is twice as great as the *cun* opening. Vacuity, on the contrary, is characterized by a *ren ying* pulse which is smaller than the *cun* opening.

BOOK SEVEN

Collated and edited by Honorary Minister Without Portfolio,
Curator of the Imperial Library,
Imperial Courier and Senior Army Protector,
Lin Yi *et al.*

Chapter One

Diseases Not Allowing Diaphoresis

If a *shao yin* disease[1] exhibits a thin, deep, and slippery pulse, the disease is internal and does not allow diaphoresis.

If the pulse is floating and tight, one would expect there to be generalized aching and pain requiring diaphoresis to resolve it. (However,) if the pulse is slow in the *chi*, then diaphoresis is not allowed. The reason for this decision is that there is an insufficiency of constructive qi or faint and scanty blood.

A *shao yin* disease with a faint pulse does not allow diaphoresis since there is absence of yang.

---

[1] The *shao yin* is one of the patterns of cold damage. Cold damage is a general term for febrile illnesses caused by external invasion. Based on Zhang Zhong-jing's methodology, cold damage is roughly classified into six patterns named after three divisions of yang and three divisions of yin. In many cases, the disease is transmuted in the order of the *tai yang* to the *yang ming* to the *shao yang* to the *shao yin*, *tai yin*, and *jue yin* respectively. The three yang patterns are characterized by heat and repletion, while the three yin ones are characterized by vacuity and cold.

The *tai yang* pattern describes evils located in the exterior. The *yang ming* pattern describes evils located in the interior. And the *shao yang* pattern describes evils located halfway between these two. Practically speaking, this means that some evils are still located in the exterior, while some evils have penetrated to the interior.

The *tai yang* pattern is mainly characterized by aversion to cold, fever, stiffness of and pain in the head and nape, a thin, white tongue fur, and a floating pulse. The *yang ming* pattern is divided into two sub-patterns: the channel and the bowel. The channel species is mainly characterized by high fever, copious sweating, burning thirst, and a large, surging pulse, while the bowel species is characterized by constipation, abdominal fullness and pain, vexation, and ravings besides fever and spontaneous sweating. The *shao yang* pattern is mainly characterized by a bitter taste in the mouth, dizziness, alternating cold and heat, fullness in the chest and lateral costal regions, no desire for food, frequent retching, slimy, white tongue fur, and a bowstring pulse. The *shao yin* pattern is mainly characterized by lethargy, somnolence, and a thin, faint pulse.

Suppose the pulse is soggy and weak, weak contrarily in the *guan* and soggy contrarily in the top (*i.e.*, the *cun*), faint contrarily in the upper (*i.e.*, the *cun*), and choppy contrarily in the lower (*i.e.*, the *chi*). In the presence of a faint (pulse), there is an insufficiency of yang qi, and, in the presence of a choppy (pulse), there is absence of blood. When yang qi contrarily becomes faint, there will be wind stroke with agitation and vexation in spite of perspiration. Since the choppiness is a result of absence of blood, there will be inversion and cold. When yang is faint but diaphoresis is employed (anyway), then agitation and insomnia will arise.

If there is a stirring (*i.e.*, palpitating) qi on the right (of the umbilicus), diaphoresis is not allowed. (In that case,) diaphoresis will produce runny snivel nosebleeding, thirst, tormenting heart vexation, and water ejection upon drinking.

If there is a stirring qi on the left (of the umbilicus), diaphoresis is not allowed. (In that case,) diaphoresis will produce dizziness, uncheckable perspiration, spasm of the sinews, and twitching of the flesh.

If there is a stirring qi above (the umbilicus), diaphoresis is not allowed. (In that case,) diaphoresis will provoke qi to surge up straight to the heart.

If there is a stirring qi below (the umbilicus), diaphoresis is not allowed. (In that case,) diaphoresis will lead to the absence of sweat and severe heart vexation, tormenting pain in the bone joints, visual dizziness, aversion to cold, vomiting upon ingestion, and inability of grain to advance [inability to transform grain in another version].

Block and constriction of the throat does not allow diaphoresis. (In that case,) diaphoresis will result in blood ejection, faint and expired qi, counterflow frigidity of the hands and feet, a desire to cuddle up, and inability to warm oneself.

In case of the various types of rapid pulse that beat faint and weak, diaphoresis is not allowed. (In that case,) diaphoresis will result in difficult defecation with dryness in the abdomen, desiccated stomach, and vexation. With these manifestations, (the *shao yin* pattern) resembles (the *yang ming* bowel pattern), but they are completely different in (disease) source.

Suppose the pulse is soggy and weak, weak contrarily in the *guan* and soggy contrarily in the top, bowstring contrarily in the upper and faint contrarily in the lower. In the presence of a bowstring (pulse), there is stirring yang, and, in the presence of a faint (pulse), there is yin cold. (This is) repletion above and vacuity below, and (the patient must) desire warmth. The faintness and bowstring combine to point to vacuity, not allowing diaphoresis. (In that case,) diaphoresis will

190

result in shivering with cold which will not stop by itself. It will exacerbate cough, producing frequent vomiting of foamy substances, invariably dryness in the throat, inhibited urination, and a hungering sensation and vexation in the heart. There are attacks once in a day which are like malaria with cold but no heat. Vacuity is responsible for shivering with cold. In the case of cough, diaphoresis will result in cuddling up and tormenting fullness in addition to abdominal tightness.

Inversion does not allow diaphoresis. (In that case,) diaphoresis will result in confused speech, hoarse voice, wilting tongue, and inability of grain to advance.

If the various cases with counterflow (frigidity) are treated by diaphoresis, a mild one will become difficult to cure, a severe one will develop confused speech, and (the one with) visual dizziness will end in death. (Then) life is impossible to save.

Eight or nine days after contraction, a *tai yang* disease may be like malaria. It manifests as fever and aversion to cold with much heat but little cold. The sick person suffers from no retching. The urination is normal and urine is clear. There are three episodes in a day. The pulse is faint and there is aversion to cold. This is due to vacuity of both yin and yang. (Therefore,) diaphoresis is no longer allowed.

If a *tai yang* disease manifests fever and aversion to cold with much heat and little cold and the pulse is faint and weak, there is absence of yang. Then diaphoresis is no longer allowed. Dryness in the throat (also) does not allow diaphoresis.

A person who suffers from loss of blood does not allow attacking the exterior. If sweat is promoted, there will be cold shudders and quivering.

A person who suffers from spontaneous external bleeding (*i.e.*, nosebleeding) does not allow attacking the exterior. If sweat is promoted, the forehead is bound to sink and the pulse[2] will become skipping, urgent, and tight. The (eyes) will keep staring straight ahead, unable to roll, and there will be insomnia.

---

[2] Here, the word pulse or vessel can also be interpreted as the sinew vessels or just the sinews. In that case, the phrase should be rendered as tension and hypertonicity of the sinews.

If a person with perspiration[3] is treated with diaphoresis, abstraction, disturbed heart (*i.e.,* agitation), and pain in the urethra at the end of urination will inevitably arise. (For this condition,) one may administer *Yu Yu Liang Wan* (Limonitum Pills).[4]

A person who suffers from strangury should not be treated with diaphoresis since diaphoresis will inevitably produce hemafecia.

A person who suffers from sores, even though there is pain all over their body, should not be treated through attacking the exterior. (In that case,) tetany will follow diaphoresis.

In winter, diaphoresis will inevitably result in vomiting, diarrhea, and ulceration and sores of the mouth.

Clear-food diarrhea does not allow attacking the exterior for diaphoresis will inevitably be followed by (abdominal) distention and fullness.

Cough with uninhibited urination or urinary incontinence does not allow attacking the exterior. (This is because) diaphoresis will produce inversion and counterflow frigidity (of the limbs). If (a person with) profuse sweating is treated by diaphoresis, (the stools) will also become hard.

One or two to four or five days after contraction of cold damage, heat will appear in the case of inversion. Inversion is invariably followed by heat. The more profound the inversion, the more profound the heat. The slighter the inversion, the slighter the heat. Inversion should be treated by precipitation. If diaphoresis is misused, there will inevitably arise ulceration and redness of the mouth. Suppose a sick person has a rapid pulse. In the presence of a rapid (pulse), there is heat, and heat will give rise to swift digestion with a large food intake. If, on the contrary, there arises vomiting, this is because the (attending) physician has applied diaphoresis. When yang is faint and the diaphragm qi is vacuous, the pulse may be rapid (nonetheless). This rapidity is (an

____

[3] This refers to any case of perspiration, for example, spontaneous sweating or perspiration induced by medication or acumoxa therapy.

[4] This formula is composed of Limonitum (*Yu Yu Liang*), Snake Bezoar (*She Huang*), Radix Et Rhizoma Notopterygii (*Qiang Huo*), Radix Auklandiae Lappae (*Mu Xiang*), Sclerotium Poriae Cocos (*Fu Ling*), Radix Ligustici Wallichii (*Chuan Xiong*), Radix Achyranthis Bidentatae (*Niu Xi*), Fructus Cardamomi (*Bai Dou Kou*), Rhizoma Curcumae Zedoariae (*E Zhu*), Fructus Foeniculi Vulgaris (*Hui Xiang*), Cortex Cinnamomi Cassiae (*Gui Xin*), Rhizoma Zingiberis (*Jiang*), Pericarpium Citri Reticulatae Viride (*Qing Pi*), Rhizoma Sparganii (*San Leng*), Fructus Tribuli Terrestris (*Bai Ji Li*), Radix Praeparatus Aconiti Carmichaeli (*Fu Zi*), and Radix Angelicae Sinensis (*Dang Gui*).

expression of) the guest yang (*i.e.*, yang vacuity). This guest yang is not able to disperse grain. Since there is vacuity cold in the stomach, there arises vomiting.

On the fourth or fifth day, cold damage may exhibit a deep pulse. There is vexation, dyspnea, and fullness. If the pulse is deep, the disease is internal. If diaphoresis is abused, fluids will be ousted and defecation will become difficult. The exterior will become vacuous, while the interior becomes replete. Over time, delirious raving will appear.

(There is a pattern of) cold damage with headache and continuous mild fever. It looks like wind stroke. If there is constant moderate perspiration accompanied by retching, precipitation will exacerbate the vexation which will (then) become a burning sensation in the heart like hunger. Diaphoresis will produce tetany. (In that case,) the body will become too rigid to contract or stretch. Fuming[5] will produce jaundice and inability to urinate, and, over time, coughing of (copious) spittle will develop.

If a *tai yang* disease is treated by diaphoresis, tetany may develop.

If cold damage exhibits a bowstring and thin pulse contrarily with headache and fever, it is categorized as a *shao yang* disease. This *shao yang* disease should not be treated by diaphoresis.

A combined disease of the *tai yang* and *shao yang* may manifest stiffness and pain in the head and nape, possibly with dizziness. If glomus and tightness below the heart like chest bind often arises, diaphoresis is not allowed.

A *shao yin* disease manifesting cough, diarrhea, and delirious speech is a result of plundering by fire qi (*i.e.*, fire therapy). There must be difficult urination. This is produced by pressing the *shao yin* for perspiration.

If diaphoresis is imposed on a *shao yin* pattern with inversion but with no sweating, the blood will inevitably be stirred up and noone will know where the blood may go. It may exit from the mouth, the nose, or the eyes. This is inversion below and (blood) exhaustion above, a condition which is difficult to treat.

---

[5] Generally speaking, fuming means steaming. However, using of hot and warm formulas is also sometimes called fuming.

There are five patterns of cold damage. All belong to the category of febrile disease. They are the same disease with different names, (possibly) presenting the same pulse (qualities) but ascribed to different channels. Although, in all cases, the disease is due to damage done by wind, since the sick persons may each have their own old troubles, they cannot be treated with the same method. If a person has had wind damage in the past and (now) sustains heat damage in addition, wind and heat will contend to give rise to wind warm which manifests as inability to contract the four limbs, headache, and bodily heat which remains unresolved in spite of constant sweating. Its treatment lies in the (foot) *shao yin* and *jue yin*. Diaphoresis is prohibited, since diaphoresis will give rise to delirious speech and soliloquy, internal vexation, agitation and restlessness causing insomnia, susceptibility to fright, and confused vision with loss of essence in the eyes (*i.e.*, dull eyes). If a physician treats this with diaphoresis in defiance of perspiration, the physician is committing murder.

The damp warm pattern of cold damage is due to constant subjection of the person to dampness in the past and, (later,) summerheat stroke. When dampness and heat contend, there will develop damp warmth. This disease gives the bitterness of counterflow frigidity of the lower legs, abdominal fullness with (arms) folded against the chest, headache, and pain in the eyes, possibly with raving. The treatment lies in the foot *tai yin*. Diaphoresis is not allowed, for diaphoresis will inevitably result in inability to speak, deafness, pain baffling location, a green-blue complexion of the body, and change in the facial complexion. This is called double summerheat stroke. Such cases will die. They are killed by the physician!

Chapter Two
Diseases Allowing Diaphoresis

The great method (*i.e.*, the general principle) is that it is appropriate to use diaphoresis in the spring and summer.

As regards the promotion of sweating, it is desirable that sweat exit all over (the body) as far as the hands and feet, and it is better still if perspiration is moderate and lasts for a watch. It is, however, undesirable that sweat should flow (copiously) like water. As long as the disease remains unresolved, it is necessary to continue diaphoresis. Because profuse sweating will cause yang to collapse, yang vacuity should not be treated with repeated diaphoresis.

When one takes a decoction of medicinals to promote perspiration, one should stop the administration once (the medicinals) have struck the disease. (In that case,) it is not necessary to finish taking all the dosage.

When diaphoresis is said to be indicated but there is no (proper formula) in decoction form, (a formula) in pill or powder form can be substituted. (In any case, successful) promotion of sweat may effect a resolution. However, (pills or powders) are not as good as decoctions in that they cannot be adjusted in accordance with the patterns.

If a *tai yang* disease has exterior signs which have not yet been resolved and the pulse is floating and weak, this requires diaphoresis for a resolution. The appropriate (formula) is *Gui Zhi Tang* (Cinnamon Twig Decoction).

A *tai yang* disease exhibiting a floating and rapid pulse allows for diaphoresis. This falls within the category indicating *Gui Zhi Tang* (Cinnamon Twig Decoction).

If a *yang ming* disease manifests a slow pulse, copious sweating, and slight aversion to cold, this shows that the exterior has not yet been resolved. It allows for diaphoresis. This falls within the category indicating *Gui Zhi Tang* (Cinnamon Twig Decoction).

Suppose the disease pulse is floating and large and, when asked, the sick person complains merely of hard stools. If diarrhea is due to vacuity, a greatly unfavorable condition, then hard (stools) are due to repletion. Once sweat is promoted, resolution will ensue. Why is this? Because, in the presence of a floating pulse, diaphoresis is required for a resolution.

Suppose cold damage exhibits a weak rather than a bowstring and tight pulse. A weak pulse must be accompanied by thirst. If (the case) is subjected to fire, there will inevitably develop delirious speech. If a weak pulse is accompanied by fever and it is (also) floating, diaphoresis is required to resolve this (disease) and recovery will never fail to follow this.

If a sick person suffers from distressing fever, resolution will ensue once sweating is promoted. If there is a malarial relapse with fever in the afternoon, this falls within the category of the *yang ming*. [It is suspected that the sentence, "If the pulse is replete, it is appropriate to apply precipitation," has been left out.] If the pulse is floating and vacuous, it is necessary to promote sweating. This falls within the category indicating *Gui Zhi Tang* (Cinnamon Twig Decoction).

If a disease manifests constant spontaneous sweating, the constructive qi is harmonious. If the constructive qi is harmonious and the exterior remains unresolved, this is disharmony of the

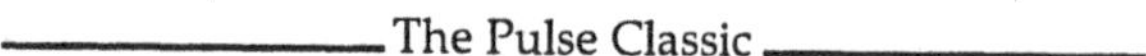

defensive (qi). The constructive circulates within the vessels, acting as yin and governing the internal, while the defensive circulates outside the vessels, acting as yang and governing the external. Nonetheless, if one employs diaphoresis, the defensive will be brought into harmony and a cure will follow. This falls within the category indicating *Gui Zhi Tang* (Cinnamon Twig Decoction).

Suppose a sick person has no illness in the viscera except for fever from time to time. There is spontaneous sweating (but this) is unable to bring about recovery. This indicates that the defensive qi is not harmonious. If sweating is (successfully) promoted before (the fever starts), a cure will ensue. This falls within the category indicating *Gui Zhi Tang* (Cinnamon Twig Decoction).

Suppose the pulse is floating and tight. In the presence of a floating (pulse), there is wind, and, in the presence of a tight (pulse), there is cold. Wind damages the defensive, while cold damages the constructive. Now that the constructive and defensive are both diseased, there is distressed aching in the bone joints. This indicates diaphoresis. The appropriate (formula) is *Ma Huang Tang* (Ephedra Decoction).

If, before a *tai yang* disease is resolved, heat is bound up in the urinary bladder, the person will suffer from a mania-like (disease). There will invariably be blood in the stools, and a cure will follow. Before the exterior is resolved, it is not yet time to attack (internally). It is first necessary to resolve the exterior. This falls within the category indicating *Gui Zhi Tang* (Cinnamon Twig Decoction).

If a *tai yang* disease develops slight dyspnea after being treated with precipitation, this is because the exterior has not yet been resolved. This falls within the category indicating *Gui Zhi Jia Hou Pi Xing Zi Tang* (Cinnamon Twig plus Magnolia & Almond Decoction).[1]

If cold damage exhibiting a floating and tight pulse is not treated by diaphoresis, there may develop spontaneous external bleeding (*i.e.,* nosebleeding). This falls within the category indicating *Ma Huang Tang* (Ephedra Decoction).

---

[1] The ingredients in this formula include Ramulus Cinnamomi Cassia (*Gui Zhi*), Rhizoma Zingiberis (*Jiang*), Radix Paeoniae Lactiflorae (*Shao Yao*), Radix Glycyrrhizae (*Gan Cao*), Cortex Magnoliae Officinalis (*Hou Po*), Semen Pruni Armeniacae (*Xing Ren*), and Fructus Zizyphi Jujubae (*Da Zao*).

196

If a *yang ming* disease exhibits a floating pulse and absence of sweating, the sick person must suffer from dyspnea. Diaphoresis will result in recovery. This falls within the category indicating *Ma Huang Tang* (Ephedra Decoction).

A *tai yin* disease[2] with a floating pulse indicates diaphoresis. This falls within the category indicating *Gui Zhi Tang* (Cinnamon Twig Decoction).

Suppose a *tai yang* disease manifests a floating and tight pulse, absence of sweating, fever, and generalized pain and aching. If it remains unresolved eight or nine days after contraction with the exterior signs still remaining, this requires promotion of sweating by taking a decoction to eliminate (the exterior signs) to a small degree. Then there will arise vexation and heavy eyes and, in severe cases, there is bound to be spontaneous external bleeding (*i.e.*, nosebleeding). Once there is spontaneous external bleeding, (a complete) resolution will ensue. This is because of the existence of heavy yang qi (*i.e.*, exuberant heat). This falls within the category indicating *Ma Huang Tang* (Ephedra Decoction).

If the pulse is floating, the disease is in the exterior and allows for diaphoresis. This falls within the category indicating *Gui Zhi Tang* (Cinnamon Twig Decoction).

Suppose cold damage (is complicated by) six or seven day long absence of bowel movement and manifests headache and fever. If *Cheng Qi Tang* (Support the Qi Decoction)[3] is administered but there arises clear urination instead (of freed defecation), this shows that (the evil) is not in the interior but (rather) in the exterior. (In that case,) it is necessary to promote sweating. If there is headache, there is invariably spontaneous external bleeding. [The preceding sentence is suspected to be an interpolation.] This falls within the category indicating *Gui Zhi Tang* (Cinnamon Twig Decoction).

If diarrhea is followed by generalized pain and aching and automatic normalization of voiding of clear urine, it is urgently necessary to salvage the exterior. The appropriate (formula) is *Gui Zhi Tang* (Cinnamon Twig Decoction).

---

[2] See note 1, Book 7, Ch. 1. The *tai yin* pattern is mainly characterized by abdominal fullness, retching and vomiting, poor appetite, diarrhea, desire for warmth, no thirst, and a slow or moderate pulse.

[3] There are three different commonly used formulas with Support the Qi (*Cheng Qi*) in their names. They are the Minor (*Xiao*), the Major (*Da*), and the Regulate the Stomach Support Qi Decoction (*Tiao Wei Cheng Qi Tang*). The translator suspects that it is the Minor that is meant here in the text. The ingredients of this formula include Radix Et Rhizoma Rhei (*Da Huang*), Fructus Immaturus Aurantii (*Zhi Shi*), and Cortex Magnoliae Officinalis (*Hou Po*).

A *tai yang* disease manifesting headache, fever, (spontaneous) sweating, and aversion to wind or aversion to cold falls within the category indicating *Gui Zhi Tang* (Cinnamon Twig Decoction).

Suppose the *tai yang* disease of wind stroke exhibits a pulse which is floating in the yang (*i.e.,* the superficial level) but soggy and weak in the yin (*i.e.,* the deep level). In the presence of a floating (pulse), there is spontaneous generation of heat, and, in the presence of a soggy and weak (pulse), there is spontaneous sweating. (In that case,) there will be quivering with aversion to cold, shivering as if after a soaking with aversion to wind, continuous mild fever, whistling of the nose, and dry retching. This falls within the category indicating *Gui Zhi Tang* (Cinnamon Twig Decoction).

If a *tai yang* disease manifests fever (in spite of) sweating, this indicates weak constructive and strong defensive. Therefore, to help the evil wind, sweating should be induced. This falls within the category indicating *Gui Zhi Tang* (Cinnamon Twig Decoction).

Suppose a *tai yang* disease is treated with precipitation. If qi then rushes upward, one may administer *Gui Zhi Tang* (Cinnamon Twig Decoction). If there is no qi rushing, one cannot administer it.

If a *tai yang* disease is treated by taking *Gui Zhi Tang* (Cinnamon Twig Decoction), but this produces vexation at first rather than resolution, one ought to first needle Wind Pool (*Feng Chi*, GB 20) and Wind Mansion (*Feng Fu*, GV 16) and then administer *Gui Zhi Tang* (Cinnamon Twig Decoction). Then recovery will ensue.

If the needled point is subject to cold while hot red needling is applied to promote sweating, this may develop a red tubercle. Then running piglet will inevitably develop with qi surging from the lower abdomen up to the heart. (To treat this,) moxa over the tubercle with one cone and then administer *Gui Zhi Jia Gui Tang* (Cinnamon Twig Plus Cinnamon Decoction).[4]

A *tai yang* disease manifesting stiffness of the nape of the neck and back contrarily with sweating and aversion to wind falls within the category indicating *Gui Zhi Jia Ge Gen Tang* (Cinnamon Twig Plus Pueraria Decoction).[5]

---

[4] This formula is composed of the same ingredients as *Gui Zhi Tang* (Cinnamon Twig Decoction) but with double the amount of Ramulus Cinnamomi Cassiae (*Gui Zhi*).

[5] The ingredients in this formula are Ramulus Cinnamomi Cassia (*Gui Zhi*), Rhizoma Zingiberis (*Jiang*), Radix Paeoniae Lactiflorae (*Shao Yao*), Radix Glycyrrhizae (*Gan Cao*), Radix Puerariae (*Ge Gen*), and Fructus Zizyphi Jujubae (*Da Zao*).

A *tai yang* disease manifesting stiffness of the nape and back, absence of sweating, and aversion to wind falls within the category indicating *Ge Gen Tang* (Pueraria Decoction).

A combined disease of the *tai yang* and *yang ming* manifesting diarrhea and no vomiting falls within the category indicating *Ge Gen Tang* (Pueraria Decoction).

A combined disease of the *tai yang* and *yang ming* manifesting no diarrhea but vomiting falls within the category indicating *Ge Gen Jia Ban Xia Tang* (Pueraria Plus Pinellia Decoction).[6]

If a *tai yang* disease categorized as indicating *Gui Zhi (Tang)* (Cinnamon Twig [Decoction]) is treated by a physician contrarily with precipitation, there may arise uncheckable diarrhea. If the pulse is skipping, the exterior is not yet resolved and there (must be) dyspnea and sweating. This falls within the category indicating *Ge Gen Huang Qin Huang Lian Tang* (Pueraria, Scutellaria & Coptis Decoction).[7]

A *tai yang* disease manifesting headache, fever, generalized aching, pain in the lower back, pain and aching in the bone joints, aversion to wind, absence of sweating, and dyspnea falls within the category indicating *Ma Huang Tang* (Ephedra Decoction).

A combined disease of the *tai yang* and *yang ming* manifesting dyspnea and fullness of the chest does not allow precipitation. This falls within the category indicating *Ma Huang Tang* (Ephedra Decoction).

A *tai yang* disease of wind stroke manifesting a floating and tight pulse, fever, aversion to cold, generalized pain and aching, sweat refusing to exit, vexation and agitation, and headache is an indication of *Da Qing Long Tang* (Major Blue-green Dragon Decoction).[8] If the pulse is faint and weak and there is (spontaneous) sweating with aversion to wind, do not take this decoction since taking it will produce inversion with spasm of the sinews and twitching of the flesh. This is a (greatly) unfavorable condition.

---

[6] This formula is composed of Ramulus Cinnamomi Cassiae (*Gui Zhi*), Rhizoma Zingiberis (*Jiang*), Radix Paeoniae Lactiflorae (*Shao Yao*), Radix Glycyrrhizae (*Gan Cao*), Radix Puerariae (*Ge Gen*), Rhizoma Pinelliae Ternatae (*Ban Xia*), and Fructus Zizyphi Jujubae (*Da Zao*).

[7] This is a formula composed of Radix Puerariae (*Ge Gen*), Radix Scutellariae Baicalensis (*Huang Qin*), and Rhizoma Coptidis Chinensis (*Huang Lian*).

[8] This formula is composed of Herba Ephedrae (*Ma Huang*), Semen Pruni Armeniacae (*Xing Ren*), Ramulus Cinnamomi Cassiae (*Gui Zhi*), Radix Glycyrrhizae (*Gan Cao*), Fructus Zizyphi Jujubae (*Da Zao*), Rhizoma Zingiberis (*Jiang*), and Gypsum (*Shi Gao*).

If cold damage exhibits a floating and moderate pulse and no generalized aching but generalized heaviness which may get better at times, and if it is devoid of (any) *shao yin* signs, *Da Qing Long Tang* (Major Blue-green Dragon Decoction) can be used to effect effusion.

Cold damage with the exterior unresolved manifesting as water qi below the heart, dry retching, fever, and cough, possible diarrhea, possible upper esophageal constriction, possible inhibited urination with lower abdominal fullness, or mild dyspnea indicates *Xiao Qing Long Tang* (Minor Blue-green Dragon Decoction).[9]

Suppose cold damage manifests as water qi below the heart, cough, mild dyspnea, fever, and no thirst. If thirst appears upon taking *Xiao Qing Long Tang* (Minor Blue-green Dragon Decoction), this shows that cold is already gone and (the other conditions) are about to be resolved. This falls within the category indicating *Xiao Qing Long Tang* (Minor Blue-green Dragon Decoction).

Suppose a *yang ming* disease of wind stroke manifests a bowstring, floating, and large pulse, shortness of breath, abdominal fullness, and pain in the lateral costal and cardiac regions. Qi becomes blocked [pain is relieved in another version] if (these regions) are pressed for a long time. There is dryness in the nose, sweat refusing to exit, somnolence, yellowing of the whole body including the eyes, difficult urination, tidal fever, occasional retching, and swelling in front and in back of the ears. Then needling may effect a cure to a small degree, but the exterior will still remain unresolved. If the pulse becomes floating again ten days after contraction of the disease, one may administer *Xiao Chai Hu Tang* (Minor Bupleurum Decoction).[10] If the pulse is floating but there are no other (pathological) signs, one may administer *Ma Huang Tang* (Ephedra Decoction). If there is absence of urination with abdominal fullness and there is also retching, (the condition) is incurable.

If a *tai yang* pattern is gone on the tenth day but the pulse is floating and thin and there is somnolence, this shows resolution of the exterior. Suppose there is chest fullness and flank pain, one may administer *Xiao Chai Hu Tang* (Minor Bupleurum Decoction). If the pulse is floating, this (however,) falls within the category indicating *Ma Huang Tang* (Ephedra Decoction).

---

[9] This formula is composed of Herba Asari Cum Radice (*Xi Xin*), Fructus Schisandrae Chinensis (*Wu Wei Zi*), Ramulus Cinnamomi Cassiae (*Gui Zhi*), Rhizoma Zingiberis (*Jiang*), Radix Paeoniae Lactiflorae (*Shao Yao*), Radix Glycyrrhizae (*Gan Cao*), Rhizoma Pinelliae Ternatae (*Ban Xia*), and Fructus Zizyphi Jujubae (*Da Zao*).

[10] The ingredients in this formula include Radix Bupleuri (*Chai Hu*), Radix Panacis Ginseng (*Ren Shen*), Rhizoma Zingiberis (*Jiang*), Radix Scutellariae Baicalensis (*Huang Qin*), Radix Glycyrrhizae (*Gan Cao*), Rhizoma Pinelliae Ternatae (*Ban Xia*), and Fructus Zizyphi Jujubae (*Da Zao*).

Suppose there is wind stroke with alternating cold and heat. From the fifth or sixth day onward, this cold damage may manifest tormenting fullness of the chest and lateral costal regions, indistinct speech, no desire for food and drink, heart vexation, and frequent retching. There is also possible vexation in the chest with no retching, possible thirst, possible abdominal pain, possible glomus and tightness in the lateral costal region, possible palpitations of the heart and inhibited urination, possible absence of thirst with presence of moderate external heat, or cough. This indicates *Xiao Chai Hu Tang* (Minor Bupleurum Decoction).

If, on the fourth or fifth day, cold damage manifests as generalized heat, aversion to wind, stiffness of the nape of the neck, fullness in the lateral costal region, warm hands and feet, and thirst, this falls within the category indicating *Xiao Chai Hu Tang* (Minor Bupleurum Decoction).

If, on the sixth or seventh day, cold damage manifests as fever, slight aversion to cold, distressed aching in the limb joints, mild retching, and propping binding below the heart — (showing that) the exterior signs remain unresolved — this falls within the category indicating *Chai Hu Gui Zhi Tang* (Bupleurum & Cinnamon Twig Decoction).[11]

(To treat) a two or three day old *shao yin* disease, one may administer *Ma Huang Fu Zi Gan Cao Tang* (Ephedra, Aconite & Licorice Decoction)[12] to promote moderate perspiration. Because there are as yet no interior signs or symptoms in this pattern on the second or third day, moderate perspiration is alright.

A floating pulse, inhibited urination, mild fever, and wasting (*i.e.*, intense) thirst (require) administering *Wu Ling San* (Five [Ingredients] Poria Powder)[13] to disinhibit urination and promote sweating.

---

[11] The ingredients in this formula are Radix Bupleuri (*Chai Hu*), Radix Panacis Ginseng (*Ren Shen*), Rhizoma Zingiberis (*Jiang*), Radix Scutellariae Baicalensis (*Huang Qin*), Radix Glycyrrhizae (*Gan Cao*), Rhizoma Pinelliae Ternatae (*Ban Xia*), Fructus Zizyphi Jujubae (*Da Zao*), and Radix Paeoniae Lactiflorae (*Shao Yao*).

[12] This formula is composed of Radix Ephedrae (*Ma Huang*), Radix Glycyrrhizae (*Gan Cao*), and Radix Praeparatus Aconiti Carmichaeli (*Fu Zi*).

[13] The ingredients in this formula include Sclerotium Polypori Umbellati (*Zhu Ling*), Sclerotium Poriae Cocos (*Fu Ling*), Rhizoma Alismatis (*Ze Xie*), and Ramulus Cinnamomi Cassiae (*Gui Zhi*).

Chapter Three
Post-Diaphoresis Diseases

The combined disease of the two yang (*i.e.*, the *tai yang* and *yang ming*) results from promoting sweating in the initial stage of a *tai yang* disease. Perspiration is induced but not adequately; so (the *tai yang* pattern) is transmuted into a *yang ming* (pattern). Then moderate spontaneous sweating continues and there is no aversion to cold. Before the *tai yang* pattern is not yet over,[1] precipitation is not allowed since it will lead to a (greatly) unfavorable condition. In such cases, one may apply diaphoresis in a small way. If the face is full red all over, yang qi (*i.e.*, heat) is depressed and bound in the exterior. It is necessary to apply effusion (*i.e.*, diaphoresis) and fuming. If sweating is promoted inadequately and quite insignificantly, it is still unable to out-thrust the depressed bound yang qi. When sweat ought to be exiting but is not, the sick person will suffer from agitation and vexation and a pain baffling location. The pain appears in the abdomen at one time but in the four limbs at another. It cannot be (exactly) located by means of palpation. The person is short of breath and can only adopt a sitting position. This is a result of inadequate diaphoresis. Continue to promote perspiration and a cure will ensue. What reveals inadequate diaphoresis? A choppy pulse.

If, before (the physician) feels the pulse, the sick person has his arms folded against his heart region and if the physician instructs him to cough but he does not do it promptly, this shows that his ears must be deaf. The cause of this deafness is vacuity due to repeated diaphoresis.

After sweating is promoted, drinking quantities of water may produce dyspnea, as may taking a bath.

If diaphoresis results in inability to take either water or medicinals through the mouth, this is a (greatly) unfavorable condition. If diaphoresis is continued, there will inevitably arise incessant vomiting and diarrhea.

If a *yang ming* disease manifests spontaneous sweating, yet the (attending) physician employs diaphoresis nonetheless, then the person will suffer from endless slight vexation though the disease is already overcome. This arises from hard stools. Because fluids are lost and the stomach is dry, the stools are hard. (At this juncture,) one should inquire about the daily frequency of

---

[1] The *tai yang* pattern is characterized by exterior signs, for example, fever and aversion to cold. Therefore, when it is said that the *tai yang* pattern is over, this means that there are no more exterior signs.

urination. If (the sick person) voided three or four times a day in the past but now (only) voids two times, then one can say that evacuation will be brought to pass soon. Now that urination has become less frequent, fluids must have returned to the stomach. Therefore, one can know that the time comes to defecate.

If diaphoresis is applied in defiance of profuse sweating, this will make yang collapse. If delirious speech appears and the pulse becomes short, this is death. If the pulse becomes harmonious on its own, this is not death.

When cold damage is treated with diaphoresis, there may develop yellowing of the body including the eyes. This is the consequence of mutual contending between cold and dampness which remain unresolved internally.

If the sick person has been suffering from cold and is now treated by diaphoresis, the stomach will become cold and, therefore, vomiting of roundworms will inevitably arise.

If following diaphoresis, a *tai yang* disease develops incessant leaking sweat and the person suffers from aversion to wind, difficult urination, and slight hypertonicity of and difficulty in contracting or stretching the four limbs, this indicates *Gui Zhi Jia Fu Zi Tang* (Cinnamon Plus Aconite Decoction).[2]

If the pulse remains surging and large after administering *Gui Zhi Tang* (Cinnamon Twig Decoction) which has induced profuse perspiration, continue administering *Gui Zhi Tang* (Cinnamon Twig Decoction). If (the illness) looks like malaria, attacking three times a day with relief following perspiration, this indicates *Gui Zhi Er Ma Huang Yi Tang* (Cinnamon Twigs Two, Ephedra One Decoction).[3]

If, after taking *Gui Zhi Tang* (Cinnamon Twig Decoction), profuse sweating results in severe vexation and unquenchable thirst and if the pulse remains surging and large, this indicates *Bai Hu Tang* (White Tiger Decoction).[4]

---

[2] This formula is composed of Ramulus Cinnamomi Cassiae (*Gui Zhi*), Radix Paeoniae Lactiflorae (*Shao Yao*), Radix Glycyrrhizae (*Gan Cao*), Rhizoma Zingiberis (*Jiang*), Fructus Zizyphi Jujubae (*Da Zao*), and Radix Praeparatus Aconiti Carmichaeli (*Fu Zi*).

[3] The ingredients in this formula are Ramulus Cinnamomi Cassiae (*Gui Zhi*), Radix Paeoniae Lactiflorae (*Shao Yao*), Radix Glycyrrhizae (*Gan Cao*), Rhizoma Zingiberis (*Jiang*), Fructus Zizyphi Jujubae (*Da Zao*), Herba Ephedrae (*Ma Huang*), and Semen Pruni Armeniacae (*Xing Ren*).

[4] This formula is composed of Rhizoma Anemarrhenae (*Zhi Mu*), Gypsum (*Shi Gao*), Radix Glycyrrhizae (*Gan Cao*), and Semen Oryzae Sativae (*Jing Mi*).

Suppose cold damage manifests as a floating pulse, spontaneous sweating, frequent urination, heart vexation, slight aversion to cold, and hypertonicity of the feet. If *Gui Zhi Tang* (Cinnamon Twig Decoction) is abused with a view to attacking the exterior, inversion will develop immediately after taking this decoction and there will be a dry throat, vexation and agitation, and counterflow vomiting. One should then prescribe *Gan Cao Gan Jiang Tang* (Licorice & Dry Ginger Decoction)[5] to recover yang. Then inversion will be cured and the feet will become warm. Furthermore, administer *Shao Yao Gan Cao Tang* (Peony & Licorice Decoction).[6] Then the feet will be able to stretch. In case of stomach qi disharmony and delirious speech, one may administer *Cheng Qi Tang* (Support the Qi Decoction). If (the sick person) has suffered double diaphoresis and red-hot needling, *Si Ni Tang* (Four Counterflows Decoction)[7] is indicated.

If cold damage has a relapse of vexation approximately a half day after being resolved by diaphoresis and the pulse is floating and rapid, diaphoresis can be continued. This indicates *Gui Zhi Tang* (Cinnamon Twig Decoction).

If, following diaphoresis, there is generalized aching and pain and the pulse is deep and slow, this indicates *Gui Zhi Jia Shao Yao Sheng Jiang Ren Shen Tang* (Cinnamon Twig Plus Peony, Fresh Ginger & Ginseng Decoction).[8]

After sweating is promoted, it is no longer permissible to administer *Gui Zhi Tang* (Cinnamon Twig Decoction). If there is sweating with dyspnea but no great heat, one may administer *Ma Huang Xing Zi Gan Cao Shi Gao Tang* (Ephedra, Almond, Licorice & Gypsum Decoction).[9]

If, following excessive diaphoresis, the person has their arms folded over their heart (because of) palpitations of the heart, desiring to suppress (those palpitations), this indicates *Gui Zhi Gan Cao*

---

[5] There are only two ingredients in this formula; namely, Radix Glycyrrhizae (*Gan Cao*) and dry Rhizoma Zingiberis (*Gan Jiang*).

[6] There are only two ingredients in this formula: Radix Albus Paeoniae Lactiflorae (*Bao Shao*) and Radix Glycyrrhizae (*Gan Cao*).

[7] This formula is composed of Radix Glycyrrhizae (*Gan Cao*), dry Rhizoma Zingiberis (*Gan Jiang*), and Radix Praeparatus Aconiti Carmichaeli (*Fu Zi*).

[8] The ingredients of this formula include Ramulus Cinnamomi Cassiae (*Gui Zhi*), Radix Paeoniae Lactiflorae (*Shao Yao*), Radix Glycyrrhizae (*Gan Cao*), Rhizoma Zingiberis (*Jiang*), Fructus Zizyphi Jujubae (*Da Zao*), and Radix Panacis Ginseng (*Ren Shen*).

[9] This formula is composed of Herba Ephedrae (*Ma Huang*), Semen Pruni Armeniacae (*Xing Ren*), Radix Glycyrrhizae (*Gan Cao*), and Gypsum (*Shi Gao*).

Tang (Cinnamon Twig & Licorice Decoction).[10]

If, following diaphoresis, the person has palpitations below the umbilicus and is inclined to develop running piglet, this indicates *Fu Ling Gui Zhi Gan Cao Da Zao Tang* (Poria, Cinnamon Twig, Licorice & Red Dates Decoction).[11]

Abdominal distention and fullness following diaphoresis indicates *Hou Po Sheng Jiang Ban Xia Gan Cao Ren Shen Tang* (Magnolia, Fresh Ginger, Pinellia, Licorice & Ginseng Decoction).[12]

If, rather than resolution, diaphoresis results in aversion to cold, this is due to vacuity and indicates *Shao Yao Gan Cao Fu Zi Tang* (Peony, Licorice & Aconite Decoction).[13] If there is no aversion to cold but there is heat, this is due to repletion. It is necessary to harmonize the stomach qi, and the appropriate (formula) is *Xiao Cheng Qi Tang* (Minor Support the Qi Decoction).[14]

If a *tai yang* disease is treated by diaphoresis and then profuse sweat is induced, the stomach will become dry and there will be vexation with inability to fall asleep. If the person desires to drink, he should drink a little to harmonize the stomach. Then there will be relief.

If, following diaphoresis, the pulse is floating and rapid and there is also distressing thirst, this indicates *Wu Ling San* (Five [Ingredients] Poria Powder).

Cold damage manifesting (spontaneous) sweating and thirst indicates *Wu Ling San* (Five [Ingredients] Poria Powder). If there is no thirst, this (then) indicates *Fu Ling Gan Cao Tang* (Poria & Licorice Decoction).[15]

---

[10] This formula is composed of only two ingredients: Ramulus Cinnamomi Cassiae (*Gui Zhi*) and Radix Glycyrrhizae (*Gan Cao*).

[11] This formula is composed of Sclerotium Poriae Cocos (*Fu Ling*), Ramulus Cinnamomi Cassiae (*Gui Zhi*), Radix Glycyrrhizae (*Gan Cao*), and Fructus Zizyphi Jujubae (*Da Zao*).

[12] The ingredients in this formula are Cortex Magnoliae Officinalis (*Hou Po*), Rhizoma Zingiberis (*Jiang*), Rhizoma Pinelliae Ternatae (*Ban Xia*), Radix Glycyrrhizae (*Gan Cao*), and Radix Panacis Ginseng (*Ren Shen*).

[13] This formula is composed of Radix Paeoniae Lactiflorae (*Shao Yao*), Radix Glycyrrhizae (*Gan Cao*), and Radix Praeparatus Aconiti Carmichaeli (*Fu Zi*).

[14] See note 3, Ch. 2 of the present book.

[15] This formula is composed of Sclerotium Poriae Cocos (*Fu Ling*), Radix Glycyrrhizae (*Gan Cao*), Ramulus Cinnamomi Cassiae (*Gui Zhi*), and Rhizoma Zingiberis (*Jiang*).

Suppose a *tai yang* disease is treated by diaphoresis which fails to effect a resolution. If the person then suffers from fever, palpitations below the heart, dizziness, convulsion of the body, and stumbling, this indicates *Zhen Wu Tang* (Turtle & Snake Decoction).[16]

If, after cold damage has been resolved by diaphoresis, there develops stomach disharmony, glomus and tightness below the heart, dry retching, a putrefying food smell (in the mouth), water qi in the lateral costal regions, thunderous rumbling in the abdomen, and diarrhea, this indicates *Sheng Jiang Xie Xin Tang* (Fresh Ginger Drain the Heart Decoction).[17]

If, after cold damage has been treated by diaphoresis, fever remains unresolved and there develops glomus and tightness in the cardiac region, retching and diarrhea, this indicates *Da Chai Hu Tang* (Major Bupleurum Decoction).

If, by the third day, a *tai yang* pattern remains unresolved in spite of diaphoresis, manifesting steaming fever, this is ascribed to the stomach and indicates *Cheng Qi Tang* (Support the Qi Decoction).

(The pattern of) heat refusing to leave in spite of profuse perspiration, abdominal urgency, aching in the four limbs, diarrhea, inversion counterflow, and aversion to cold indicates *Si Ni Tang* (Four Counterflows Decoction).

Massive perspiration causing yang collapse and delirious speech does not allow for precipitation. It should be treated with *Chai Hu Gui Zhi Tang* (Bupleurum & Cinnamon Twig Decoction) to harmonize the constructive and defensive and to the free flow of fluids and humors. Then a cure will ensue by itself.

———————————

[16] The ingredients in this formula include Sclerotium Poriae Cocos (*Fu Ling*), Radix Paeoniae Lactiflorae (*Shao Yao*), Rhizoma Zingiberis (*Jiang*), Rhizoma Atractylodis Macrocephalae (*Bai Zhu*), and Radix Praeparatus Aconiti Carmichaeli (*Fu Zi*).

[17] This formula is composed of uncooked Rhizoma Zingiberis (*Sheng Jiang*), Radix Glycyrrhizae (*Gan Cao*), Radix Panacis Ginseng (*Ren Shen*), dry Rhizoma Zingiberis (*Gan Jiang*), Rhizoma Coptidis Chinensis (*Huang Lian*), Radix Scutellariae Baicalensis (*Huang Qin*), Rhizoma Pinelliae Ternatae (*Ban Xia*), and Fructus Zizyphi Jujubae (*Da Zao*).

Diseases Not Allowing Ejection

A *tai yang* disease should manifest aversion to cold with fever. Suppose now there is spontaneous sweating contrarily accompanied by no aversion to cold and no fever and the pulse is thin and rapid in the *guan*. This is the fault of the (attending) physician who has abused ejection. If ejection is applied one or two days after contraction of disease, hungering in the abdomen will develop yet the mouth will be unable to take in food. If it is applied three or four days (after contraction), then hating (hot) gruel, desire for cold food, and vomiting in the evening of the food taken in the morning will develop. All this is impugned to the (attending) physician who has abused ejection. This is a minor unfavorable condition.

If treated by ejection, a *tai yang* disease which was characterized by aversion to cold manifests no aversion to cold but (so high a fever that the sick person) does not want their clothes on, this is due to internal vexation caused by ejection.

Suppose a *shao yin* disease is characterized by vomiting of food and drink immediately upon ingestion and distressing desire of the heart but inability to vomit (when no food is taken in). If this is repletion in the chest, it does not allow precipitation at the onset if the hands and feet are cold and the pulse is bowstring and slow. If there is cold rheum over the diaphragm causing dry retching, ejection is not allowed. It is necessary to apply a warming (therapy).

The various cases of counterflow frigidity of the four limbs do not allow ejection, neither does a person suffering from vacuity.

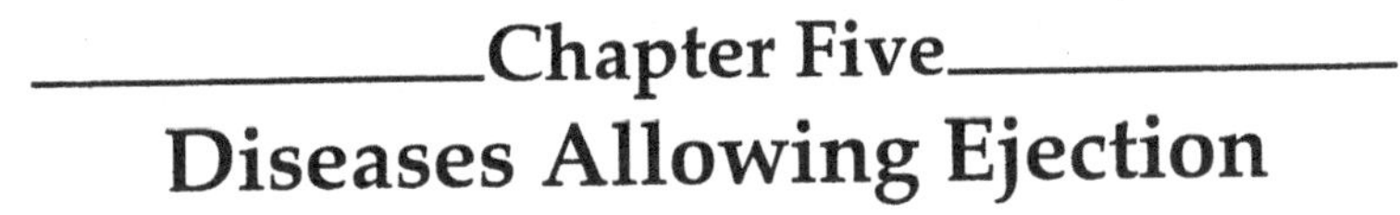

Diseases Allowing Ejection

The great method (*i.e.*, general principle) is, in spring, ejection is appropriate.

When taking a decoction to induce vomiting, once the disease has been struck, (the sick person) should take it no further. It is not necessary to finish up all the (prescribed) dosage.

Suppose a disease is like a pattern indicating *Gui Zhi Tang* (Cinnamon Twig Decoction). If there is no headache or stiffness of the nape, the *cun* opening pulse is slightly floating, and there is glomus and tightness in the chest with qi surging up into the throat causing inability to breathe, then there is cold in the chest. It is necessary to apply ejection (to treat this).

The various diseases of repletion in the chest manifesting as oppression and pain in the chest, inability to take in food, desire to have someone press (the chest), spitting of foul sputum, more than ten bowel movements per day, and a slow pulse which is faint and slippery in the *cun* necessitate ejection. Diarrhea will be relieved upon ejection.

A *shao yin* disease manifesting vomiting immediately upon ingestion and a distressing desire of the heart but inability to vomit requires ejection.

If there is food retention in the upper venter, ejection is required.

If the sick person suffers from inversion frigidity of the hands and feet and the pulse becomes suddenly tight, then there are evils bound up in the chest. There is fullness below and vexation of the heart and inability to take in food in spite of hunger. Since the disease is located in the chest, ejection is required.

Chapter Six
Diseases Not Allowing Precipitation

Suppose the pulse is soggy and weak, weak contrarily in the *guan* and soggy contrarily in the top (*i.e.*, the *cun*), faint contrarily in the upper (*i.e.*, the *cun*) and choppy contrarily in the lower (*i.e.*, the *chi*). In the presence of a faint (pulse), there is an insufficiency of yang qi, and, in view of the choppiness, there is absence of blood. When yang qi contrarily becomes faint, there will be wind stroke with perspiration contrarily accompanied by agitation and vexation. Because the choppiness is a result of absence of blood, there will be inversion and cold. When yang is faint, precipitation is not allowed since precipitation will produce glomus and tightness below the heart.

If there is a stirring qi to the right (of the umbilicus), precipitation is not allowed. (In that case,) precipitation will exhaust the fluids internally, giving rise to dry throat and nose, dizziness, and palpitations.

If there is a stirring qi to the left (of the umbilicus), precipitation is not allowed. (In that case,) precipitation would produce hypertonicity in the abdomen, inability to take in food, exacerbation of the stirring qi, and cuddling up in spite of generalized heat.

If there is a stirring qi above (the umbilicus), precipitation is not allowed. (In that case,) precipitation will produce distressing heat in the palms, cold on the surface of the body, spontaneous sweating due to (internal) heat, and a desire to drink to quench (this heat).

If there is a stirring qi below (the umbilicus), precipitation is not allowed. (In that case,) precipitation will produce abdominal fullness, dizziness arising on attempt to rise up, (evacuation of) clear grain (immediately) after eating, and glomus and tightness below the heart.

Block and constriction of the throat does not allow for precipitation. (In that case,) precipitation will produce top-heaviness, failure (even) of water to descend, cuddling up, generalized hypertonicity and pain, and more than ten bowel movements per day.

The various cases of external repletion do not allow for precipitation since precipitation will result in mild fever. If the pulse disappears, there will arise inversion and heat around the umbilicus.

The various cases of vacuity do not allow for precipitation since precipitation will produce thirst. Those who drink are easy to recover. Those who are averse to water are serious.

Suppose the pulse is soggy and weak, weak contrarily in the *guan* and soggy contrarily in the top, bowstring contrarily in the upper and faint contrarily in the lower. In the presence of a bowstring (pulse), there is stirring yang, and, in the presence of a faint (pulse), there is yin cold. This is repletion above and vacuity below. (The sick person must) have a desire for warmth. The faintness and bowstring (images) combine to indicate vacuity, and vacuity does not allow for precipitation. In the presence of this faint (pulse), there is coughing, and coughing gives rise to vomiting of foamy substances. If precipitation is employed, coughing will stop, but incessant diarrhea will arise and there will be a sensation of worms eating in the chest, vomiting upon ingestion of gruel, inhibited urination, hypertonicity of the lateral costal regions, difficult dyspneic breathing, a contracting discomfort between the nape and upper back, insensitivity of the upper arms, sweating contrarily accompanied by excessive cold, ice-cold body, dim vision, talkativeness, and entrance of much grain qi (*i.e.*, a large food intake). This threatens bankruptcy of the center (*chu zhong*).[1] Bankruptcy of the center is characterized by a desire to speak but inability to move the tongue.

Suppose the pulse is soggy and weak, weak contrarily in the *guan* and soggy contrarily in the top, floating contrarily in the upper and rapid contrarily in the lower. In the presence of a floating (pulse), there is yang vacuity, and, in the presence of a rapid (pulse), there is absence of blood. If the floating points to vacuity, the rapidity suggests generation of heat. Since floating means vacuity, there is spontaneous sweating and aversion to cold. The rapidity suggests pain with cold shuddering. When the pulse is faint and weak in the *guan,* there is hypertonicity under the chest with dyspnea, fullness, copious sweating, and inability to breathe. Pain in the flanks arises with breathing. When cold shuddering starts, it resembles (an episode) of malaria. If the physician abuses precipitation, the pulse will be made urgent and rapid and fever, manic walking, the illusion of ghosts, glomus under the heart, dribbling urination, extreme tightness of the lower abdomen, and hematuria will develop.

Suppose the pulse is soggy and tight. In the presence of a soggy (pulse), yang qi is faint, and, in the presence of a tight (pulse), there is cold in the constructive (*i.e.,* the blood). Faint yang and wind stroke of the defensive give rise to fever and aversion to cold. Tight (*i.e.,* cold) constructive and cold qi in the stomach give rise to mild retching and heart vexation. If the physician mistakes this for (a case of) great heat and applies diaphoresis to resolve the muscles, then there will be collapse of yang giving rise to vacuity vexation and agitation and tormenting glomus and tightness below the heart. (Now) both the exterior and the interior are exhausted. There will be dizziness on attempt to rise up, guest (*i.e.,* vacuity) heat in the skin, and vexation causing inability to fall asleep. Unaware of the cold qi in the stomach and tight (*i.e.,* severe) cold in the Origin Pass, (the physician), who is at a loss as to what technique and therapy to employ, may pump water (*i.e.,* treats with diaphoresis) to pour (sweat) onto the body (of the sick person. As a result,) the guest heat may come to a temporary halt, but cold shuddering will reappear. Then (the sick person) is covered with layers of quilts. Perspiration is induced and dizziness, tugging of the body, recurring cold shuddering, and slightly difficult urination develop. Because the cold qi is provoked by water, clear grain is not allowed to stay for a moment (in the stomach and intestines. Thus) there will arise vomiting, prolapse of the rectum, turning about restlessly (on the bed), slight counterflow frigidity of the hands and feet, a cold trunk, and internal vexation. If (the physician) intends to put off rescuing (for a moment), it will be impossible to recover the chance (to save the sick person).

---

[1] This term refers to the central qi or the stomach qi bordering on expiry yet with suddenly enlarged food intake. This is a dangerous case. Expiration of the central qi often manifests as frigidity of the four limbs and incessant diarrhea for example.

Suppose the pulse is floating and large. In the presence of a floating (pulse), there is qi repletion, and, in the presence of a large (pulse), there is blood vacuity. Blood vacuity is absence of yin. (In that case,) solitary yang has to descend into the yin (*i.e.*, genitalia) part, and there should arise difficult urination and a vacuous bladder. Suppose now, on the contrary, urination is uninhibited with sweating copious. The defensive should be faint. If now it is, on the contrary, the more replete, it will make fluids issue out in every direction. Because the constructive is already exhausted and the blood has run out, vacuity vexation, insomnia, thin blood, and wasted flesh develop. Fluids are now boiled away. If the physician continues to administer toxic medicinals to attack the stomach, this will produce dual vacuity. (Then) the departure of the guest (*i.e.*, vacuous) yang is not far off and death will inevitably come with evacuation of filthy sludge-like stools.

If the instep pulse is slow and moderate, the stomach qi is in good order. If the instep pulse is floating and rapid, the floating (quality) points to a damaged stomach and the rapidity to a disturbed spleen. This was not originally a disease but is the result of the (attending) physician's (use of) precipitation. When the constructive and defensive are sunken internally, a faint (pulse image) should precede the rapidity. (Now,) however, the pulse is floating all the time. Therefore, the person must suffer from hard (stools), and belching will result in relief. Why is this? The spleen pulse ought to be moderate, but now it is rapid. This reveals a disturbed spleen. Since the rapid (pulse image) should have been preceded by faintness, it is known that the spleen qi fails to exercise its government, thus giving rise to hard stools and relief by belching. Now the pulse is contrarily floating, and rapidity has substituted for faintness. (Therefore,) evil qi has lodged predominantly, giving rise to a hungry (sensation) in the heart. This evil heat, (however,) does not disperse grain, (but is capable of producing) tidal fever and thirst. The rapid pulse should become slow and moderate, and the pulse should be restored to the same rate as before. (Then) the sick person will feel hungry (and be able to take in food). If a rapid pulse frequently appears, malign sores will break out.

The rapid pulse should keep up its rate without interruption. If there is interruption, there are evils bound up. Then the righteous qi not only cannot be restored but will (also) be bound up in the viscera. In consequence, the evil qi is upborne to engage the skin and hair. The rapid pulse does not allow for precipitation, for precipitation will inevitably produce vexation and incessant diarrhea.

A *shao yin* disease with a faint pulse does not allow for diaphoresis since there is absence of yang (in this case). If there is vacuity of yang and the pulse is weak and choppy in the *chi*, precipitation is also not allowed.

If the pulse is floating and large, it is necessary to employ diaphoresis. If, on the contrary, the physician employs precipitation, this will cause a greatly unfavorable condition.

Suppose the pulse is floating and large, and contrarily there is tightness below the heart. Then there is heat which is ascribed to the viscera. One may attack (internally, *i.e.*, precipitate) but should not employ diaphoresis. Suppose (there is heat) which is ascribed to the bowels. Then frequent urination will be accompanied by hard stools, profuse sweating will bring relief, but scanty perspiration will be accompanied by difficult defecation. If the pulse is slow, it is not yet time to attack (internally).

A combined disease of the two yang (*i.e.*, the *tai yang* and *yang ming*) is a result of diaphoresis at the initial stage of a *tai yang* pattern. Sweat is promoted but not adequately. Therefore, the *tai yang* is transmuted into the *yang ming* which is disposed to give rise to spontaneous sweating with no aversion to cold. Before the *tai yang* pattern has come to an end, precipitation is not allowed since precipitation would bring to pass a (greatly) unfavorable condition.

The disease of chest binding with a floating and large pulse does not allow for precipitation, for precipitation will be followed by instant death.

A combined illness of the *tai yang* and *yang ming* manifesting dyspnea and chest fullness does not allow for precipitation.

For a combined disease of the *tai yang* and *shao yang* manifesting glomus and tightness below the heart, stiffness of the nape of the neck, and dizziness, do not employ precipitation.

The various cases of counterflow inversion of the four limbs do not allow for precipitation. Neither does the case of vacuity.

The disease of desire to vomit does not allow for precipitation.

A *tai yang* disease with exterior manifestations unresolved does not allow for precipitation since precipitation will produce a (greatly) unfavorable condition.

If a disease that starts in the yang (*i.e.*, the exterior) is treated contrarily by precipitation, heat will penetrate deeply giving rise to chest binding. If an illness that starts in the yin (*i.e.*, the interior) is treated contrarily by precipitation, glomus will develop. If the glomus [the word glomus is suspected to be a mistaken redundancy] pulse is floating and tight and precipitation is used contrarily, then the tight (quality) will contrarily come into (the internal)[2] and consequently glomus will develop.

If a disease of abundance of yang manifesting heat is treated by precipitation, tightness will develop (below the heart).

If there has been vacuity and one uses (precipitation) to attack the heat (that there is), retching will inevitably develop.

If there is absence of yang with strong yin accompanied by hard (stools), precipitation will inevitably produce clear grain (diarrhea) and abdominal fullness.

If a *tai yin* disease manifesting abdominal fullness, vomiting, and inability of food to descend is treated by precipitation, it will become worse. Abdominal pain will arise from time to time with binding and tightness under the chest.

A *jue yin*[3] disease manifesting wasting thirst, qi surging up, aching and heat in the heart, hunger with no desire for food, and, in the extreme, a desire to vomit will not be stopped by precipitation.

(Taken with) a *shao yin* disease, the person may suffer from vomiting upon ingestion of food and drink and a distressing desire of the heart but inability to vomit (when no food is taken in). At its onset, the hands and feet are cold and the pulse is bowstring and slow. This is due to repletion in the chest. It does not allow for precipitation.

If, on the fifth or sixth day, cold damage manifests no chest binding with a soft abdomen and the pulse is vacuous in addition to inversion, precipitation is not allowed. (In that case,) precipitation will bring about collapse of the blood and (hence) death.

Suppose cold damage manifests fever, headache all the time, and mild perspiration. If it is treated by diaphoresis, inability to recognize people will develop. If it is treated by fuming, inability to urinate, and cardiac and abdominal fullness will develop. If it is treated by precipitation, shortness of breath, abdominal fullness, difficult urination, headache, and rigidity of the back will develop. If it is treated with red-hot needling, spontaneous external bleeding (*i.e.*, nosebleeding) will inevitably arise.

---

2   This means that the pulse becomes deep and taut.

3   See note 3, Ch. 2, this present book. The *jue yin* pattern is the last stage of cold damage characterized by extreme vacuity. The distinctive manifestation of the *jue yin* pattern is counterflow frigidity of the extremities

If cold damage manifests a tight pulse in both the yin and yang (*i.e.*, from the *cun* to the *chi*) accompanied by aversion to cold and a fever, the pulse is inclined towards an inversion (pulse). An inversion (pulse) is a pulse coming large at first and then gradually becoming small. Later it gradually becomes large again. This is the feature (of the inversion pulse). In the case of severe aversion to cold, there is continuous mild perspiration with sore throat. In the case of abundance of heat, there is reddening of the eyes with dim vision. If the physician employs effusion (*i.e.*, diaphoresis), the throat will be damaged. If precipitation is employed, there will be shut closed eyes. If there is abundance of cold, there will arise (diarrhea) with clear grain; or in case of abundance of heat, there will be (diarrhea) with pus and blood in the stools. Fuming will result in jaundice, and ironing will result in a dry throat. Those with uninhibited urination are savable, but those with difficult urination are in danger.

Suppose cold damage manifests fever, blowing out rough hot qi from the mouth, headache, yellowing of the eyes, and uncheckable runny snivel nosebleeding. Those who are greedy for water will invariably develop retching. Those who are averse to water will suffer from inversion. If this is treated with precipitation, sores in the throat will develop. If the hands and feet are warm, there is pressure in the rectum with pus and blood in the stools.[4] In the case of headache and yellowing of the eyes, precipitation will ensue in shut closed eyes. If those who are greedy for water are treated with precipitation, the pulse will inevitably become an inversion (pulse) and the voice will become chirpy (*i.e.*, confused and obscure) with constriction of the throat. If this is treated with diaphoresis, cold shuddering and vacuity of both yin and yang will arise. If those who are averse to water are treated with precipitation, internal cold will arise with no desire for food and untransformed grain in the stools. If they are treated with diaphoresis, damage will be done to the mouth. The tongue fur will become glossy, and there will be vexation and agitation. If the pulse is rapid and replete and there has been no evacuation of stools for six or seven consecutive days, there will inevitably be blood in the stools. If diaphoresis is employed nonetheless, urination will become disinhibited automatically.

Suppose two or three days after contraction (of cold damage), the pulse is weak with no signs of the *tai yang* indicating *Chai Hu Tang* (Bupleurum Decoction) but with vexation and agitation and tightness below the heart. On the fourth day, even though there is ability to eat, one should administer a small dose of *Cheng Qi Tang* (Support the Qi Decoction) to harmonize (the stomach) to a small degree in order to effect some sort of relief. On the sixth day, one may administer one *sheng* (*i.e.*, liter) of *Cheng Qi Tang* (Support the Qi Decoction). Suppose there has been no defecation for six or seven consecutive days. If there is scant urine, though there has been no

---

[4] The translator suspects there is a typographical error in this sentence in the original text and that the sentence should accordingly be rendered as follows: If the hands and feet are warm, precipitation will produce pressure in the rectum and pus and blood in the stools.

defecation (for days), only the beginning end (of the stool) is hard but the rest is thin liquid. Before the stool is set hard (completely), attacking (internally) will inevitably result in thin stool diarrhea. One may attack only after urination is disinhibited and the stool is set hard.

When visceral binding[5] manifests no yang signs, (that is to say,) there is cold but no heat, if the person is contrarily quiet with glossy tongue fur, attacking (internally) is not allowed.

Cold damage manifesting frequent vomiting cannot be treated with attacking (therapy) even though there are manifestations of a *yang ming* disease.

A *yang ming* disease with tidal fever can be treated with *Cheng Qi Tang* (Support the Qi Decoction) if (the stool) is slightly hard. If (the stool) is not hard, (this formula) cannot be administered. If there has been absence of defecation for six or seven consecutive days, there is possibly dry stool. The method to determine this is to try administering a little *Cheng Qi Tang* (Support the Qi Decoction).

If there is flatus turning in the abdomen, this betrays dry stool. Only then can one attack (internally). If there is no flatus turning, this shows that only the beginning end (of the stool) is hard but the rest is thin liquid. This prohibits attacking, for attacking (in that case) would inevitably produce abdominal fullness and inability to take in food. Those who desire to drink will develop retching. If fever arises later, the stool is bound to become hard again. Then one may administer *Xiao Cheng Qi Tang* (Minor Support the Qi Decoction) to harmonize (the stomach). If there is no turning of flatus, one should be careful not to attack (internally).

If a *yang ming* disease manifests a red complexion all over the body, attacking (therapy) is not allowed. (Otherwise,) fever, yellowing (of the skin), and inhibited urination will arise.

A *yang ming* disease manifesting tightness and fullness right under the heart does not allow attacking (internally) since attacking will produce incessant diarrhea and (hence) death. If the diarrhea is checked, (there is hope of) recovery.

If a *yang ming* disease with spontaneous sweating is treated by diaphoresis, urination will remain uninhibited. This will cause (the fluids) to become exhausted internally. Even though (the stool) is hard, one cannot attack (internally). Only when (the sick person) has a desire to defecate is it appropriate to conduct and free (the stool) with boiled honey. Radix Trichosanthis Curcumeroidis (*Tu Gua Gen*) or pig bile are (also) able to conduct (the stool).

---

5   Visceral binding is a species of the *tai yang* pattern of cold damage characterized by pain and fullness in the chest and frequent diarrhea. The pulse is floating in the *cun* but deep in the *chi*.

Diarrhea with a floating, large pulse is due to vacuity. This is a result of forced (*i.e.,* mistaken) precipitation. If the pulse is floating and drumskin and there is rumbling in the intestines, this indicates *Dang Gui Si Ni Tang* (Dang Gui Four Counterflows Decoction).[6]

---

[6] This formula is composed of Radix Angelicae Sinensis (*Dang Gui*), Ramulus Cinnamomi Cassiae (*Gui Zhi*), Radix Paeoniae Lactiflorae (*Shao Yao*), Herba Asari Cum Radice (*Xi Xin*), Radix Glycyrrhizae (*Gan Cao*), Caulis Akebiae Mutong (*Mu Tong*), and Fructus Zizyphi Jujubae (*Da Zao*).

_______________Chapter Seven_______________
Diseases that Indicate Precipitation

The great method (*i.e.,* the general principle) is, in autumn, precipitation is appropriate.

When precipitation is indicated, (a formula in) the shape of a decoction excels that in the shape of a pill or powder. Once the disease has been struck, (the decoction) should be discontinued. It is not necessary to finish the (prescribed) three doses [dosage instead of three doses in the *Qian Jin*].

A *yang ming* disease manifesting fever and copious (spontaneous) sweating should be treated with precipitation without delay. *Da Chai Hu Tang* (Major Bupleurum Decoction) is indicated.

A *shao yin* disease, if manifesting a dry mouth and throat two or three days after contraction, should be treated with precipitation without delay. *Cheng Qi Tang* (Support the Qi Decoction) is indicated.

A *shao yin* disease manifesting abdominal fullness and absence of defecation six or seven days after contraction should be treated with precipitation without delay. It falls within the category indicating *Cheng Qi Tang* (Support the Qi Decoction).

If a *shao yin* disease manifests watery diarrhea and a green-blue facial complexion, there will invariably be pain below the heart. If the mouth is dry, (the disease) allows for precipitation. It falls within the category indicating *Da Chai Hu Tang* (Major Bupleurum Decoction) and *Cheng Qi Tang* (Support the Qi Decoction).

Diarrhea can be treated with precipitation if the pulse is normal in all its three positions and if the infra-cardiac region feels tight when pressed. This falls within the category indicating *Cheng Qi Tang* (Support the Qi Decoction).

A combined disease of the *yang ming* and *shao yang* with diarrhea is favorable if the pulse shows no inferiority, but it is unfavorable if the pulse shows inferiority. Inferiority means mutual restraint (between the *yang ming* and *shao yang*).[1]

A slippery and replete pulse points to food retention which requires precipitation. This falls within the category indicating *Da Chai Hu Tang* (Major Bupleurum Decoction) and *Cheng Qi Tang* (Support the Qi Decoction).

Suppose the pulse is deep after cold damage. In the presence of a deep (pulse), there is internal repletion. If resolution follows precipitation, (the disease) falls within the category indicating *Da Chai Hu Tang* (Major Bupleurum Decoction). [The *Yu Han (Jade Cabinet)*[2] says: "Suppose the pulse is deep and replete...The deepness and repleteness indicate precipitation ..."]

If, on the sixth or seventh day, cold damage manifests as blurred vision with the eyes not in good shape and there exists neither exterior nor interior manifestations except for difficult defecation and slight fever, this is (a case of) repletion and should be treated with precipitation without delay. It falls within the category indicating *Da Chai Hu Tang* (Major Bupleurum Decoction) and *Cheng Qi Tang* (Support the Qi Decoction).

Suppose a *tai yang* disease remains unresolved. If the pulses in the yin and yang (*i.e.*, from the *cun* to the *chi*) are in proportion, there is invariably cold shuddering and relief will follow perspiration. If the yang (*i.e.*, the *cun*) pulse alone is faint, one should promote sweating to realize relief. If the yin (*i.e.*, the *chi*) pulse alone is faint, one should employ precipitation to realize relief. (The latter case) falls within the category indicating *Da Chai Hu Tang* (Major Bupleurum Decoction).

Suppose the pulse is bowstring and slow on both hands. If there is tightness below the heart and if the pulse is large and tight (in addition), there is yin within yang. This necessitates precipitation. It falls within the category indicating *Cheng Qi Tang* (Support the Qi Decoction).

---

[1] The *yang ming* pulse is reflected in the *guan* position, while the *shao yang* pulse reflected in the *chi*. In the normal or favorable case, the *yang ming* pulse is stronger than the *shao yang* pulse. Should the *shao yang* pulse be stronger than the *yang ming* pulse, however, this means that the *shao yang* is superior to the *yang ming*. That is to say, liver wood overwhelms spleen earth. Hence it is a critical condition.

[2] I.e., *Guang Cheng Zi Yu Han Jing (Master Guang-cheng's Classic of the Jade Cabinet)* in full. This is also a work on the pulse written by Du Guang-ting of the Tang dynasty.

Suppose there is chest binding with rigidity of the nape like soft tetany. Then precipitation may immediately soften (this rigidity).

Suppose a patient suffers from no exterior or interior pattern except for fever which has run for seven or eight days. Even though the pulse is floating and rapid, one may employ precipitation. This falls within the category indicating *Da Chai Hu Tang* (Major Bupleurum Decoction).

Suppose on the sixth or seventh day, the *tai yang* still manifests an exterior pattern. If the pulse is faint and deep and if, contrarily, there is no chest bind and the sick person is running around manically, this shows existence of heat in the lower burner. There must be abdominal tightness and fullness. If the urination is uninhibited, cure will follow discharging of blood in the stools. This is because (the evils in) the *tai yang* follow the channel and heat is depressed internally. This indicates *Di Dang Tang* (Flushing Decoction).[3]

A *tai yang* disease manifesting generalized yellowing, a deep and bound pulse, lower abdominal tightness, and inhibited urination is due to absence of blood. If urination is disinhibited and the patient looks as if mad, the disease of blood (amassment) is verified. It falls within the category indicating *Di Dang Tang* (Flushing Decoction).

Suppose cold damage manifests fever and lower abdominal fullness, the urination should be inhibited. If now, on the contrary, the urination is uninhibited, this is due to blood (amassment) requiring precipitation. It falls within the category indicating *Di Dang Wan* (Flushing Pills).[4]

If a *yang ming* disease manifests fever with (spontaneous) sweating, this shows that heat is passing outward and is incapable of yellowing (the body). If sweat appears only on the head, is absent from the trunk, and is confined to above the neck and if there is inhibited urination and thirst with massive drinking, this shows there is depressed heat internally. Generalized yellowing will inevitably arise, indicating *Yin Chen Hao Tang* (Artemisia Capillaris Decoction).[5]

A *yang ming* disease is invariably accompanied by blood amassment if the sick person suffers from impaired memory. The explanation is that blood stasis of long duration produces impaired memory. The stool, though hard, must be black. This falls within the category indicating *Di Dang Tang* (Flushing Decoction). Delirious speech in spite of sweating suggests dry stool in the stomach.

---

[3] This formula is composed of Hirudo (*Shui Zhi*), Tabanus (*Meng Chong*), Semen Pruni Persicae (*Tao Ren*), and Radix Et Rhizoma Rhei (*Da Huang*).

[4] This formula is composed of the same ingredients as in the decoction. See note 3 above.

[5] The ingredients in this formula include Herba Artemisiae Capillaris (*Yin Chen Hao*), Radix Et Rhizoma Rhei (*Da Huang*), and Fructus Gardeniae Jasminoidis (*Zhi Zi*).

This is due to wind. Only when the channel is outreached or passed[6] can precipitation be employed. If precipitation is carried out earlier than necessary, confused speech will develop, for there is vacuity of the exterior and repletion in the interior. When precipitation is capable of effecting a cure, this falls within the category indicating *Da Chai Hu Tang* (Major Bupleurum Decoction) and *Cheng Qi Tang* (Support the Qi Decoction).

Suppose the sick person is immediately relieved of distressing fever by diaphoresis but then has a relapse as if in malaria, experiencing an episode in the late afternoon. This is categorized as a *yang ming* disease. If the pulse is replete, this requires precipitation. It falls within the category indicating *Da Chai Hu Tang* (Major Bupleurum Decoction) and *Cheng Qi Tang* (Support the Qi Decoction).

If a *yang ming* disease manifests delirious speech and tidal fever contrarily with inability to take in food, there must be five or six pieces of dry feces (retained). If (the sick person) is able to take in food, (the trouble is merely) hard stools, falling within the category indicating *Cheng Qi Tang* (Support the Qi Decoction).

The *tai yang* disease of wind stroke with diarrhea and counterflow retching cannot be treated through attacking (internally) before the exterior is resolved. If the sick person suffers from continuous mild sweating and if there are attacks at regular intervals of headache, glomus, tightness and fullness below the heart sending a dragging pain to the flanks, retching with shortness of breath, sweating, and no aversion to cold, this shows that the exterior is resolved but the interior is still out of harmony. This indicates *Shi Zao Tang* (Ten Dates Decoction).[7]

If heat is bound in the urinary bladder before a *tai yang* disease is resolved and the patient looks as if mad, blood will discharge from below by itself (*i.e.*, hemafecia). Cure will follow this discharge. Before the exterior is resolved, one should not attack (internally). It is necessary to resolve the exterior first. Only when the exterior is resolved and there is hypertonicity and

---

[6] This phrase is often boiled down to the term channel passage or out-reaching (*guo jing*). Cold damage has several stages or is transmuted in a certain order. At first, it manifests as the *tai yang* pattern. Then it develops into the *yang ming* pattern and then into the *shao yang* pattern, etc. This is called channel transmutation (*chuan jing*). When cold damage is transmuted from one stage, the *tai yang* to the *yang ming*, for example, this is called channel passage or out-reaching. In other words, channel passage is the ending of one pattern and the beginning of the succeeding pattern. In most cases, channel passage happens in a fixed number of days. If the course of a channel pattern, the *tai yang*, for example, is over, but part of or all the signs and symptoms typical of it still linger, this is called failure of resolution beyond the channel passage.

[7] This formula is composed of Flos Daphnis Genkwae (*Yuan Hua*), Radix Euphorbiae Kansui (*Gan Sui*), Herba Cirsii Japonici (*Da Ji*), and Fructus Zizyphi Jujubae (*Da Zao*).

binding in the lower abdomen can one employ attacking. *Tao Ren Cheng Qi Tang* (Persica Support the Qi Decoction)[8] is indicated.

Seven or eight day old cold damage manifesting as generalized yellowing like the orange (color), inhibited urination, and slight lower abdominal fullness falls within the category indicating *Yin Chen Hao Tang* (Artemisia Capillaris Decoction).

More than ten day old cold damage with heat binding internally (giving rise to) alternating cold and heat falls within the category indicating *Da Chai Hu Tang* (Major Bupleurum Decoction).

Chest binding alone with no great heat is due to water bound in the chest and lateral costal regions. If there is moderate sweating on the head, administer *Da Xian Xiong Tang* (Major Sunken Chest Decoction).[9]

If six or seven day old cold damage manifests as chest binding due to heat repletion, a deep, tight pulse, and pain below the cardiac region which feels as hard as rock, administer *Da Xian Xiong Tang* (Major Sunken Chest Decoction).

Suppose there is a *yang ming* disease. If the sick person suffers from copious perspiration, fluids will exit and the stomach will become dry, then there must be hard stools. Hard stools will give rise to delirious speech. This falls within the category indicating *Cheng Qi Tang* (Support the Qi Decoction).

A *yang ming* disease manifesting no vomiting or diarrhea but heart vexation can be treated with *Cheng Qi Tang* (Support the Qi Decoction).

If a *yang ming* disease manifests with a slow pulse and no aversion to cold despite exiting of sweat, there must be generalized heaviness, shortness of breath, abdominal fullness, dyspnea, and tidal fever. Such a case has already had the exterior resolved, allowing attacking of the interior. If the hands and feet are wet with sweat, the stools are already hardened, indicating *Cheng Qi Tang* (Support the Qi Decoction). If there is fever but it is not tidal, it is not yet time to administer this decoction. If the abdomen is full and enlarged with absence of defecation, *Xiao Cheng Qi Tang* (Minor Support the Qi Decoction) is indicated. This is used to harmonize the stomach qi to a small

---

[8] The ingredients in this formula are Semen Pruni Persicae (*Tao Ren*), Radix Et Rhizoma Rhei (*Da Huang*), Radix Glycyrrhizae (*Gan Cao*), Cortex Cinnamomi Cassiae (*Rou Gui*), and Rhizoma Zingiberis (*Jiang*).

[9] This formula is composed of Radix Euphorbiae Kansui (*Gan Sui*), Radix Et Rhizoma Rhei (*Da Huang*), and Mirabilitum (*Mang Xiao*).

degree. One should avoid causing great (*i.e.*, drastic) precipitation.

A *yang ming* disease may manifest delirious speech, tidal fever, and a slippery and rapid pulse. If so, it indicates *Cheng Qi Tang* (Support the Qi Decoction). Then administer one *sheng* of *Cheng Qi Tang* (Support the Qi Decoction). When flatus turns in the abdomen, administer one more *sheng*. In case no flatus turns, one should not administer more. If there is still absence of defecation the next day and the pulse contrarily turns to become faint and choppy, this shows vacuity of the interior. It is difficult to treat, and one should not administer *Cheng Qi Tang* (Support the Qi Decoction) anymore.

If a combined disease of the two yang (*i.e.*, the *tai yang* and *yang ming*) is stripped of the *tai yang* pattern and merely manifests tidal fever, hands and feet wet with sweat, difficult defecation, and delirious speech, precipitation will effect recovery. This falls within the category indicating *Cheng Qi Tang* (Support the Qi Decoction).

If the sick person suffers from inhibited urination with defecation difficult at one time but easy at another and there are at times moderate fever, dyspnea, dizziness, and insomnia, then there is hard stool. This falls within the category indicating *Cheng Qi Tang* (Support the Qi Decoction).

Chapter Eight
Diseases Following Diaphoresis, Ejection & Precipitation

The master explained:

If the sick person has a faint and choppy pulse, it is the (attending) physician who is the producer of the disease. Carrying out great (*i.e.*, drastic) diaphoresis and then repeated great precipitation causes the patient loss of blood. Then there should be an disease of aversion to cold and a fever. It will go on without an end. In the exuberant heat of the summer months, there is a desire to wear clothes that are lined (*i.e.*, heavy, warm clothes), but, in the exuberant cold of the winter months, there is the desire to be naked. The explanation for this is that faint yang is responsible for aversion to cold, while weak yin is responsible for fever.

Diaphoresis has made yang qi faint, and additional great precipitation has made yin qi weak. In the fifth month, yang qi is in the exterior. (Therefore,) there is vacuity cold in the stomach. Since yang qi is faint internally, it is unable to resist (external) cold. Thus there is a desire to wear lined clothes. In the eleventh month, yang qi is in the interior. (Therefore,) there is distressing heat in the stomach. Since yin qi is weak internally, it is unable to resist (internal) heat. Thus there is the desire to be naked. Again, since the yin pulse (*i.e.*, pulse in the *chi*) is slow and choppy, blood is known to be lost.

If, on the third day, a *tai yang* disease still remains unresolved though already treated with diaphoresis, ejection, precipitation, and warm needling, this is a nasty disease. It is no longer appropriate to administer *Gui Zhi Tang* (Cinnamon Twig Decoction). One should examine the pulse and (other) signs to determine what is the offence, and then mete out a treatment in accordance with the pattern.

If the pulse is floating and rapid, recovery is expected to follow perspiration. If precipitation is carried out instead, generalized heaviness and heart palpitations will arise. One should not employ diaphoresis (now) but let sweat spontaneously exit to effect a resolution. The reason is that the pulse is faint in the *chi*. This suggests vacuity internally. One should wait till the exterior and the interior are replenished and the fluids come into harmony. Then sweat will exit of its own and healing will ensue.

If, following diaphoresis, ejection, precipitation, or loss of blood, the fluids run out but yin and yang can restore harmony by themselves, the disease is certain to heal by itself.

Following drastic precipitation, diaphoresis may make the patient suffer from inhibited urination which is a result of loss of fluids. This requires no treatment. When urination becomes disinhibited, healing is certain to ensue of itself.

Following precipitation, diaphoresis will inevitably result in cold shuddering. Besides, the pulse will become faint and thin. The reason why this arises is that the interior and the exterior are both (already) made vacuous.

If a *tai yang* disease is first treated with precipitation but has not recovered and subsequently is treated with diaphoresis, the exterior and the interior will both be made vacuous. The patient should feel dizzy. A patient suffering from dizziness will recover automatically following (spontaneous) sweating. The reason is that, following perspiration, the exterior becomes harmonious. After the exterior becomes harmonious, one may carry out precipitation.

Suppose that six or seven days after contraction of an illness, the pulse is slow, floating, and weak and there is aversion to wind and cold with warm hands and feet. If the (attending) physician repeatedly carries out precipitation, inability to take in food will arise and the sick person will suffer from fullness in the lateral costal regions, yellowing of the whole body including the face and eyes, stiffness of the nape of the neck, and difficult urination. If *Chai Hu Tang* (Bupleurum Decoction) is administered, there will be pressure in the rectum. Although there was thirst, (desire to) drink, and retching in the past,[1] *Chai Hu Tang* (Bupleurum Decoction) can be administered no longer. There is dry retching upon ingestion of food.

If, on the second or third day, a *tai yang* disease manifests inability to fall asleep at all with desire to rise up, there must be binding below the heart. If the pulse is faint and weak, this shows that there has been cold in the past and that precipitation was abused. When diarrhea is stopped (by precipitation), chest binding unavoidably arises. If diarrhea is not checked, one can carry out precipitation again four or five days later. This is contained heat diarrhea.

Suppose a *tai yang* disease is treated with precipitation. If then the pulse becomes skipping and there arises no chest binding, this shows a tendency to resolution. If the pulse is floating, there must be chest binding. If the pulse is tight, there must be sore throat. If the pulse is bowstring, there must be hypertonicity of the lateral costal regions. If the pulse is thin and rapid, headache is not yet at an end. If the pulse is deep and tight, there must be a desire to retch. If the pulse is deep and slippery, there is contained heat diarrhea. If the pulse is floating and slippery, there must be hemafecia.

If a combined disease of the *tai yang* and *shao yang* is treated contrarily with precipitation and chest binding, tightness below the heart, uncheckable diarrhea, and (even) water refusing to descend develop, then the sick person must suffer from heart vexation.

If the pulse is floating and tight but precipitation is carried out, the tight (pulse quality) will contrarily enter internally.[2] Then there will arise glomus which feels soft when palpated. It is but a glomus of qi.

Suppose cold damage is treated by ejection, precipitation, and diaphoresis and there arises vacuity vexation with a very faint pulse. If, on the eighth or ninth day, glomus and tightness below the heart, pain in the lateral costal region, qi surging up into the throat, dizziness, and twitching of the channel vessels arises, then, over time, atony will develop.

A *yang ming* disease manifesting inability to take in food may remain unresolved after being treated by precipitation. The sick person may (still) be unable to take in food. If (cool and cold

---

[1] This phrase is ambiguous. It may also be rendered as, "Retching will take the place of the original thirst and (desire) to drink."

[2] This means that the floating and tight pulse becomes deep and tight.

medicinals are used to) attack heat, retching will invariably arise. This is because there is vacuity cold in the stomach.

If a *yang ming* disease is characterized by a slow pulse, difficulty in eating to the full, and vexation and dizziness arising upon eating to the full, then there must be difficult urination. There is a tendency towards grain jaundice.[3] In spite of precipitation, abdominal fullness will remain as before. This is because the pulse is slow.

If a *tai yang* disease exhibits a pulse which is slow in the *cun*, floating in the *guan*, and weak in the *chi* and the patient suffers from fever, aversion to cold in spite of sweating, no retching, and glomus below the heart, this is caused by the (attending) physician using precipitation.

After cold damage is treated by great (*i.e.*, drastic) ejection and great precipitation, there may be the severest of vacuity. If great diaphoresis is carried out in addition, the sick person's exterior qi will become depressed. If the sick person is given water (to drink) for the purpose of perspiration, there will be retching. This is because there is vacuity cold in the stomach.

If, following ejection, precipitation, and diaphoresis, the sick person has a pacific pulse but suffers from slight vexation, this is because grain qi (*i.e.*, a large food intake) is too much (for the stomach) which has just undergone evacuation.

Suppose a *tai yang* disease is treated by a physician who employs diaphoresis and then develops fever and aversion to cold. If it is (then) furthermore treated by precipitation, glomus below the heart will arise. This is due to vacuity of both the exterior and interior, exhaustion of both yin qi and yang qi, and absence of yang with solitary yin.[4] If red-hot needling is applied in addition, vexation, yellowish green-blue facial complexion, and twitching of the skin will arise. Such a case is difficult to treat. If the facial complexion is slightly yellow and the hands and feet are warm, the case is easy to cure.

If, following administration of *Gui Zhi Tang* (Cinnamon Twig Decoction) and employment of precipitation, stiffness and pain in the head and the nape, continuous mild fever, absence of sweating, fullness and slight pain below the heart, and inhibited urination arise, this indicates *Gui*

---

[3] This is a kind of jaundice characterized by alternating fever and chills, inability to take in food, dizziness arising upon ingestion, distention of the chest and abdomen, yellowing, and inhibited urination.

[4] The translator suspects that the ideogram *du* for the word solitary may be a typographical error. The part, "yang qi, and absence of yang with solitary yin" might be better translated as, "yang qi. Absence of yang results in turbid yin." Turbid yin implies superabundance of yin which may cause untransformed grain in the stools, cold diarrhea, etc.

Zhi Qu Gui Jia Fu Ling Zhu Tang (Cinnamon Twig Minus Cinnamon Plus Poria & Atractylodes Decoction).[5]

Suppose a *tai yang* disease remains unresolved after first being treated with diaphoresis. When precipitation is subsequently applied, cure will not be effected (either) if the pulse is floating. Since a floating pulse points to (evils) in the exterior, precipitation is contrary and, therefore, will not effect a cure. Since the pulse is floating, (the evil) is in the exterior. (Therefore,) it is necessary to resolve the exterior to realize a cure. This indicates *Gui Zhi Tang* (Cinnamon Twig Decoction).

Suppose precipitation is followed by diaphoresis. Then vexation and agitation with sleeplessness during the day but tranquility at night will arise. There is no retching and no thirst. The exterior pattern is absent, the pulse becomes deep and faint, and there is no high fever. This indicates *Gan Jiang Fu Zi Tang* (Dry Ginger & Aconite Decoction).[6]

After cold damage is treated by ejection, precipitation, and diaphoresis, counterflow fullness below the heart, qi surging up into the chest, dizziness arising on attempt to rise up, and a deep, tight pulse may develop. If diaphoresis is (now) used, the channels will be stirred up so that the body will tremble. This indicates *Fu Ling Gui Zhi Zhu Gan Cao Tang* (Poria, Cinnamon Twig, Atractylodes & Licorice Decoction).[7]

Suppose diaphoresis, ejection, and precipitation fail to effect a resolution. If vexation and agitation then arise, this indicates *Fu Ling Si Ni Tang* (Poria Four Counterflows Decoction).[8]

After cold damage is treated by diaphoresis, ejection, and precipitation, if vacuity vexation with sleeplessness and, in severe cases, turning about (restlessly on the bed) develop with a burning sensation in the heart, this indicates *Zhi Zi Tang* (Gardenia Decoction). If there is diminished qi,

---

[5] This formula is composed of Radix Paeoniae Lactiflorae (*Shao Yao*), Rhizoma Zingiberis (*Jiang*), Rhizoma Atractylodis Macrocephalae (*Bai Zhu*), Sclerotium Poriae Cocos (*Fu Ling*), Radix Glycyrrhizae (*Gan Cao*), and Fructus Zizyphi Jujubae (*Da Zao*).

[6] This formula is composed of only two ingredients: dry Rhizoma Zingiberis (*Gan Jiang*) and Radix Praeparatus Aconiti Carmichaeli (*Fu Zi*).

[7] This formula is composed of Sclerotium Poriae Cocos (*Fu Ling*), Cortex Cinnamomi Cassiae (*Gui Zhi*), Radix Glycyrrhizae (*Gan Cao*), and Rhizoma Atractylodis Macrocephalae (*Bai Zhu*).

[8] The ingredients in this formula include Sclerotium Poriae Cocos (*Fu Ling*), Radix Glycyrrhizae (*Gan Cao*), Radix Panacis Ginseng (*Ren Shen*), Radix Praeparatus Aconiti Carmichaeli (*Fu Zi*), and Rhizoma Zingiberis (*Jiang*).

it indicates *Zhi Zi Gan Cao Tang* (Gardenia & Licorice Decoction).[9] If there is retching, it indicates *Zhi Zi Sheng Jiang Tang* (Gardenia & Fresh Ginger Decoction).[10] If there is abdominal fullness, it indicates *Zhi Zi Hou Po Tang* (Gardenia & Magnolia Decoction).[11]

Suppose diaphoresis is succeeded by precipitation. If distressed heat and congestion in the chest then arises, this falls within the category indicating *Zhi Zi Tang* (Gardenia Decoction).

Suppose, more than ten days after the channel passage or out-reaching, a *tai yang* disease develops a distressed sensation below the heart with desire to vomit and pain in the chest. (In addition,) there is contrarily duck-stool diarrhea, slight abdominal distention, depression, and slight vexation. If it has been treated by great (*i.e.,* drastic) ejection and precipitation in the past, then administer *Cheng Qi Tang* (Support the Qi Decoction). If it has not, do not administer this decoction. Desire to vomit, pain in the chest, and slight duck-stool diarrhea, these are not a pattern indicating *Chai Hu Tang* (Bupleurum Decoction). Vomiting reveals (the past) great ejection and precipitation.

After a *tai yang* disease is treated with repeated diaphoresis succeeded by precipitation, there may be absence of defecation for five or six consecutive days, a dry tongue, thirst, and moderate tidal fever in the late afternoon. There may be fullness, tightness, and pain from below the heart through the lower abdomen. (These troubles may be so severe that they) daunt one from touching (the affected parts) with the hand. This indicates *Da Xian Xiong Tang* (Major Sunken Chest Decoction).

Suppose on the fifth or sixth day of cold damage, the sick person has already been treated with diaphoresis but is (now) furthermore treated with precipitation. If fullness and slight binding in the chest and lateral costal region, inhibited urination, thirst, no retching, sweating confined to the head, alternating cold and heat, and heart vexation develop, this shows (that the cold damage) has not yet been resolved, indicating *Chai Hu Gui Zhi Gan Jiang Tang* (Bupleurum, Cinnamon Twig & Dry Ginger Decoction).[12]

---

[9] This formula is composed of Fructus Gardeniae Jasminoidis (*Zhi Zi*), Radix Glycyrrhizae (*Gan Cao*), and Semen Praeparatus Sojae (*Dou Chi*).

[10] This formula is composed of Fructus Gardeniae Jasminoidis (*Zhi Zi*), Rhizoma Zingiberis (*Jiang*), and Semen Praeparatus Sojae (*Dou Chi*).

[11] This formula is composed of Fructus Gardeniae Jasminoidis (*Zhi Zi*), Cortex Magnoliae Officinalis (*Hou Po*), and Fructus Immaturus Aurantii (*Zhi Shi*).

[12] The ingredients in this formula are Radix Bupleuri (*Chai Hu*), Ramulus Cinnamomi Cassiae (*Gui Zhi*), Radix Scutellariae Baicalensis (*Huang Qin*), Rhizoma Zingiberis (*Jiang*), calcined Concha Ostreae (*Mu Li*), Radix Glycyrrhizae (*Gan Cao*), and Radix Trichosanthis Kirlowii (*Tian Hua Fen*).

Suppose cold damage is treated by diaphoresis or ejection and precipitation. If a resolution is effected but glomus and tightness below the heart and belching are left, this indicates *Xuan Fu Dai Zhe Tang* (Inula & Hematite Decoction).[13]

Following drastic precipitation, one should not further administer *Gui Zhi Tang* (Cinnamon Twig Decoction). If there is (spontaneous) sweating with dyspnea but no high fever, one may administer *Ma Huang Xing Zi Gan Cao Shi Gao Tang* (Ephedra, Armeniaca, Licorice & Gypsum Decoction).

After cold damage is treated by drastic precipitation and then by diaphoresis, there may be glomus below the heart and aversion to cold. This shows that the exterior has not yet been resolved. One should not attack the glomus. It is necessary to resolve the exterior first. Only after the exterior is resolved can one attack the glomus. Resolution of the exterior indicates *Gui Zhi Tang* (Cinnamon Twig Decoction). Attacking the glomus indicates *Da Huang Huang Lian Xie Xin Tang* (Rhubarb & Coptis Drain the Heart Decoction).[14]

Suppose, seven or eight days after ejection and precipitation, cold damage remains unresolved. There is heat bound internally and there exists heat in both the exterior and interior. (This heat) produces aversion to wind at times, fierce thirst, a distressingly dry tongue, and a desire to drink several *sheng* of water. This indicates *Bai Hu Tang* (White Tiger Decoction).

Suppose, following ejection and precipitation, cold damage remains unresolved. There is no defecation for five or six or even up to ten days. The sick person suffers from tidal fever in the afternoon but no aversion to cold. They speak to themselves as if meeting with ghosts. And, in severe cases, during spells, there is failure to recognize people, carphologia, apprehension, restlessness, slight dyspnea, and staring straight ahead. Those who have a bowstring pulse may survive, but those who have a choppy one will die. Slight cases with only fever and delirious speech indicate *Cheng Qi Tang* (Support the Qi Decoction). If precipitation has already been induced, one should not administer more (of this decoction).

Suppose a combined disease of the three yang manifests as abdominal fullness, generalized heaviness, difficulty in turning over, insensitivity of the mouth, a grimy facial complexion, delirious speech, and enuresis. If diaphoresis is carried out, delirious speech will arise. If

---

[13] The ingredients in this formula include Flos Inulae (*Xuan Fu Hua*), Hematitum (*Dai Zhe Shi*), Radix Panacis Ginseng (*Ren Shen*), Rhizoma Zingiberis (*Jiang*), Radix Glycyrrhizae (*Gan Cao*), Rhizoma Pinelliae Ternatae (*Ban Xia*), and Fructus Zizyphi Jujubae (*Da Zao*).

[14] This formula is composed of Radix Et Rhizoma Rhei (*Da Huang*) and Rhizoma Coptidis Chinensis (*Huang Lian*).

precipitation is carried out, sweating on the forehead, inversion frigidity of the hands and feet, and spontaneous perspiration will arise. This falls within the category indicating *Bai Hu Tang* (White Tiger Decoction).

Suppose a *yang ming* disease manifests with a floating, tight pulse, a dry throat, a bitter taste in the mouth, abdominal fullness, dyspnea, fever, sweating, aversion to heat rather than cold, and generalized heaviness. If this is treated by diaphoresis, agitation, confused heart (*i.e.*, mind), and delirious speech will develop. If this is treated with red-hot needling, apprehension in addition to vexation, agitation, and insomnia will inevitably develop. If it is treated with precipitation, the stomach will become empty and vacuous with the guest qi (*i.e.*, vacuity heat) stirring the diaphragm accompanied by a burning sensation of the heart and fur growing over the tongue. This falls within the category indicating *Zhi Zi Tang* (Gardenia Decoction).

If, following precipitation, a *yang ming* disease manifests heat in the exterior, warm hands and feet, no chest binding, and a burning sensation in the heart, (constant) hunger without ability to take in food, and sweating confined to the head, this falls within the category indicating *Zhi Zi Tang* (Gardenia Decoction).

If, following precipitation, a *yang ming* disease manifests a burning sensation in the heart with vexation and dry stools staying in the stomach, one may attack (internally). If the sick person suffers from slight abdominal fullness and (the stools) are hard at the beginning but the rest is thin liquid, one should not attack (internally). The case with dry stool falls within the category indicating *Cheng Qi Tang* (Support the Qi Decoction).

After a *tai yang* disease has been treated with ejection, precipitation, and diaphoresis, if slight vexation and frequent urination giving rise to hard stools arise, one may administer *Xiao Cheng Qi Tang* (Minor Support the Qi Decoction) to harmonize (the stomach). Then a cure will ensue.

Inversion frigidity (of the four limbs) following great (*i.e.*, drastic) diaphoresis or great precipitation falls within the category indicating *Si Ni Tang* (Four Counterflows Decoction).

After a *tai yang* disease has been treated with precipitation, if a skipping pulse and fullness of the chest appear, this falls within the category indicating *Gui Zhi Qu Shao Yao Tang* (CinnamonTwig

Minus Peony Decoction).[15] If there is slight cold, this indicates *Gui Zhi Qu Shao Yao Jia Fu Zi Tang* (Cinnamon Twig Minus Peony & Plus Aconite Decoction).[16]

Suppose, on the fifth or sixth day, cold damage is treated with drastic precipitation. If generalized heat is still lingering with binding and pain in the heart, this shows no tendency towards resolution and falls within the category indicating *Zhi Zi Tang* (Gardenia Decoction).

After cold damage is treated with precipitation, if vexation, abdominal fullness, and restlessness either when lying down or on arising occur, this indicates *Zhi Zi Hou Po Tang* (Gardenia & Magnolia Decoction).

After cold damage is treated by a physician who uses pills to induce great precipitation, if generalized heat still lingers with slight vexation, this indicates *Zhi Zi Gan Jiang Tang* (Gardenia & Dry Ginger Decoction).[17]

Suppose, after cold damage is treated by a physician with precipitation, there develops incessant diarrhea of clear grain. If there is generalized pain and aching, it is urgently necessary to rescue the interior. If there is generalized pain and aching with normal voidings of clear urine, it is urgently necessary to rescue the exterior. To rescue the interior, the appropriate (formula) is *Si Ni Tang* (Four Counterflows Decoction). To rescue the exterior, the appropriate (formula) is *Gui Zhi Tang* (Cinnamon Twig Decoction).

Suppose, more than ten days after the channel passage or out-reaching, a *tai yang* disease is treated with repeated precipitation. If, four or five days after, indications of *Chai Hu Tang* (Bupleurum Decoction) still are manifesting, one should administer *Xiao Chai Hu Tang* (Minor Bupleurum Decoction) first. Then vomiting will be checked and relief will be realized to a small extent. If the sick person (now) suffers from depression and slight vexation, this shows that (the illness) has not been resolved. One may administer *Da Chai Hu Tang* (Major Bupleurum Decoction) and recovery will follow precipitation.

----

[15] This formula is composed of Ramulus Cinnamomi Cassiae (*Gui Zhi*), Rhizoma Zingiberis (*Jiang*), Radix Glycyrrhizae (*Gan Cao*), and Fructus Zizyphi Jujubae (*Da Zao*).

[16] This formula is composed of Ramulus Cinnamomi Cassiae (*Gui Zhi*), Rhizoma Zingiberis (*Jiang*), Radix Glycyrrhizae (*Gan Cao*), Fructus Zizyphi Jujubae (*Da Zao*), and Radix Praeparatus Aconiti Carmichaeli (*Fu Zi*).

[17] This formula is composed of Fructus Gardeniae Jasminoidis (*Zhi Zi*) and dry Rhizoma Zingiberis (*Gan Jiang*).

Suppose cold damage has remained unresolved for thirteen days manifesting as fullness in the chest and lateral costal region, retching, tidal fever in the late afternoon, and moderate diarrhea. This (illness) should have been treated with *Chai Hu Tang* (Bupleurum Decoction) to precipitate, and there should not have been diarrhea before. Now, on the contrary, there is diarrhea. Thus, one can know that the (attending) physician has used pills for the purpose of precipitation. This was not the correct treatment. Tidal fever is due to repletion. One should first administer *Xiao Chai Hu Tang* (Minor Bupleurum Decoction) to resolve the exterior. Then the later (development) will indicate *Chai Hu Jia Mang Xiao Tang* (Bupleurum Plus Mirabilitum Decoction).[18]

If, on the thirteenth day, cold damage develops delirious speech following channel passage or out-reaching,[19] this shows that there is heat internally requiring an (appropriate) decoction to precipitate (it). Suppose urination is uninhibited, the stools should (then) be hard. If, on the contrary, there is diarrhea and the pulse is harmonious and pacific, one can know that the (attending) physician has used pills to precipitate. This was not the correct treatment. If there is diarrhea, the pulse should be faint and there is inversion. Now, on the contrary, (the pulse) is harmonious. This points to internal repletion. This falls within the category indicating *Cheng Qi Tang* (Support the Qi Decoction).

Suppose, on the eighth or ninth day, cold damage is treated by precipitation. If fullness of the chest, vexation, susceptibility to fright, inhibited urination, delirious speech, and inability to turn the body over develop, this indicates *Chai Hu Jia Long Gu Mu Li Tang* (Bupleurum Plus Dragon Bone & Oyster Shell Decoction).[20]

Vexation and agitation arising as a result of malpractice of a fire modality and precipitation or due to red-hot needling indicates *Gui Zhi Gan Cao Long Gu Mu Li Tang* (Cinnamon Twig, Licorice, Dragon Bone & Oyster Shell Decoction).[21]

---

[18] The ingredients in this formula include Radix Bupleuri (*Chai Hu*), Radix Scutellariae Baicalensis (*Huang Qin*), Radix Panacis Ginseng (*Ren Shen*), Radix Glycyrrhizae (*Gan Cao*), Rhizoma Zingiberis (*Jiang*), Rhizoma Pinelliae Ternatae (*Ban Xia*), Mirabilitum (*Mang Xiao*), and Fructus Zizyphi Jujubae (*Da Zao*).

[19] This implies that the *tai yang* pattern is already resolved and a *yang ming* pattern then appears.

[20] The ingredients of this formula include Radix Bupleuri (*Chai Hu*), Radix Scutellariae Baicalensis (*Huang Qin*), Radix Panacis Ginseng (*Ren Shen*), Rhizoma Zingiberis (*Jiang*), Rhizoma Pinelliae Ternatae (*Ban Xia*), Mirabilitum (*Mang Xiao*), Fructus Zizyphi Jujubae (*Da Zao*), Os Draconis (*Long Gu*), Concha Ostreae (*Mu Li*), Radix Et Rhizoma Rhei (*Da Huang*), Ramulus Cinnamomi Cassiae (*Gui Zhi*), Sclerotium Poriae Cocos (*Fu Ling*), and Acetale of Lead (*Qian Dan*).

[21] The ingredients in this formula are Ramulus Cinnamomi Cassiae (*Gui Zhi*), Radix Paeoniae Lactiflorae (*Shao Yao*), Radix Glycyrrhizae (*Gan Cao*), Rhizoma Zingiberis (*Jiang*), Concha Ostreae (*Mu Li*), Os Draconis (*Long Gu*), and Fructus Zizyphi Jujubae (*Da Zao*).

Suppose a *tai yang* disease manifests a floating, stirring, and rapid pulse. In the presence of a floating (pulse), there is wind. In the presence of a rapid (pulse), there is heat. In the presence of a stirring (pulse), there is pain. And in the presence of a rapid (pulse), there is vacuity. Headache, fever, moderate night sweats, and aversion to cold show that the exterior has not yet been resolved. If the (attending) physician contrarily uses precipitation, the stirring, rapid pulse will become a slow pulse and headache will be accompanied by dizziness. The stomach will become empty and vacuous with guest qi stirring the diaphragm. Shortness of breath, agitation, vexation, and a burning sensation in the heart will arise. Because yang qi is sunken internally, tightness below the heart will appear which will develop into chest bind. This indicates *Da Xian Xiong Tang* (Major Sunken Chest Decoction). If there is no chest bind but there is sweating only on the head but absent from the rest of the body and confined to above the neck, and if urination is inhibited, there will inevitably develop generalized yellowing which is an indication of *Chai Hu Zhi Zi Tang* (Bupleurum & Gardenia Decoction).[22]

Suppose, on the fifth or sixth day, cold damage manifests retching and fever and there exists all the manifestations indicating *Chai Hu Tang* (Bupleurum Decoction). If another (formula) is used instead to precipitate, then the manifestations indicating *Chai Hu Tang* (Bupleurum Decoction) will still exist. (In this case,) one may administer *Chai Hu Tang* (Bupleurum Decoction) all the same. Although precipitation has been carried out, this is not a (greatly) unfavorable (condition). Then there will invariably arise steaming (fever) and quivering (with cold). Later, heat will induce sweat and then a resolution will ensue. If there is fullness below the heart with tightness and pain, this is chest binding, indicating *Da Xian Xiong Tang* (Major Sunken Chest Decoction). If there is fullness but no pain, this is glomus. At this point, one should administer *Chai Hu (Tang)* (Bupleurum [Decoction]) no longer. (Now) *Ban Xia Xie Xin Tang* (Pinellia Drain the Heart Decoction)[23] is indicated.

Suppose it is because of precipitation that there is glomus below the heart. After a heart-draining decoction is administered, if the glomus remains unresolved and the sick person suffers from thirst, a dry mouth, and inhibited urination, this indicates *Wu Ling San* (Five [Ingredients] Poria Powder). There is another instruction, which says that if one tolerates this for one day, recovery will ensue.

---

[22] This formula is composed of Radix Bupleuri (*Chai Hu*), Fructus Gardeniae Jasminoidis (*Zhi Zi*), Cortex Radicis Moutan (*Dan Pi*), Radix Ligustici Wallichii (*Chuan Xiong*), Radix Paeoniae Lactiflorae (*Shao Yao*), Sclerotium Poriae Cocos (*Fu Ling*), Radix Angelicae Sinensis (*Dang Gui*), Rhizoma Atractylodis Macrocephalae (*Bai Zhu*), Semen Arctii Lappae (*Niu Bang Zi*), and Radix Glycyrrhizae (*Gan Cao*).

[23] This formula is composed of Rhizoma Coptidis Chinensis (*Huang Lian*), Radix Scutellariae Baicalensis (*Huang Qin*), Rhizoma Zingiberis (*Jiang*), Radix Panacis Ginseng (*Ren Shen*), Radix Glycyrrhizae (*Gan Cao*), and Fructus Zizyphi Jujubae (*Da Zao*).

If a wind stroke (pattern of) cold damage is treated by a physician contrarily with precipitation, the sick person will suffer from tens of bowel movements in a day with untransformed grain in the stools and thunderous rumbling in the abdomen. There will be glomus below the heart with tightness and fullness, dry retching, vexation, and inability to quiet down (for a moment). If, seeing the glomus below the heart which shows that the illness is not yet been exterminated, the (attending) physician repeats precipitation, then the glomus will become exacerbated. This is not a case of bound heat but of stomach vacuity. Since the guest qi (*i.e.*, vacuity qi) counterflows upward, tightness arises. This indicates *Gan Cao Xie Xin Tang* (Licorice Drain the Heart Decoction).[24]

Suppose a decoction is administered for cold damage but incessant diarrhea with glomus and tightness below the heart develop. Then one takes a heart-draining decoction and, later, another (formula of) medicinals to precipitate. The diarrhea, (however,) still persists. Now, if the (attending) physician administers (medicinals) to rectify the center, the diarrhea will become worse. It is the middle burner which is rectified by a center-rectifying (formula), while this kind of diarrhea is ascribed to the lower burner. This indicates *Chi Shi Zhi Yu Yu Liang Tang* (Halloysitum & Limonitum Decoction).[25] If diarrhea (still) persists (after taking this decoction), it is necessary to disinhibit urination.

If a *tai yang* disease is treated with repeated precipitation before the exterior manifestations are resolved, incessant contained heat diarrhea and glomus and tightness below the heart may arise. Since neither the exterior nor the interior has been resolved, this indicates *Gui Zhi Ren Shen Tang* (Cinnamon Twig & Ginseng Decoction).[26] After cold damage is treated with precipitation, if abdominal fullness arises, one may administer *Cheng Qi Tang* (Support the Qi Decoction).

If the sick person suffers from no exterior or interior pattern but has had fever for seven or eight days, one may prescribe precipitation even though the pulse is floating and rapid. Suppose the pulse is still rapid after precipitation and there is heat resulting in swift digestion with rapid hungering. If there has been no defecation for six or seven days running, there is blood stasis, indicating *Di Dang Tang* (Flushing Decoction). If, (after taking this decoction,) the pulse still

---

[24] The ingredients in this formula include Radix Scutellariae Baicalensis (*Huang Qin*), Rhizoma Zingiberis (*Jiang*), Rhizoma Pinelliae Ternatae (*Ban Xia*), Radix Glycyrrhizae (*Gan Cao*), and Fructus Zizyphi Jujubae (*Da Zao*).

[25] There are only two ingredients in this formula: Halloysitum Rubrum (*Chi Shi Zhi*) and Limonitum (*Yu Yu Liang*).

[26] This formula is composed of Ramulus Cinnamomi Cassiae (*Gui Zhi*), Radix Glycyrrhizae (*Gan Cao*), Rhizoma Atractylodis Macrocephalae (*Bai Zhu*), Radix Panacis Ginseng (*Ren Shen*), and Rhizoma Zingiberis (*Jiang*).

remains rapid and there is incessant (diarrhea), then there must be contained heat producing pus and blood in the stools.

If a *tai yang* disease is contrarily treated by a physician with precipitation, there may arise abdominal fullness with oft-occurring pain. This is (now) a case of the *tai yin* pattern, indicating *Gui Zhi Jia Shao Yao Tang* (Cinnamon Twig Plus Peony Decoction).

Severe (abdominal) repletion pain indicates *Gui Zhi Jia Da Huang Tang* (Cinnamon Twig Plus Rhubarb Decoction).[27]

If, on the sixth or seventh day of cold damage, after the sick person has been treated with great (*i.e.*, drastic) precipitation, the pulse is deep and slow and there is inversion counterflow (frigidity) of the hands and feet, absence of a pulse in the lower (*i.e.*, the *chi*), inhibited throat, spitting of pus and blood, and incessant diarrhea, this is difficult to treat. It indicates *Ma Huang Sheng Ma Tang* (Ephedra & Cimicifuga Decoction).[28]

If cold damage originally manifesting diarrhea due to cold is treated by a physician with ejection and precipitation, cold may constitute obstruction (to the heart) and hence result in vomiting and refluxing of food upon ingestion. This indicates *Gan Jiang Huang Qin Huang Lian Ren Shen Tang* (Dry Ginger, Scutellaria, Coptis & Ginseng Decoction).[29]

---

[27] This formula is composed of Ramulus Cinnamomi Cassiae (*Gui Zhi*), Radix Glycyrrhizae (*Gan Cao*), Rhizoma Et Radix Rhei (*Da Huang*), Radix Paeoniae Lactiflorae (*ShaoYao*), and Rhizoma Zingiberis (*Jiang*).

[28] The ingredients in this formula are Herba Ephedrae (*Ma Huang*), Rhizoma Cimicifugae (*Sheng Ma*), Radix Angelicae Sinensis (*Dang Gui*), Rhizoma Anemarrhenae (*Zhi Mu*), Radix Scutellariae Baicalensis (*Huang Qin*), Rhizoma Polygonati Odorati (*Wei Rui*), Radix Paeoniae Lactiflorae (*Shao Yao*), Tuber Asparagi Cochinensis (*Tian Dong*), Ramulus Cinnamomi Cassiae (*Gui Zhi*), Sclerotium Poriae Cocos (*Fu Ling*), Radix Glycyrrhizae (*Gan Cao*), Gypsum (*Shi Gao*), Rhizoma Atractylodis Macrocephalae (*Bai Zhu*), and Rhizoma Zingiberis (*Jiang*).

[29] This formula is composed of dry Rhizoma Zingiberis (*Gan Jiang*), Radix Scutellariae Baicalensis (*Huang Qin*), Rhizoma Coptidis Chinensis (*Huang Lian*), and Radix Panacis Ginseng (*Ren Shen*).

Diseases Allowing Warming

The great method (*i.e.*, general principle) is, in winter, it is appropriate to administer warm and hot medicinals and to moxa.

The master explained:

If a disease manifesting as fever and headache contrarily with a deep pulse remains unrelieved (for a long time), there will be more severe generalized pain and aching. This requires rescuing the interior, and the appropriate (formula of) medicinals is a warming one, (namely,) *Si Ni Tang* (Four Counterflows Decoction).

Diarrhea, abdominal fullness, and generalized pain and aching should be first treated by warming the interior. The appropriate (formula) is *Si Ni Tang* (Four Counterflows Decoction).

Diarrhea with no thirst is categorized as a *tai yin* disease. It is caused by cold in the viscus (*i.e.*, the spleen) requiring warming. The appropriate (formulas) are *Si Ni Tang* (Four Counterflows Decoction) and its like.

(If taken with) a *shao yin* disease, the sick person may suffer from vomiting immediately upon ingestion of food or drink and a distressing desire of the heart yet with inability to vomit (when no food is taken). At the onset of its contraction, the hands and feet are cold and the pulse is bowstring and slow. If there is cold rheum above the diaphragm giving rise to dry retching, one should not carry out ejection. This requires warming, and the appropriate (formula) is *Si Ni Tang* (Four Counterflows Decoction).

A *shao yin* disease exhibiting a deep pulse should be treated with warming without delay. The appropriate (formula) is *Si Ni Tang* (Four Counterflows Decoction).

Diarrhea with desire for food is rightly a case requiring warming.

When diarrhea is accompanied by a slow and tight pulse and (abdominal) pain does not tend to end, this requires warming. When subjected to chill, there will be (abdominal) fullness and discharge of filthy substances in the stool.

Diarrhea with a floating and large pulse is due to vacuity, a result of forced (*i.e.*, wrongful) application of precipitation. If the pulse is floating and drumskin and there is rumbling in the intestines, it is necessary to apply warming and the appropriate (formula) is *Dang Gui Si Ni Tang* (Dang Gui Four Counterflows Decoction.)[1]

If a *shao yin* disease manifests diarrhea and a faint and choppy pulse, there must be vomiting and (spontaneous) sweating. (If really so,) there must be frequent bowel movements. If, on the contrary, defecation is infrequent, warming is required.

Suppose cold damage is treated by a physician who uses precipitation. Then incessant diarrhea of clear grain and generalized pain and aching will develop. (In that case,) it is urgently necessary to rescue the interior. It is appropriate to warm (internally) with *Si Ni Tang* (Four Counterflows Decoction).

---

[1] This formula is composed of Radix Angelicae Sinensis (*Dang Gui*), Ramulus Cinnamomi Cassiae (*Gui Zhi*), Radix Paeoniae Lactiflorae (*Shao Yao*), Herba Asari Cum Radice (*Xi Xin*), Radix Glycyrrhizae (*Gan Cao*), Caulis Akebiae Mutong (*Mu Tong*), and Fructus Zizyphi Jujubae (*Da Zao*).

_________________Chapter Ten_________________
Diseases Not Allowing Moxibustion

If the pulse is faint and rapid, one should be careful not to apply moxibustion. When fire works as an evil, it will produce vexation and (qi) counterflow. It leads to (yin) vacuity, is in pursuit of (yang) repletion, and disperses blood in the vessels. Faint as a fire qi may be, it is mighty in attacking internally. It may parch the bones, damage the sinews, and makes it difficult to restore the blood.

If the pulse is floating, it is necessary to effect a resolution by means of diaphoresis. If, on the contrary, moxibustion is used, evils will have no way to leave and, by dint of the fire (from moxaing), they will become superabundant. (In consequence,) a disease of heaviness and *bi* from the lumbus down will inevitably arise. This is fire counterflow. Before there is a tendency towards a natural resolution, there should first appear vexation. With vexation, there will be perspiration, and following perspiration, a resolution will ensue. What shows (this resolution)? The pulse is floating. It tells that there should be perspiration which will effect a resolution.

Suppose the pulse is floating and there is severe fever, but moxibustion is used. This is a repletion case (originally). If repletion is treated as vacuity, fire will stir up (yin blood), inevitably resulting in a dry throat and spitting of blood.

Chapter Eleven
Diseases Allowing Moxibustion

If the needled point catches cold in the process of red-hot needling to promote perspiration, a red tubercle (over the point) will arise. In consequence, running piglet (*ben tun*) with qi surging up from the lower abdomen will inevitably develop. (In that case,) moxa over the tubercle with one cone and administer *Gui Zhi Jia Gui Tang* (Cinnamon Twig Plus Cinnamon Decoction).

A *shao yin* disease manifesting on the first or second day with harmony within the mouth[1] and aversion of the back to cold requires moxibustion.

If people who are taken with a *shao yin* disease suffer from vomiting, diarrhea, and fever rather than counterflow frigidity of the hands and feet, they will not die. If the pulse is impalpable, moxa the *shao yin* channel[2] with seven cones.

If a *shao yin* disease manifests diarrhea and a faint and choppy pulse, there must be vomiting and (spontaneous) sweating. (In that case,) there must be frequent bowel movements. If, on the contrary, defecation is infrequent, it is necessary to warm the upper by moxibustion.

---

[1] According to Hong-yen Hsu and William G. Peacher in *Shang Han Lun, The Great Classic of Chinese Medicine*, Oriental Healing Arts Institute, Los Angeles, 1981, p. 48, harmony within the mouth should be interpreted as no dryness in the mouth.

[2] This refers to the point Great Ravine (*Tai Xi*, Ki 3).

The various cases of diarrhea can be treated by moxaing Great Metropolis (*Da Du*, Sp 2) with five cones and Shang Hill (*Shang Qui*, Sp 5) and Yin Mound Spring (*Yin Ling Quan*, Sp 9) both with three cones.

Suppose diarrhea is accompanied by inversion frigidity of the hands and feet and absence of the pulse. If this is treated with moxibustion but (the hands and feet) do not become warm but rather slight dyspnea arise, this is death. If the *shao yin* (pulse) is inferior to the instep (pulse),[3] this is favorable.

If, on the sixth or seventh day, cold damage manifests as a faint pulse, inversion frigidity of the hands and feet, and vexation and agitation, then moxa the *jue yin* channel. If this inversion is not overcome, this is death.

Cold damage manifesting a skipping pulse and inversion counterflow (frigidity) of the hands and feet allows for moxibustion. One may moxa the *shao yin* and *jue yin* channels. They are the ruling (channels) for counterflow.

---

[3] In other words, the pulse at the point Surging Yang (*Chong Yang*, St 42) is stronger than the pulse at the point Great Ravine (*Tai Xi*, Ki 3).

______Chapter Twelve______
Diseases Not Allowing Needling

Do not needle (someone) while they are in a great rage, and do not become angry immediately after having been needled.

Do not needle (someone) immediately after sexual intercourse, and do not engage in sexual intercourse immediately after having been needled.

Do not needle (someone) who is greatly taxed (*i.e.*, fatigued), and do not tax oneself (*i.e.*, labor) immediately after having been needled.

Do not needle (someone) while they are intoxicated, and do not become intoxicated immediately after having been needled.

Do not needle (someone) when they have overeaten, and do not overeat immediately after having been needled.

Do not needle (someone) when they are very hungry, and do not go hungry immediately after having been needled.

Do not needle (someone) while they are thirsty, and do not become thirsty immediately after having been needled.

Do not needle (someone) immediately after they have experienced violent fright.

Do not needle (when someone has) great (*i.e.*, intense) heat.

Do not needle if there is prodigious sweating. Do not needle if there is a deranged pulse. Do not receive needling when there is severe generalized heat and both the yin and yang (pulses) are bellicose.[1] For those indicating needling, do it without delay and (the treatment will) drain (the evils) even if it fails to promote sweating. The reason why some cases are said to prohibit needling is that there are signs and symptoms of death. One should not needle if the disease and the pulse are mutually incongruous. The superior practitioner will needle without the engenderment (of disease, *i.e.*, before the disease arises). Secondly, he will needle a disease before it is fully developed. And finally, he will needle a disease when it is on the wane. (Conversely,) an inferior practitioner acts to the contrary. (Such a physician) is said to be felling the form (*i.e.*, the body).

---

[1]   This means that the pulse feels exuberant in both the superficial and deep levels.

_____________Chapter Thirteen_____________
Diseases Allowing Needling

A *tai yang* disease manifesting headache will heal by itself on the seventh day since, (by that time, the evil) has out-passed the (*tai yang*) channel. If there is a tendency (for the evil) to work up the next channel,[1] it is necessary to needle the foot *yang ming* channel to avert channel transmission. Then a cure will ensue.

Suppose *Gui Zhi Tang* (Cinnamon Twig Decoction) has first been administered for a *tai yang* disease. If this results in vexation rather than resolution, it is necessary first to needle Wind Pool (*Feng Chi*, GB 20) and Wind Mansion (*Feng Fu*, GV 16), and then administer *Gui Zhi Tang* (Cinnamon Twig Decoction). Then a cure will ensue.

If cold damage manifests abdominal fullness, delirious speech, and a floating and tight *cun* opening pulse, this is the liver overwhelming the spleen and is known as sequential advance (*cong*).[2] It requires needling Cycle Gate (*Qi Men*, Liv 14).

If cold damage manifests fever and aversion to cold as after a soaking and the sick person is intensely thirsty, desiring to drink vinegar, then abdominal fullness will inevitably arise. If there is spontaneous sweating and the urination is disinhibited, the disease is tending towards resolution. This is liver overwhelming the lungs and is called rebellion (*heng*).[3] It (also) requires needling Cycle Gate (*Qi Men*, Liv 14).

If a *yang ming* disease manifests hemafecia and delirious speech, this is due to heat entering the blood chamber. If perspiration is confined to the head, it is necessary to needle Cycle Gate (*Qi Men*, Liv 14), draining it in accordance with repletion. When moderate sweat exits, a cure will ensue.

---

[1] After the *tai yang* comes the *yang ming*. Therefore, this section refers to the appearance of the *yang ming* pattern.

[2] From the point of view of five phase theory, it is natural, for instance, when metal restrains wood or earth restrains water. Therefore, this term in this context means that wood (*i.e.*, the liver) restrains earth (*i.e.*, the spleen).

[3] Metal should restrain wood, but now, on the contrary, wood (*i.e.*, the liver) is restraining metal (*i.e.*, the lungs). Therefore wood is being rebellious.

Suppose a woman is taken with wind stroke, suffering from fever and aversion to cold when her menstrual water comes. Seven or eight days later, fever is eliminated and the pulse becomes slow with a cool body. If fullness in the chest and flanks like chest binding arises with delirious speech, this shows that heat has entered the blood chamber. It requires needling Cycle Gate (*Qi Men*, Liv 14), performing whatever manipulation is appropriate for vacuity or repletion. It is said in the *Ping Bing (Discussion on Disease)*[4] that, when heat has entered the blood chamber, one should avoid offending the stomach qi and the two upper burners. In terms of violation (of this principle) how can medication alone be spoken of and needling be excluded?

If a combined disease of the *tai yang* and *shao yang* manifests headache, stiffness of the nape, dizziness, and, at times, glomus and tightness below the heart like chest binding, it is necessary to needle the first vertebral interspace, (*i.e.*, Great Shuttle (*Da Zhui*, Bl 11), Lung Shu (*Fei Shu*, Bl 13), and Liver Shu (*Gan Shu*, Bl 18). One should be careful not to promote sweating, for diaphoresis will produce delirious speech. With delirious speech, the pulse is bowstring. If delirious speech does not come to an end in five days, it is necessary to needle Cycle Gate (*Qi Men*, Liv 14).

A *shao yin* disease manifesting diarrhea with pus and blood in the stools allows needling.

Suppose a woman who is taken with cold damage in pregnancy suffers from abdominal fullness and inability to urinate besides heaviness from the lumbus down as if there were water (inside. This is due to the fact that,) in the seventh month of pregnancy, it is the turn of the *tai yin* to nourish (the fetus) but, (in this case,) it fails to do so.[5] This arises from heart qi repletion, requiring needling Palace of Toil (*Lao Gong*, Per 8) and Origin Pass (*Guan Yuan*, CV 4) with draining. Once urination is disinhibited, a cure will ensue.

(To treat) cold damage with throat *bi*, needle the hand *shao yin* channel. (The point) of the *shao yin* (to be needled) is located at the wrist on the stirring (*i.e.*, pulsating) vessel aligned with the small finger (*i.e.*, Spirit Gate, [*Shen Men*, Ht 7]), needling to a depth of three *fen* with supplementation.

(The Yellow Emperor) asked:

Suppose there is a disease of (spontaneous) sweating, generalized heat, vexation, and (chest) fullness. What kind of disease is it if vexation and fullness are unresolvable by perspiration?

---

[4] This is a long-lost medical classic.

[5] This suggests the theory that each of the five viscera and six bowels are responsible for the nourishment of the fetus during certain months of gestation.

The master answered:

Sweating with generalized heat is wind. Vexation and fullness remaining unresolved in spite of perspiration is inversion. This disease is named wind inversion. The *tai yang* governs the qi. Therefore, it is the first that is subject to (wind cold) evils. Because the *shao yin* stands in an interior/exterior relationship with it, when possessed by the heat (transformed from cold wind in the *tai yang*, the *shao yin*) ascends. When (the *shao yin*) ascends, inversion arises. To treat this, needle the exterior and the interior (*i.e.*, the *shao yin* and the *tai yang* channels) and administer an (appropriate) decoction.

On the third day of a febrile disease, if the qi opening (pulse) is tranquil but the *ren ying* (pulse) is agitated, one should select from the points of the various yang channels (on the list of) the fifty-nine needling (points) to drain heat, induce perspiration, and replenish yin in order to supplement insufficiency.[6] The so-called fifty-nine needling (points) include three points on either side of each hand, totaling twelve in all;[7] a point between each of the five fingers, eight in all;[8] the same number in the feet;[9] three points on the head bilateral (to the midline of the head, beginning) one *cun* into the hairline, six in all;[10] five points in the hair, three *cun* (bilateral to the midline of the head), ten in all;[11] one point anterior and one point posterior to the auricle, one point below the mouth, one point in the nape of the neck, six in all;[12] and one point on the vertex.[13]

---

[6] The qi opening or *cun* opening pulse is a yin pulse in comparison to the *ren ying* pulse which is located in the neck and is, therefore, a yang pulse. A tranquil qi opening pulse suggests that the febrile disease remains lodged within the three yang channels and has not entered the yin channels.

[7] These are Lesser Shang (*Shao Shang*, Lu 11), Central Hub (*Zhong Chong*, Per 9), and Lesser Thoroughfare (*Shao Chong*, Ht 9) on the radial aspect of the fingers and Lesser Marsh (*Shao Ze*, SI 1), Passage Hub (*Guan Chong*, TB 1), and upper Yang (*Shang Yang*, LI 1) on the ulnar aspect. Counting these points bilaterally, there are twelve in all.

[8]

[9] These are Bundle Bone (*Shu Gu*, Bl 65), Foot on the Verge of Tears (*Zu Lin Qi*, GB 41), Sunken Valley (*Xian Gu*, St 43), and Supreme White (*Tai Bai*, Sp 3).

[10] These are Fifth Space (*Wu Chu*, Bl 5), Light Guard (*Cheng Guang*, Bl 6), and Celestial Connection (*Tong Tian*, Bl 7).

[11] These are Head On the Verge of Tears (*Tou Lin Qi*, GB 15), Eye Window (*Mu Chuang*, GB 16), Upright Nutrition (*Zheng Ying*, GB 17), Spirit Support (*Cheng Ling*, GB 18), and Brain Hollow (*Nao Kong*, GB 19).

[12] These are Auditory Convergence (*Ting Hui*, GB 2), Completion Bone (*Wan Gu*, GB 12), Nectar Receptacle (*Cheng Jiang*, CV 24), and Mute's Gate (*Ya Men*, GV 15).

[13] This is Hundred Convergence (*Bai Hui*, GV 20).

If a febrile disease is first characterized by pain in the skin, nasal congestion, and puffiness of the face, one should treat at the level of the skin with the first type of needle,[14] choosing from the fifty-nine needling (points). In the case of depressed heat causing a rash on the nose, one should appeal to the skin on behalf of the lungs.[15] If this does not work, appeal to fire, fire being the heart.[16]

If a febrile disease is characterized by a dry throat, copious drinking, susceptibility to fright, and disturbed sleep, one should treat at the level of the flesh using the sixth type of needle[17] and choosing from the fifty-nine needling (points). In the case of red canthi, one should appeal to the flesh on behalf of the spleen. If this does not work, appeal to wood, wood being the liver.

For a febrile disease with pain in the chest and lateral costal region and fidgeting of the hands and feet, one should treat between the sinews, puncturing the four extremities with the fourth type of needle.[18] In the case of sinew limpness and soaked eyes, one should appeal to the sinews on behalf of the liver. If this does not work, appeal to metal, metal being the lungs.

For a febrile disease with susceptibility to fright, tugging and slackening, and mania, one should treat at the level of the vessels, promptly draining the surplus (vessel) using the fourth type of needle.[19] In the case of madness and loss of hair, one should appeal to the blood on behalf of the heart. If this does not work, appeal to water, water being the kidneys.

---

[14] This refers to the arrowhead needle.

[15] Appealing to the skin on behalf of the lungs means that one should just puncture through the skin to balance the qi of the lungs. Similar expressions appear below which should all be understood in the same way.

[16] Heat in the skin is due to evils lodging in the surface and is associated with the lungs. Thus the lungs should be treated through needling the skin. This means shallow insertion of the needle, not allowing the needle to go deeper than the skin. It also means that one should choose points specifically effective for the skin from the fifty-nine points. If this fails, it is because there is a surplus of metal. In that case, the restraining phase of metal (*i.e.*, fire) must be supplemented to restrain metal. Therefore, in that case, the heart channel should be needled with a supplementing manipulation. When the heart is replenished, lung metal will be restored to normal.

[17] This refers to the round-sharp needle.

[18] This refers to the sharp needle.

[19] This refers to the round end needle.

For a febrile disease with generalized heaviness, painful bones, deafness and heavy eyes, one should needle at the level of the bones using the fourth type of needle and choosing from the fifty-nine needling (points). For bone disease with tooth decay and green-blue auricles, one should appeal to the bones on behalf of the kidneys. If this does not work, appeal to earth, earth being the spleen.

(To treat) a febrile disease characterized at first by extensive rough (skin of the) body, vexation, oppression, and dry lips and dry throat, needle choosing from among the fifty-nine needling (points) with the first type of needle. Skin distention, dry mouth, and cold sweat [there is something left out here].

Febrile disease with headache, tense temples, tense ocular vessel, and frequent nosebleeding is due to inverted heat. (To treat this,) choose the third type of needle, (supplementing or draining) in accordance with vacuity or repletion. Cold and heat disease [these four words seem to be superfluous].

(To treat) a febrile disease with generalized heaviness and heat in the intestines, puncture with the fourth type of needle the points of the channels (*i.e.,* those of the spleen and stomach) and the points between the toes, appealing to qi on behalf of the stomach connecting vessel network. The qi must be obtained (when needling).

(To treat) a febrile disease with periumbilical pain and tension and propping fullness of the chest and lateral costal regions, puncture Gushing Spring (*Yong Quan,* Ki 1) and (the points) of the (foot) *tai yin* and *yang ming* with the fourth type of needle. Also (puncture) Throat Interior (*Yi Li,* CV 23).

(To treat) a febrile disease with (spontaneous) sweating or one with a propitious pulse allowing diaphoresis, needle Fish Border (*Yu Ji,* Lu 10), Great Abyss (*Tai Yuan,* Lu 9), Great Metropolis (*Da Du,* Sp 2), and Supreme White (*Tai Bai,* Sp 3). Draining (manipulation) eliminates the heat, while supplementing (manipulation) promotes perspiration. In the case of excessive perspiration, needle the crease above the (medial) malleolus (*i.e.,* Three Yin Intersection, *San Yin Jiao,* Sp 6) to stop it.

(To treat) a febrile disease with a stirring pulse, dyspnea, and dizziness on the seventh or eighth day, needle without delay to promote sweating, puncturing at the thumb (*i.e.,* Lesser Shang, *Shao Shang,* Lu 11) to a superficial depth.

(To treat) a febrile disease with pain in the chest and lateral costal region and fidgeting of the hands and feet, needle the foot *shao yang* (and the hand *tai yin*), supplementing at the hand *tai yin*. In severe cases, puncture choosing from among the fifty-nine needling (points).

(To treat) a febrile disease with pain first in the forearms, needle the hand *yang ming* and *tai yin*. Once sweat exits, relief will ensue.

(To treat) a febrile disease first involving the head and face, needle the *tai yang* at the nape. Once sweat exits, relief ensues.

(To treat) a febrile disease at first manifesting generalized heaviness, painful bones, deafness, and heavy eyes, needle the foot *shao yin*. In severe cases, puncture choosing from the fifty-nine needling (points).

(To treat) a febrile disease at first manifesting dizziness, fever, and fullness in the chest and lateral costal region, needle the foot *shao yin* and *shao yang*.

(To treat) a febrile disease initially involving the lower legs, first needle the foot *yang ming* to promote sweating.

Chapter Fourteen
Diseases Not Allowing Water Therapy

After diaphoresis, copious drinking will inevitably result in dyspnea. So will a bath.

After cold damage is treated by drastic ejection and drastic precipitation, there will be the severest of vacuity. If drastic diaphoresis is then furthermore carried out, the sick person's exterior qi will become depressed. If the sick person is given water (to drink) for the purpose of perspiration, there will arise retching. This is because there is cold in the stomach.

A *yang ming* disease with tidal fever can be treated with *Cheng Qi Tang* (Support the Qi Decoction) if (the stool) is slightly hard. If (the stool) is not hard, this formula cannot be administered. If there has been absence of defecation for six or seven consecutive days, there is possibly dry stool. The method to determine this is to try administering *Xiao Cheng Qi Tang* (Minor Support Qi Decoction). If there is no flatus turning in the abdomen, this shows that only the (beginning) end of the stool is hard and that the rest is thin liquid. Attacking (internally in that case) is not allowed since attacking would inevitably produce abdominal fullness and inability to take in food. Those who desire to drink will develop retching.

Suppose there is a *yang ming* disease with vacuity cold in the stomach and the sick person suffers from inability to take in food. Then drinking will immediately produce retching.

Diarrhea with a floating and large pulse is due to vacuity, a result of forced (*i.e.*, wrong) use of attacking. Suppose the pulse is floating and drumskin and there is rumbling in the intestines, warming is required. If water is given (to drink), there will be retching.

Illness in the yang (exterior) requires diaphoresis to effect a resolution. If, on the contrary, one performs water spraying or water bathing, heat will not be eliminated but rather vexation, gooseflesh, and a desire to drink yet with no thirst will arise. It is appropriate (to administer) *Wen He San* (Clam Shell Powder).[1] If no relief is effected (nonetheless), administer *Wu Ling San* (Five [Ingredients] Poria Powder). For chest binding due to cold repletion accompanied by no signs of heat, administer *San Wu Xiao Xian Xiong Tang* (Three Materials Minor Sunken Chest Decoction).[2] *Bai San* (White Powder)[3] is also appropriate. Suppose generalized fever and gooseflesh are not resolved (after taking these) and (the sick person) desires to pull quilts over himself. If (the physician) performs water spraying or bathing, this will make heat retreat. Because (the heat) will not be able to come out, sweat will refuse to exit when it should exit, thus resulting in vexation. If, following perspiration, there is abdominal pain, administer three *liang* (1 *liang* = approximately 30 grams) of Radix Paeoniae Lactiflorae (*Shao Yao*) as instructed above.

If the *cun* opening pulse is floating and large but the (attending) physician contrarily uses precipitation, this is a great error. In the presence of a floating (pulse), there is absence of blood, and, in the presence of a large (pulse), there is cold. When cold qi is contending, there is rumbling in the intestines. If the physician is unaware of this and (makes the sick person) drink to promote copious sweating, water will meet cold qi. Then (water) must contend with cold and the sick person will unavoidably suffer from esophageal constriction.

Suppose the *cun* opening pulse is soggy and weak. In the presence of a soggy (pulse), there is aversion to cold, and, in the presence of a weak (pulse), there is fever. The sogginess and the weakness combine to show that the visceral qi is debilitated and faint, giving rise to tormenting vexation. This is not a case of bound heat. If (the sick person) is treated with cold compresses with a wet cloth or a cold water container, then yang qi is made fainter and the various viscera have

---

[1] This formula is composed of a single ingredient: Concha Meretricis (*Wen He*).

[2] This formula, also known simply as *Xiao Xian Xiong Tang* (Minor Sunken Chest Decoction), is composed of Rhizoma Coptidis Chinensis (*Huang Lian*), Rhizoma Pinelliae Ternatae (*Ban Xia*), and Fructus Trichosanthis Kirlowii (*Gua Lou*).

[3] The ingredients in this formula include Radix Platycodi Grandiflori (*Jie Geng*), Bulbus Fritillariae (*Bei Mu*), and Semen Crotonis Tiglii (*Ba Dou*).

nothing to hang on to. The yin (*i.e.*, blood) vessels become congealed, bound below the heart, and refuse to move. With vacuity cold in the stomach, water and grain are incapable of being transformed. Even though urination is uninhibited, urine is scanty. Such a case, if mild, is savable, but, when cold gathers below the heart, there is no help.

_______________Chapter Fifteen_______________
Diseases Allowing Water Therapy

Suppose a *tai yang* disease is treated with diaphoresis or there is copious (spontaneous) sweating, then the stomach will become dry and vexation causing inability to sleep arises. If the sick person desires to drink, it is necessary to drink a little to harmonize the stomach. Then recovery will ensue.

A *jue yin* disease with thirst and desire to drink will be overcome when water is drunk.

If a *tai yang* disease exhibits a moderate pulse in the *cun*, is small and floating in the *guan*, and is weak in the *chi* and the sick person suffers from fever and (spontaneous) perspiration in addition to aversion to cold with no retching or glomus below the heart, this is produced by the (attending) physician using precipitation. If no precipitation has been used and the sick person suffers from no aversion to cold but is thirsty, this is transmutation (of the *tai yang*) into the *yang ming* (pattern). If urination is frequent, the stool must be hard. Absence of defecation (even) for ten days will give rise to no bitterness (*i.e.*, suffering). To those who desire to drink, just give them water. To assist this, it is necessary to mete out an (appropriate) formula. For thirst, *Wu Ling San* (Five [Ingredients] Poria Powder) is appropriate.

Suppose the *cun* opening pulse is surging and large, rapid and slippery. In the presence of a surging and large (pulse), there is fulminant constructive qi, and, in the presence of slipperiness and rapidity, there is stomach qi repletion. Fulminant constructive qi means exuberance of yang (or heat) which is depressed and unable to leave the body. With stomach repletion, the stool is hard and difficult to evacuate, (*i.e.*, the stool is dry). The triple burner is blocked and congested, and the circulation of fluids is at a standstill. When the physician uses diaphoresis, yang (heat) is too exuberant to let (sweat) exit thoroughly. Then (the physician) may further carry out precipitation. This will make the stomach dry with heat accumulating. In consequence, the stool becomes bound up, while urination is inhibited. The constructive and defensive contend with one another, producing heart vexation, fever, eyes glaring like two fires, a dry nose, and a red facial complexion. The tongue is dry and the teeth are parched and yellow colored. Therefore, intense thirst arises. The result of channel passage or out-reaching is a nasty disease which will not yield to needling or medication. If one gives the languishing (body) a bath, the yang qi will become slightly dispersed and the body will become cold. Then (the sick person) has to be dressed in warm clothes. (As a result,) sweat exits and the exterior and interior may be freed. However, although the disease (seems) to be eliminated, the form and the pulse are (still) incongruous in most cases. This kind of recovery is not achieved through proper treatment. A physician should be prudent (in treatment) and not recklessly commit the blunder of damaging the constructive and defensive.

Sudden turmoil (*i.e.*, choleraic disease) accompanied by headache, fever, generalized pain and aching, and a desire to drink in high fever indicates *Wu Ling San* (Five [Ingredients] Poria Decoction).

Suppose there is retching and vomiting with the disease located above the diaphragm. If later there arises a desire for water, it is urgently necessary to administer *Zhu Ling San* (Polyporous Powder).[1] Drinking water will also effect (relief).

---

[1]   This formula is composed of Sclerotium Poriae Cocos (*Fu Ling*), Sclerotium Polypori Umbellati (*Zhu Ling*), and Rhizoma Atractylodis Macrocephalae (*Bai Zhu*).

_______________Chapter Sixteen_______________
Diseases Not Allowing Fire Therapy[1]

If a *tai yang* disease of wind stroke is treated with fire to force sweat out, the evil wind will be heated by this fire. (Then) blood and qi will spill over and flood, keeping no measure. The two yang (*i.e.*, wind and fire-heat) mutually fume and act upon one another, producing generalized yellowing. Yang exuberance produces a tendency to nose bleeding, while yin vacuity (*i.e.*, scanty

---

[1]   In its narrow sense, fire therapy includes ironing, red-hot needling, fire cupping and steaming, etc. However, in a broader sense, it may also include moxibustion or even formulas of hot nature or of medicinals processed with fire.

fluids) result in difficult urination. If there is vacuity and exhaustion of both yin and yang, the body will become dry and desiccated with perspiration only seen on the head and confined to above the neck. Abdominal fullness, slight dyspnea, a dry mouth, and ulceration of the throat will arise. There will be absence of defecation which, over time, will produce delirious speech. In severe cases, there will be retching, agitation and fidgeting of the hands and feet, and carphologia. If urination can be disinhibited, the sick person can be treated.

Suppose a *tai yang* disease is treated by a physician with diaphoresis and subsequently there arises fever and aversion to cold. If it is further treated with precipitation, glomus below the heart will arise because there is vacuity of both the exterior and interior and exhaustion of both yin and yang qi. With absence of yang, yin is left solitary. If this is further treated with red-hot needling, vexation, yellowish green-blue facial complexion, and twitching of the flesh will arise. Such a case is difficult to treat. Those with a slightly yellow facial complexion and warm hands and feet can be cured.

Cold damage, if treated with warm needling, will inevitably develop susceptibility to fright.

If the pulse is floating in the yang (*i.e.,* the *cun*) and weak in the yin (*i.e.,* the *chi*), there is blood vacuity. With blood vacuity, the sinews are damaged. If the pulse is deep, the constructive is faint. If the pulse is floating and sweat exits (copiously) like rolling pearls, the defensive qi is debilitated. If the constructive qi is faint and red-hot needling is applied, blood will stop circulating, fever will become higher, and vexation and agitation will arise.

If cold damage with a floating pulse is treated by a physician with fire to force (sweat) out, there will be yang collapse with susceptibility to fright, mania, and restlessness either in lying down or rising up. This indicates *Gui Zhi Qu Shao Yao Jia Shu Qi Mu Li Long Gu Jiu Ni Tang* (Cinnamon Twig Minus Peony & Plus Dichroa, Oyster Shell & Dragon Bone Rescue Counterflow Decoction).[2]

(The Yellow Emperor) asked:

Fifteen or sixteen days after contraction, a disease manifested as generalized yellowing, diarrhea, and mania with a desire to run about. You, Master, examined the pulse, saying that a cure would follow a discharge of clear blood the color of pig's liver (with the stools). Later your words turned out to be true. How did you arrive at that prognosis?

The master answered:

---

[2] This formula is composed of Ramulus Cinnamomi Cassiae (*Gui Zhi*), Rhizoma Zingiberis (*Jiang*), Herba Dichroae Febrifugae (*Shu Qi*), Fructus Zizyphi Jujubae (*Da Zao*), Concha Ostreae (*Mu Li*), Os Draconis (*Long Gu*), and Radix Glycyrrhizae (*Gan Cao*).

The *cun* opening pulse was floating in the yang (*i.e.*, the *cun*) and soggy and weak in the yin (*i.e.*, the *chi*). Floating in the yang pointed to wind, and sogginess and weakness in the yin pointed to scant blood. The floating and vacuity (pulse qualities) indicated subjection to wind. (Together with wind) scanty blood produced fever, aversion to cold as after a soaking, stiffness of the nape, and dizziness. The (attending) physician had used fire fuming to drive sweat outward. In consequence, aversion to cold was exacerbated. The guest (*i.e.*, vacuity) heat was wrought up by the strength of the fire. (This heat) was depressed, steaming the flesh and skin, yellowing the body, including the eyes. Slightly difficult urination, shortness of breath, and nosebleeding also arose. Then further (treatment with) precipitation deprived the stomach of fluids. As a result, there was incessant diarrhea. Since the heat was depressed within the urinary bladder, settling and binding there to develop (blood) gatherings and accumulations like pig's liver. Because of the precipitation (of the gathering and accumulation), the heart was disturbed with confusion. (The sick person) ran about and could not control himself (from his desire to) plunge himself into water. If the blood amassment could be removed, then the eyes would become bright and the heart would be pacified. All this was entirely due to the work of the (attending) physician rather than a (natural) calamity. As long as such a case is mild or slight, relief can be effected, but severe cases are incurable.

Cold damage is invariably accompanied by thirst if the pulse is not bowstring, tight, or weak. It will be accompanied by delirious speech if treated with fire. It will be accompanied by fever if the pulse is weak. If the pulse is floating, it requires diaphoresis for resolution. Then a cure will follow.

If a *tai yang* disease is treated with fire fuming but no perspiration is induced, then the sick person must be agitated. If resolution is not realized after the channel is run through,[3] there will invariably be clear blood (in the stools).

If a *yang ming* disease is treated with fire, there will be moderate perspiration on the forehead and inhibited urination. Then there will invariably be yellowing (of the body).

Suppose a *yang ming* disease manifests a floating and tight pulse, a dry throat, a bitter taste in the mouth, abdominal fullness, dyspnea, fever, sweating, aversion to heat rather than cold, and generalized heaviness. If it is treated with diaphoresis, agitation, confused heart, and delirious speech will arise. If it is further treated with red-hot needling, apprehension as well as vexation

---

[3] If there is no aberration, cold damage takes a fixed number of days to transmit from one channel to another. Usually the *tai yang* pattern is finished in six or seven days. Then the *yang ming* pattern appears. Therefore, in this context, the expression "the channel is run through" means the end of the *tai yang* pattern.

and agitation causing sleeplessness will inevitably occur.

A *shao yin* disease with cough, diarrhea, and delirious speech is the result of forcing (sweat) out (erroneously) with fire. There is invariably difficult urination which is due to pressing the *shao yin* for sweat.

If, on the second day, a *tai yang* disease is treated by means of ironing the back with a heated tile and copious perspiration is (hence) induced, the fire qi will enter the stomach. Then the stomach will be exhausted and dry up, and inevitably there will be delirious speech. After more than ten days, if there is cold shuddering contrarily with (spontaneous) sweating, this shows a tendency to resolution.

Suppose sweat is absent from below the lumbus and the sick person suffers from a desire but inability to urinate, urinary incontinence occurring while retching, and aversion of the underside of the feet to wind. If the stool is hard, there should be frequent urination. If, however, there is (practically) infrequent voiding of scant urine with headache arising on finishing defecation, the sick person must have heat in the soles of the feet. This is because the grain qi is flowing downward.

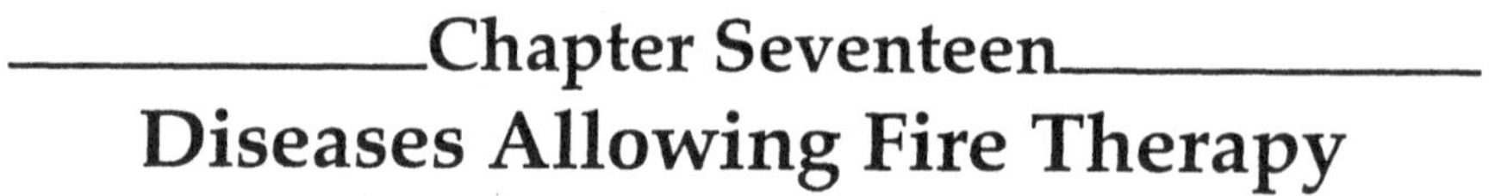

Chapter Seventeen
Diseases Allowing Fire Therapy

(To treat) diarrhea with pain inside the grain duct (*i.e*, the anus), it is necessary to warm with fire, the appropriate (method) being to iron with heated powdered salt. Another method is to iron with fried Fructus Immaturus Aurantii (*Zhi Shi*).

Signs of Life & Death in Relation to the Febrile Diseases of Yin-Yang Conjunction, *Shao Yin* (Patterns), Inversion Counterflow & Yin-Yang Exhaustion

(The Yellow Emperor) asked:

There is a warm disease characterized by heat returning immediately after perspiration and a pulse refusing to be less agitated and less racing in spite of perspiration. It manifests manic speech and inability to take in food. What is the name of this disease?

(The master) answered:

This is called yin-yang conjunction which means death. Sweat from human beings is generated from grain which is the producer of essence. The evil qi joins and contends (with the righteous qi) within the bones and flesh, and, when sweat is produced, the evil should be retreating, while the essence should becoming triumphant. When the essence is triumphant, there should be ability to take in food and there should be no more heat. Heat is an evil qi, while sweat is an essential qi. (In this case,) perspiration is immediately succeeded by heat; so the evil is the triumphant one. (In addition,) inability to take in food leads to no recruitment of the essence. With heat persisting in spite of perspiration, longevity goes to ruin in no time.

If the pulse remains agitated and exuberant in spite of perspiration, death is a certainty. Since the pulse does not respond to the perspiration, this shows that (the essence) is unable to triumph over the disease. Manic speech shows loss of orientation. Loss of orientation ends in death. Since there are three (signs) of death without one (sign) of life, death is inevitable even though there is (temporary) relief.

If, in a febrile disease, perspiration has already been induced but the pulse remains agitated and exuberant, this is a most exaggerated yang pulse[1] portending death. If the pulse becomes tranquil

---

[1] This does not merely mean a very exuberant pulse. Since the word *mai* can mean vessels as well as the pulse, this sentence implies that the yang vessels, or channels, of the hand and foot are all affected by excessive heat.

following perspiration, there is life (*i.e.*, hope of survival).

If, in a febrile disease, the pulse remains agitated and exuberant and sweat refuses to exit, this is a most exaggerated yang pulse. This is death. If the pulse is agitated and exuberant but sweat is induced, there is life.

If, in a febrile disease, sweat is already induced, the pulse is still agitated, and there is dyspnea with recurring fever, one should not perform needling at the superficial level. If dyspnea is severe, this is death.

A febrile disease with yin-yang conjunction will end in death.

If a febrile disease manifests vexation after perspiration, the pulse ought to become tranquil.

A *tai yang* disease contrarily with an agitated, exuberant pulse is a yin-yang conjunction and will end in death. If sweat is induced and the pulse becomes tranquil, there is life.

If there is a febrile disease with yin-yang conjunction, there will be fever and vexation and agitation of the body. If the *cun* opening pulse on the (hand) *tai yin* is surging on both hands, remaining agitated and exuberant, this shows a yin-yang conjunction. There is death. If, following perspiration, the pulse becomes tranquil, there is life.

In terms of a febrile disease, when yang is advancing while yin is retreating, sweat will exit only from the head. This portends death. If yin is advancing while yang is retreating, sweat exits from the lumbus down to the feet. This also portends death. If yin and yang are both advancing, heat will remain the same as before (even) after perspiration. This also portends death. If both yin and yang are retreating, following perspiration there will be endless cold shuddering with cold qi at the nose and mouth. This also portends death.

A febrile disease with so-called yin merging (*bing yin*) is a febrile disease where sweat is already induced and, following it, there arises diarrhea. This is what yin merging means. It is curable.

A febrile disease with so-called yang merging (*bing yang*) is a febrile disease where sweat is already induced but the pulse remains agitated and exuberant with a high fever. (Further) promotion of sweating fails to induce perspiration or results in nosebleeding. This is what yang merging means. It is curable.

A *shao yin* pattern manifesting aversion to cold, cuddling up, diarrhea, and counterflow frigidity of the hands and feet is beyond cure.

A *shao yin* pattern manifesting dizziness following diarrhea and, at times, cloudedness will end in death.

If people who are taken with a *shao yin* disease suffer from vomiting, diarrhea, agitation, and counterflow (frigidity of the limbs), they will die. If a *shao yin* disease manifests counterflow frigidity of the four limbs, aversion to cold, cuddling up, and absence of the pulse and the sick person suffers from no vexation but from agitation, (the sick person) will die.

If, on the sixth or seventh day of a *shao yin* disease, the sick person has high breathing, then they will die.

Suppose a *shao yin* disease manifests as a faint, thin, and deep pulse, (the sick person) desiring for nothing but to lie down, and there is (spontaneous) sweating, no vexation, and desire to vomit. If, on the fifth or sixth day, there arises diarrhea in addition to vexation and agitation and inability to lie down and sleep, this will end in death.

Suppose a *shao yin* disease manifests diarrhea. If the diarrhea is stopped and there arises aversion to cold and cuddling up and if the hands and feet are warm, this is curable.

A *shao yin* disease with aversion to cold and cuddling up is curable if at times there arises vexation with a desire to remove one's clothes and quilts.

Suppose a *shao yin* disease manifests inversion counterflow (frigidity of the limbs), absence of the pulse, and dry vexation [dry retching in another version] after the diarrhea is checked. If the pulse suddenly appears fulminant after taking a decoction, there is death. If the pulse appears faint and thin, there is life.

If, on the sixth or seventh day of cold damage, the pulse is faint and there is inversion (frigidity) of the hands and feet with vexation and agitation, moxa the *jue yin* (channel). If the inversion is not overcome, there is death.

Cold damage with diarrhea, inversion counterflow (frigidity of the limbs), and agitation causing sleeplessness will end in death.

Suppose cold damage manifests fever and diarrhea. If (diarrhea) provokes endless inversion (frigidity of the extremities), there is death.

Suppose cold damage with inversion counterflow (frigidity of the extremities) has had no diarrhea for six or seven days. If then fever followed by diarrhea occurs, there is life. If the sick person has perspiration and endless diarrhea, they will die, for there is exclusively yin without yang.

If, on the fifth or sixth day, cold damage manifests no chest binding but a soft abdomen, inversion, and a vacuous pulse, it does not allow precipitation. (In this case,) precipitation would cause loss of blood and (hence) death.

Cold damage with fever and inversion will end in death if diarrhea occurs on the seventh day.

If a febrile disease is characterized by pain baffling location, inability to contract (the limbs), a dry mouth, and excessive heat in the yang (*i.e.,* the skin) but much cold in the yin (*i.e.,* the flesh), then there is heat in the (bone) marrow. There is death without a remedy.

If a febrile disease is in the kidneys, it will cause the sick person thirst, a dry mouth, and a parched tongue with a yellow or red color. There will be such an endless desire for water day and night (that even when) the abdomen becomes enlarged and distended, no boredom with drinking will arise. If the eyes have lost their essence brightness (*i.e.,* have become dull), there is death without a remedy.

If the spleen is damaged, wind stroke will make yin and yang qi separate. Since the yin (qi) no longer follows the yang (qi), one has to determine death or survival through the three divisions (of the wrist pulse).

Cold damage with counterflow coughing and qi ascent will end in death if the pulse is dissipated. This refers to a sick person of a reduced form (*i.e.,* an emaciated body).

Cold damage with diarrhea of more than ten bowel movements per day will end in death if the pulse is contrarily replete.

Suppose a sick person has had glomus in the lateral costal region in the past. If the glomus (now) has developed downward to the region lateral to the umbilicus with pain radiating to the lower abdomen and penetrating the genitals and their sinews, this is visceral binding. This is death.

Repletion gives rise to delirious speech, and vacuity to mussitation. Mussitation is (confused) repetition. If there is staring straight ahead, delirious speech, and dyspnea with (chest) fullness, there is death. If there is diarrhea (in addition), death is also certain.

If all the manifestations of chest binding are present, agitation portends death.

Protrusion of a curled tongue portends death. Sputum as sticky as glue signifies difficult resolution. If the sides of the tongue gradually (become wet with) fluid, this shows a tendency towards resolution. When a disease has run through the channel,[2] if the upper lip is (a normal) color and the pulse becomes harmonious by itself, this shows a tendency towards resolution. If the facial complexion is urgent (*i.e.*, the face is screwed up as in pain), resolution is yet to be.

____

[2] This means that a pattern, the *tai yang* for example, has reached its succeeding pattern, the *yang ming* in this case. However, since cold damage is also classified into channels, viscera, and bowel sub-patterns, this line may also be interpreted as "the disease has come to the channel."

Chapter Nineteen
Signs of Life & Death in Relation to Dual Repletion, Dual Vacuity & Yin-Yang Mutual Subjugation

(The Yellow Emperor) asked:

What is vacuity and repletion?

(The master) answered:

Exuberance of evil qi is repletion, and retrenchment of essence qi is vacuity. Dual repletion refers to a disease of great heat. Hot qi (*i.e.*, fever) and a full pulse are indications of dual repletion.

(The Yellow Emperor) asked:

What is repletion of both the channels and their vessel networks?

(The master) answered:

Repletion of both the channels and their vessel networks is characterized by an urgent *cun* (opening) pulse and lax cubit (skin. In this case,) both the channels and the vessel networks should be treated. It is reasonable to say that slipperiness (*i.e.*, smoothness) is a favorable indication, while roughness is an unfavorable one. Vacuity and repletion can be introduced (in an analogous way) to (various) kinds of things. It follows that when the five viscera, the bones, and the flesh are slippery (or smooth) and uninhibited, a long life is maintained.[1] If cold qi ascends abruptly, the pulse will become full and replete. If the pulse is not only replete but slippery, this is a favorable sign prognosticating life. If the pulse is replete but choppy, this is an unfavorable indication prognosticating death. The form may be full all over with an urgent, large, and hard pulse and rough cubit skin. This is an incongruity. Given (the following) favorable indicators, such cases may survive, but given the (following) unfavorable indicators, they will die. What is considered favorable are warm hands and feet, and what is considered unfavorable are cold hands and feet.

(The Yellow Emperor) asked:

What is dual vacuity?

(The master) answered:

A vacuous pulse, qi vacuity, and vacuous (*i.e.*, lax) cubit (skin) comprise dual vacuity. What is called qi vacuity is manifested by erratic speech (*i.e.*, soft, broken speech). Cubit vacuity is manifested by a timid and unsteady step. And a vacuous pulse is a pulse devoid of yin.[2] In such cases, a slippery pulse indicates life, while a choppy one portends death.

Qi vacuity is lung vacuity, and qi counterflow means cold feet. If this does not occur in the (lung-restrained) season, (the sick person) may survive. But, if it happens in the (lung-restrained) season, the condition is fatal. This is true of other viscera as well.[3] Those with a replete and full pulse as well as cold hands and feet and a hot head may survive if it is spring or autumn, but will die if it is winter or summer. If the pulse is floating and choppy and if there is generalized fever in spite of the choppy pulse, this is death.

---

[1] This implies that, since vacuity and repletion are concepts applicable in an analogous way to everything and smoothness or slipperiness is a normal state of a replenished condition, smooth viscera, smooth bowels, etc. are a guarantee for smooth life or health. Hence, if there are smooth viscera and bowels, a long life will be secured.

[2] The *cun* opening is the pulse of the *tai yin*, reflecting yin, *i.e.*, the internal viscera. Therefore, when the pulse is vacuous, it reflects exhausted yin or viscera. This is what is meant by a pulse devoid of yin.

[3] Vacuity of the visceral qi with qi counterflow, *i.e.*, cold hands and feet, is always critical, but the sick person may survive when this does not occur in the season of the restrained phase of the affected viscus. The lungs, for example, are metal. Therefore, summer/fire which restrains metal is the most unfavorable season for lung disease. If a lung disease happens in some other season than summer, there is hope of recovery. In the same, one can prognose diseases of the other viscera in terms of five phase theory.

If there is an insufficiency of the vessel network qi with a surplus of the channel qi, there will be a hot pulse with cold cubit (skin).[4] This is unfavorable in autumn and winter but favorable in spring and summer.

Vacuous channels and full vessel networks manifest as hot and full cubit (skin) with a cold choppy (pulse). This is fatal in autumn or winter. In the case of full vessel networks with vacuous channels, moxa the yin (channel) and needle the yang (channel). In the case of full channels with vacuous vessel networks, needle the yin and moxa the yang.

(The Yellow Emperor) asked:

In autumn and winter, yin should not be forced to the extreme, while, in spring and summer, yang should not be forced to the extreme. What is the meaning of this statement?

(The master) answered:

Not forcing yang to the extreme is a prohibition against repeatedly evacuating the *yang ming* during spring and summer. Evacuation of the *yang ming* leads to mania. Not forcing yin to the extreme is a prohibition against repeatedly evacuating the *tai yin* during the autumn and winter. Evacuation of the *tai yin* leads to death.

In relation to febrile disease, so-called yang subjugated by yin is (a condition where) there is heat from the lumbus down to the feet with cold from the lumbus up. The yin qi is contending below. If (the victorious yin qi) comes back up to the cardiac and abdominal region giving rise to fullness (there), it will cause death. So-called yin subjugated by yang is (a condition where) there is heat from the lumbus up to the head with cold from the lumbus down. The yang qi is contending above. If (yin and yang) are restored to normal so as to induce perspiration, there is life.

---

[4] A hot pulse is a rapid and/or slippery pulse. One should note that this is a case of exuberant yin and vacuity of yang since the *cun* opening pulse reflects the interior/channel and the cubit skin reflects the exterior/vessel networks.

The Signs & Date of Life & Death
in Relation to Febrile Diseases

In connection with the *tai yang* vessel, the appearance of a brilliant color in the zygomatic region indicates a febrile disease. If the brilliance is not perished, (the condition) will heal by itself when (the vessel) has its day provided perspiration is induced. If the *jue yin* vessel vies for an appearance,[1] death is expected to come in less than three days. This is because the qi of the febrile disease has already linked with the kidneys.[2] In connection with the *shao yang* vessel, the appearance of a brilliant color anterior to the cheek indicates a febrile disease. If the brilliance is not perished, (the condition) will heal by itself when (the vessel) has its day provided perspiration is induced. If the *shao yin* vessel vies for an appearance,[3] death is expected to come in less than three days. If, on the seventh or eighth day, the febrile disease exhibits a faint and small pulse and the sick person suffers from hematuria with dryness in the mouth, death will occur in one and a half days. If the pulse is regularly interrupted, death will occur in one day.

If, on the seventh or eighth day, a febrile disease exhibits a pulse which is not agitated or gasping-like and is not rapid (either), sweat will exit three days later. If sweat does not exit then, death will occur on the fourth day. Before sweat exits, do not needle at the superficial depth [another version simply says do not needle].

Suppose, on the third or fourth day, a febrile disease exhibits a pulse which is not gasping-like but beating evenly. Even though there is vexation with fever, perspiration will come out by itself and this will be followed by survival. An old classic says, "(Evils) start in the bowels and then enter the

---

[1] The brilliant color referred to here is a red color and a perished color is a dull, ghastly color. If a green-blue color appears in the area, this indicates that the *jue yin* is vying with the *tai yang*. However, since the word *mai* in this sentence is ambiguous, possibly referring to the pulse rather than the vessel, vying for an appearance may have another interpretation. In that case, the *jue yin* pulse, *i.e.*, a bowstring pulse, appears instead of a floating one.

[2] If a green-blue complexion, representing the liver or the *jue yin*, appears in the zygomatic region instead of a red color, this indicates that the *jue yin* channel is vying for control of the situation. In this case, wood is insulting water which, in turn, is the *shao yin* and *tai yang*. Therefore, the author says that the disease qi has involved the kidneys.

[3] See note 1 above. This might mean a black color appearing anterior to the cheek.

viscera. After they have finished with the yin (interior), they will come back to the yang (exterior). As a result, there will be perspiration."

If, on the seventh or eighth day, a febrile disease exhibits a pulse which is not gasping-like but beating evenly, there is life. Since there is (only) slight heat in the yang which is unable to enter the yin, there is now spontaneous sweating.

If, on the seventh or eighth day, a febrile disease exhibits a pulse which is not gasping-like but beating rapidly at a constant pace, there ought to arise a disease of loss of voice. Perspiration is expected to come in three days. If it fails (to come) then, death will occur on the fourth day.

If a febrile disease is characterized by yellowing and swelling of the whole body including the face, heat in the heart, a dry mouth, a curled tongue with a blackish yellow, parched color, and numbness and rancid (odor) of the whole body, then there are hidden toxins which have damaged the lungs. If these hidden toxins strike the spleen, they will cause death.

Suppose a febrile disease is characterized by tugging and slackening, manic speech, and sweat refusing to exit. If the tugging and slackening continues endlessly, the liver is damaged by hidden toxins. If these toxins strike the gallbladder, they will cause death.

If a febrile disease is characterized by sweat refusing to exit or sweating not reaching the feet, retching of gall, ejection of blood, and susceptibility to fright causing sleeplessness, then hidden toxins have settled in the liver. If they settle in the bowel of the foot *shao yang*, they will cause death.

_______________Chapter Twenty-One_______________
The Ten Unfavorable Death
Patterns in Febrile Disease

In febrile disease, abdominal fullness and distention, generalized heat, inability to defecate and urinate, and a choppy, small, racing pulse are the first unfavorable pattern. Its appearance prognosticates death.

In febrile disease, rumbling in the intestines, abdominal fullness, frigidity of the four limbs, outpour diarrhea, and a persistent floating, large, surging pulse are the second unfavorable pattern. Its appearance prognosticates death.

In febrile disease, incessant massive nosebleeding, abdominal pain, a floating, large, interrupted pulse, and dyspnea with shortness of breath are the third unfavorable pattern. Its appearance prognosticates death.

In febrile disease, retching and hemafecia retrenching the body's flesh, severe fever, and an extremely stirring and racing pulse are the fourth unfavorable pattern. Its appearance prognosticates death.

In febrile disease, cough, dyspnea, palpitations, dizziness, fever, a small, racing pulse, and retrenched bodily flesh are the fifth unfavorable pattern. Its appearance prognosticates death.

In febrile disease, an enlarged abdomen with distention, frigidity of the four limbs, retrenched bodily flesh, and shortness of breath are the sixth unfavorable pattern. Its appearance prognosticates death within ten days.

In febrile disease, abdominal distention, hemafecia, a large pulse which at times becomes small and expired, sweating with dyspnea, a dry mouth, parched tongue, and inability to recognize people are the seventh unfavorable pattern. Its appearance prognosticates death in ten days.

In febrile disease, high fever, a pulse gradually becoming small, cough, hemafecia, sunken eyesockets, ravings, carphologia, a dry mouth, and agitation and fidgeting causing sleeplessness are the eighth unfavorable pattern. Its appearance prognosticates death in one watch.

In febrile disease, tugging and slackening, frenetic walking about, inability to take in food, abdominal fullness, chest pain radiating to the lower back, umbilicus, and upper back, and retching of blood are the ninth unfavorable pattern. Its appearance prognosticates death in one watch.

In relation to febrile disease, retching of blood, dyspnea, cough, vexation, fullness, generalized yellowing, abdominal drum-distention, incessant diarrhea, and an expiring pulse are the tenth unfavorable pattern. Its appearance prognosticates death in one watch.

The Signs & Date of Death in Febrile Disease With Expiry of Qi of the Five Viscera

In febrile disease, lung qi expiry is characterized by counterflow dyspnea, coughing and spitting of blood, swelling of the hands, feet, and abdomen, a yellow facial complexion, shivering, and inability to speak. It will end in death. When the corporeal soul (*po*) is gone together with the skin and hair, the lungs are already dead. Exacerbation occurs on the *bing* day and death on the *ding* day.

In febrile disease, spleen qi expiry is characterized by headache, retching of old juice, inability to take in food, counterflow retching and vomiting of blood, inability to take in (even) water, manic speech, ravings, an enlarged and full abdomen, inability to contract the four limbs, and melancholy. It will end in death. When the qi of the pulse and the flesh are both gone, the spleen is already dead. Exacerbation occurs on the *jia* day and death on the *yi* day.

In febrile disease, heart-governor qi expiry is characterized by vexation, fullness, painful bones, a swollen throat with inability to swallow, desire but inability to cough, and singing, crying, and laughing (*i.e.*, emotional lability). It will end in death. When the spirit is gone together with the constructive and the (blood) vessels, the heart is already dead. Exacerbation occurs on the *ren* day and death on the *gui* day.

In febrile disease, liver qi expiry is characterized by sudden collapse, inability to stand steadily, retching of blood, apprehension, aversion to cold as after a soaking, frenetic exiting of blood, and fecal and urinary incontinence. It will end in death. When the ethereal soul (*hun*) is gone together with the sinews and the blood, the liver is already dead. Exacerbation happens on the *geng* day and death on the *xin* day.

In febrile disease, kidney qi expiry is characterized by dyspnea, palpitations, counterflow vomiting, *ju* in the heel, *yong* in the coccygeal region, dim vision, pain in the bones, shortness of breath, dyspnea with (chest) fullness, and sweat flowing like pearls. It will end in death. When the essence and the marrow are both gone, the kidneys are already dead. Exacerbation happens on the *wu* day and death on the *ji* day.

If it is observed externally that the pupils of the eyes are smaller (than usual) and a green-blue color and that there are dry nails, loss of hair, rough body (skin), grimy, (seemingly) lengthened teeth, a thick, dusty black face, coughing and spitting of blood, thirst with desire to drink frequently, and great fullness [of the abdomen may be left out here], these are exterior illnesses due to expiry of the five viscera.

Chapter Twenty-Three
Prognosis of the Date of Death in Terms of the Augmented (*i.e.*, Quickened) Pulse Pattern in Febrile Diseases

The febrile disease of four pulse beats will end in death in three days. Four pulse beats is said when, during the time it takes a normal person to have one pulse beat, the sick person's pulse beats four times.

The febrile disease of five pulse beats will end in death in one day. If the pulse has a big strike from time to time, death will come in half a day. If there is abstraction, oppression, and agitation, this is death.

The febrile disease of six pulse beats will end in death in half day. When the pulse suddenly becomes racing and large, death is coming in awhile.

Chapter Twenty-Four
Prognosis of the Date of Death in Terms of the Damaged (*i.e.*, Slowed-Down) Pulse Pattern in Febrile Disease

The febrile disease with a fourfold reduction pulse will end in death in three days. Fourfold reduction is said when, during the time that takes a normal person to have four pulse beats, the sick person's pulse beats once. This is the meaning of fourfold reduction.

The febrile disease with a fivefold reduction pulse will end in death in one day. Fivefold reduction is said when, during the time that takes a normal person to have five pulse beats, the sick person's pulse beats once. This is the meaning of fivefold reduction.

The febrile disease with a sixfold reduction pulse will end in death in one watch. Sixfold reduction is said when, during the time that takes a normal person to have six pulse beats, the sick person's pulse beats once. This is the meaning of sixfold reduction. If the pulse is expired, not coming at all, or it comes (only) after a long pause, death is imminent.

BOOK EIGHT

Collated & Edited by Honorary Minister Without Portfolio,
Curator of the Imperial Library,
Imperial Courier and Senior Army Protector,
Lin Yi *et al.*

Chapter One
A Discussion on the Pulse (& Other) Signs of Sudden Death-like Inversion

Suppose the pulse is deep, large, and slippery. In the presence of a deep (pulse), there is [blood is suspected to be left out here] repletion, and, in the presence of a slippery (pulse), there is qi [repletion is suspected to be left out here]. Since (blood and) qi repletion act upon one another, blood and qi (evils) invade the viscera. Then death is imminent. If, (however,) they invade the bowels, there is life (*i.e.*, hope of survival). This is known as sudden inversion. Inability to recognize people accompanied by green-blue lips and a cold body is (an indication of) invasion of the viscera. This causes imminent death. If the body is warm and harmonious with spontaneous sweating, (this shows) invasion of the bowels. Cure will ensue by itself later.

Chapter Two
A Discussion on the Pulse (& Other) Signs of Tetany, Dampness & Summerheat Stroke

A *tai yang* disease manifesting fever, absence of sweat, and aversion to cold is known as hard tetany.

A *tai yang* disease manifesting fever, sweating, and no [the word no is suspected to be an erroneous addition] aversion to cold is known as soft tetany.

A *tai yang* disease manifesting fever and a deep, thin pulse is developing towards tetany.

A *tai yang* disease may develop into tetany as a result of promoting sweating.

If a sick person suffers from body heat (*i.e.*, generalized fever) with cold in the feet, stiffness of the nape of the neck, aversion to cold, occasional heat in the head, a red facial complexion with the eye's veins [the preceding word is suspected to be a redundancy] red, and shaking head, tetany is developing.

If a *tai yang* disease manifests absence of sweating contrarily with scanty urine, qi surging up into the chest, clenched teeth, and inability to speak, hard tetany is about to start. (For this,) *Ge Gen Tang* (Pueraria Decoction) is the ruling formula.

The disease of hard tetany is characterized by chest fullness, clenched jaw, arched-back rigidity, and hypertonicity of the feet. The sick person must have grinding of the teeth (To treat this,) administer *Da Cheng Qi Tang* (Major Support the Qi Decoction).

After the disease of tetany is treated with diaphoresis, if the pulse becomes slippery like a snake and the abdomen suddenly becomes distended and enlarged, this shows a tendency towards resolution. If the pulse remains as before or rather becomes hidden and bowstring, there is bound to be (another attack of) tetany.

The pulse of tetany feels rigidly bowstring, beating straight all the way from the upper to the lower positions.

A sick person with tetany has a pulse which is hidden and hard, beating straight all the way from the upper to the lower positions.

Wind disease if treated with precipitation will develop tetany. If it is further treated with diaphoresis, there is bound to be hypertonicity.

If all the manifestations of a *tai yang* disease are present, rigidity of the body with a deep, slow pulse is tetany. The ruling formula is *Gua Lou Gui Zhi Tang* (Trichosanthes & Cinnamon Twig Decoction).[1]

A sick person with tetany and moxibustion sores is difficult to treat. A sick patient with sores should not be treated with diaphoresis even though there is generalized pain and aching. (In this case,) diaphoresis will lead to tetany.

A *tai yang* disease with distressed aching in the joints and a deep, moderate pulse is dampness stroke. [It is said in the *(Shang Han) Lun (Za Bing) (Treatise [on Cold Damage & Miscellaneous*

---

[1] This formula is composed of Radix Trichosanthis Kirlowii (*Hua Fen*), Ramulus Cinnamomi Cassiae (*Gui Zhi*), Radix Paeoniae Lactiflorae (*Shao Yao*), Rhizoma Zingiberis (*Jiang*), and Fructus Zizyphi Jujubae (*Da Zao*).

Diseases])[2] that dampness stroke is a pattern of damp *bi*. The sick person suffers from inhibited urination contrarily with smooth defecation. It is necessary to disinhibit urination (for a resolution).]

If the sick person has pain all over the body and fever which worsens in the late afternoon, this is wind dampness. It is caused by perspiration. [It is said in the *Lun (Treatise)* that this disease is caused by damage done by sweating in a draft or injury done by protracted subjection to cold.]

The disease of dampness may manifest as aching all over the body, fever, and a dull yellow complexion of the body.

The sick person suffering from dampness will have diseases such as sweating confined to the head, rigidity of the back, and a desire to be covered with quilts and be near to a fire. If it is treated with precipitation earlier (than necessary), retching or chest fullness with uninhibited [inhibited in another version] urination, and a tongue as if with fur will arise. This is due to heat in the Cinnabar Field (*i.e.*, the lower abdomen) and cold in the chest. Because there is inability to drink in spite of a desire to, the mouth is dry.

Suppose a sick person who is taken with dampness is treated with precipitation. If then sweating on the forehead, slight dyspnea, and uninhibited [inhibited in another version] urination arise, (the sick person) will die. If there is incessant diarrhea, this is also death.

(The Yellow Emperor) asked:

When wind and dampness contend, there is generalized pain and aching. Then diaphoresis is expected to effect a resolution. If it happens to be wet weather, raining continuously, your Sir instructs that this allows for diaphoresis. In case (diaphoresis) should fail to cure the disease, then what is the explanation?

(The master) answered:

If diaphoresis is carried out and massive sweating is induced, the wind qi may be eliminated, but the dampness qi persists. Therefore, (the treatment) fails to effect recovery. To treat wind dampness, one should perform diaphoresis to such a degree that only moderate sweating appears. Then both wind and dampness will be gone.

---

[2] This is the older version of the *Shang Han Lun (Treatise on Cold Damage)* and the *Jin Gui Yao Lue (Essential Outline of the Golden Cabinet)* written by Zhang Zhong-jing and originally published combined together into one work. It was the author of the present work, Wang She-he, who separated these into two individual books.

For a sick person with dampness suffering from distressing generalized aching, one may administer *Ma Huang Tang* (Ephedra Decoction) with four *liang* of Rhizoma Atractylodis Macrocephalae (*Bai Zhu*) added. It is appropriate to promote sweating. One should be careful not to apply fire attacking.

For wind dampness manifesting as a floating pulse, generalized heaviness, (spontaneous) sweating, and aversion to wind, the ruling formula is *Fang Ji Tang* (Stephania Decoction).[3] Suppose a sick person suffers from dyspnea, headache, nasal congestion, and vexation, but they have a large pulse, ability to take in food (as usual), and harmony in the abdomen which is not diseased. The disease is in the head. It is stroke by cold and dampness. Therefore, there is nasal congestion. Insert some (appropriate) medicinals into the nose and a cure will ensue.

Suppose that on the eighth or ninth day of cold damage, wind and dampness are contending with one another, giving rise to generalized pain and aching, inability to turn over, no retching, no thirst, and a floating, vacuous, and choppy pulse. The ruling formula is *Gui Zhi Fu Zi Tang* (Cinnamon Twig & Aconite Decoction).[4] If the sick person has hard stools and uninhibited urination, *Zhu Fu Zi Tang* (Atractylodes & Aconite Decoction)[5] is the ruling formula.

Wind and dampness contending with one another will give rise to vexing ache in the bone joints with a contracting pain and inability to bend or stretch. The pain will be exacerbated by the slightest touch. (In addition,) there will be sweating, shortness of breath, inhibited urination, and aversion to wind with desire never to be undressed or slight swelling of the body. The ruling formula is *Gan Cao Fu Zi Tang* (Licorice & Aconite Decoction).[6]

A *tai yang* disease of heat stroke is just summerheat stroke. The sick person suffers from (spontaneous) sweating, aversion to cold, fever, and thirst. The ruling formula is *Bai Hu Tang* (White Tiger Decoction).

---

[3] The ingredients in this formula include Radix Stephaniae Tetrandrae (*Fang Ji*), Sclerotium Poriae Cocos (*Fu Ling*), Rhizoma Atractylodis Macrocephalae (*Bai Zhu*), Cortex Cinnamomi Cassiae (*Gui Xin*), Rhizoma Zingiberis (*Jiang*), Radix Aconiti (*Wu Tou*), Radix Panacis Ginseng (*Ren Shen*), and Radix Glycyrrhizae (*Gan Cao*).

[4] This formula is composed of Ramulus Cinnamomi Cassiae (*Gui Zhi*), Radix Praeparatus Aconiti Carmichaeli (*Fu Zi*), Rhizoma Zingiberis (*Jiang*), Radix Glycyrrhizae (*Gan Cao*), and Fructus Zizyphi Jujubae (*Da Zao*).

[5] This formula is composed of Radix Praeparatus Aconiti Carmichaeli (*Fu Zi*), Rhizoma Zingiberis (*Jiang*), Radix Glycyrrhizae (*Gan Cao*), Fructus Zizyphi Jujubae (*Da Zao*), and Rhizoma Atractylodis Macrocephalae (*Bai Zhu*).

[6] The ingredients in this formula are Rhizoma Atractylodis Macrocephalae (*Bai Zhu*), Radix Praeparatus Aconiti Carmichaeli (*Fu Zi*), Ramulus Cinnamomi Cassiae (*Gui Zhi*), and Radix Glycyrrhizae (*Gan Cao*).

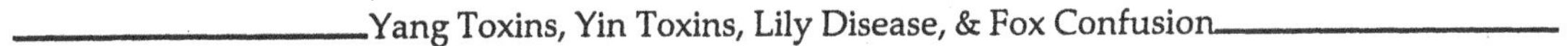

If a *tai yang* disease of summerheat stroke is characterized by fever and generalized aching and heaviness yet their pulse is faint and weak, this is due to cold water damage in the summer months resulting in water trespassing in the skin. The ruling formula is *Gua Di Tang* (Melon Peduncle Decoction).[7]

A *tai yang* disease of summerheat stroke may be characterized by fever, aversion to cold, generalized heaviness, and pain and aching. The pulse is bowstring, thin, scallion-stalk, and slow. Shuddering with gooseflesh on voiding urine may appear. There may be counterflow frigidity of the hands and feet, generalized heat arising on the slightest taxation, the mouth kept open (to facilitate breathing), and dry teeth. If this is treated with diaphoresis, aversion to cold will become worse. If it is treated with warm needling, fever will become worse. If it is treated with repeated precipitation, strangury will become worse.

---

[7] This formula is composed of only one ingredient: Pedunculus Melonis (*Gua Di*).

_______________Chapter Three_______________

A Discussion on the Pulse (& Other) Signs of Yang Toxins, Yin Toxins, Lily Disease & Fox Confusion

The disease of yang toxins is characterized by generalized heaviness, pain in the upper and lower back, vexation, oppression, restlessness, and manic speech, possible frenetic walking about, possible alleging to have seen ghosts, or ejection of blood with dysentery. The pulse is floating, large, and rapid. The face is red with colorful maculas. (In addition,) there is sore throat and spitting of pus and blood. Before the fifth day, the case is curable, but, on the seventh day, the case is beyond cure. There are cases where it takes only one or two days for cold damage to develop into yang toxins and cases where (cold damage) develops into yang toxins after administration of medicinals for the purpose of ejection or precipitation. The ruling formula is *Sheng Ma Tang* (Cimicifuga Decoction).[1]

---

[1] This formula is composed of Rhizoma Cimicifugae (*Sheng Ma*), Sclerotium Pararadicis Poriae Cocos (*Fu Shen*), Radix Panacis Ginseng (*Ren Shen*), Radix Ledebouriellae Divaricatae (*Fang Feng*), Cornu Rhinocerotis (*Xi Jiao*), Cornu Antelopis Saiga-tatarici (*Ling Yang Jiao*), Radix Et Rhizoma Notopterygii (*Qiang Huo*), and Ramulus Cinnamomi Cassiae (*Gui Zhi*).

The disease of yin toxins is characterized by generalized heaviness, rigidity of the back, gripping pain in the abdomen, inhibited throat, toxic qi attacking the heart,[2] tightness and tension below the heart, qi too short for breath, counterflow retching, green-blue lips with a black facial complexion, and inversion frigidity of the four limbs. The pulse is deep, thin, tight, and rapid. The body is (painful) as if beaten. Before the fifth or sixth day, the case is curable, but, on the seventh day, the case is beyond cure. Cold damage may develop into yin toxins on the first or second day or may transmute into it six or seven to ten days after administration of some medicinals. The ruling formula is *Gan Cao Tang* (Licorice Decoction).[3]

Lily disease manifests as always keeping silent and desire but inability to sleep. (The sick person) sometimes looks like a healthy, strong person. They desire but are unable to go out for a trip. They intend to have but are unable to take in food. They have a good appetite at one time but, at another, they do not feel like eating when they smell food. They feel cold yet there is no cold. They feel hot yet there is no heat. In the morning, there is a bitter taste in the mouth with yellow or reddish urine. The bodily form seems to be harmonious. The pulse is faint and rapid. Because the hundred vessels are from the same and one source, all of them are involved in this disease. This should be treated in accordance with the (particular) pattern.

If lily disease manifests as a yin pattern, then one should help it with a yang method (*i.e.,* yang supplementation). If it manifests as a yang pattern, then one should help it with a yin method (*i.e.,* yin enrichment). If a yang pattern is observed but one attacks yin and further treats it with diaphoresis, this will lead to an unfavorable condition and the illness will become difficult to treat. If a yin pattern is observed but one attacks yang and further treats it with precipitation, this, too, will lead to an unfavorable condition and the illness will become difficult to treat.

The disease of fox confusion (*hu huo*)[4] has the manifestations of cold damage. These consist of taciturnity, a desire to sleep but the eyes unable to shut (*i.e.,* drowsiness but inability to fall asleep), and restlessness either in lying down or on rising up. If corrosion occurs to the throat, this is called confusion. If corrosion occurs to the genitals, this is called fox. The disease of fox confusion is accompanied by no desire for food or drink, [aversion to is suspected to be left out here] the smell of food, and the face and eyes turning red at one time, white at another, and black at yet another. When the toxins corrode the upper (*i.e.,* the throat), the voice becomes hoarse. When the toxins

---

2   Toxins attacking the heart is a syndrome of mental disorders. There are, for instance, confusion, sudden collapse, and loss of voice.

3   There is only one ingredient in this formula: Radix Glycyrrhizae (*Gan Cao*).

4   This is an illness characterized mainly by ulceration occurring to either the throat or the genitals, but often both.

corrode the lower (*i.e.*, the genitals), the throat becomes dry. When there is corrosion in the upper, *Xie Xin Tang* (Drain the Heart Decoction) is the ruling formula. When there is corrosion in the lower, wash (the affected area) with *Ku Shen Tang* (Sophora Decoction).[5] If corrosion occurs to the anus, fumigate it with Realgar (*Xiong Huang*).

Suppose a sick person has a rapid pulse, no fever, slight vexation, taciturnity, drowsiness, and sweating. On the third or fourth day of contraction, the eyes will be red like the eyes of a turtledove, and, on the seventh or eighth day, the four canthi will be all blackish yellow. If now (the sick person) is able to take in food, purulence is mature. The ruling formula is *Chi Xiao Dou Dang Gui San* (Aduki Bean & Dang Gui Powder).[6]

The sick person may have their throat corroded through respiration or have their anus and genitals corroded through the lower burner. Corrosion of the upper (part) is called fox, while corrosion of the lower (part) is confusion. For the disease of fox confusion, *Zhu Ling San* (Polyporus Powder) is the ruling formula.

---

[5]   This formula is composed of Radix Sophorae Flavescentis (*Ku Shen*), Radix Sanguisorbae (*Di Yu*), Rhizoma Coptidis Chinensis (*Huang Lian*), Semen Vaccariae Segetalis (*Wang Bu Liu Xing*), Radix Angelicae Pubescentis (*Du Huo*), Folium Artemisiae Argyii (*Ai Ye*), and Herba Lophatheri Gracilis (*Zhu Ye*).

[6]   This formula is composed of Semen Phaseoli Calcarati (*Chi Xiao Dou*) and Radix Angelicae Sinensis (*Dang Gui*).

_______________Chapter Four_______________
A Discussion on the Pulse (& Other) Signs of Sudden Turmoil & Cramps

(The Yellow Emperor) asked:

What is sudden turmoil like?

The master answered:

Retching and vomiting with diarrhea, this is sudden turmoil.

(The Yellow Emperor) asked:

If a sick person suffers from fever, headache, generalized aching, and aversion to cold, and, later, vomiting and diarrhea, what kind of disease should this be?

The master answered:

This should be sudden turmoil. Sudden turmoil is an illness where fever arises after vomiting and diarrhea have stopped. Cold damage with a faint and choppy pulse is, in essence, sudden turmoil. Now that it is cold damage, on the fourth or fifth day, it may reach the yin channels. When it is transmitted into yin, there will inevitably arise vomiting and diarrhea.

The disease of cramps is characterized by straightened arms and legs. The pulse is straight from the upper to the lower positions, slightly bowstring. When cramps involve the abdomen, *Ji Shi Bai San* (Chicken Droppings White Powder)[1] is the ruling formula.

---

[1] There is only one ingredient in this formula, namely, the white part of the droppings from the chicken.

Chapter Five
A Discussion of the Pulse (& Other) Signs of Wind Stroke & Articular Wind

The disease of wind ought to develop hemiplegia. Paralysis of only one arm is *bi*. A faint and rapid pulse is a product of wind stroke.

Headache with a slippery pulse is wind stroke. The pulse of wind is vacuous and weak.

Suppose the *cun* opening pulse is floating and tight. In the presence of the tightness, there is (external) cold, and, in the presence of the floating, there is vacuity. When vacuity and cold are contending with one another, the evil is in the skin (and flesh). The floating (pulse quality) is a revelation of blood vacuity. Since the vessel networks are empty and vacuous, the murderous evil is impossible to drain away. Therefore, it lodges either in the left or right side. The evil qi slackens (the affected part), while the righteous qi makes (the opposite part) tense. The righteous qi tries to draw the evil. Thus there arises deviation (of the eyes and mouth) and hemiplegia. When the evil lies in the vessel networks, there is insensitivity of the muscles and skin. When the evil is in the channels, there is unsurmountable heaviness (of the limbs). If the evil enters the bowels, (the sick person) will be unable to recognize people. If the evil enters the viscera, (the sick person) will suffer from difficult tongue in speaking and drooling at the mouth.

Suppose the *cun* opening pulse is slow and moderate. In the presence of the slowness, there is (external) cold, and, in the presence of the moderateness, there is (internal) vacuity. When the constructive is moderate,[1] the blood collapses. When the defensive is slow, wind stroke will arise. When evil qi strikes the channel, generalized itching and dormant papules arise. If there is an insufficiency of heart qi, the evil qi will enter the center, giving rise to fullness of the chest and shortness of breath.

Suppose the instep pulse is floating and slippery. In the presence of the slipperiness, there is repletion of grain qi,[2] and, in the presence of the floating, there is spontaneous sweating.

Suppose the *shao yin* pulse[3] is floating and weak. In the presence of the weakness, there is insufficiency of blood, and, in the presence of the floating, there is wind. When wind and blood (vacuity) contend with one another, a generalized contracting pain and aching arise.

In an exuberant (*i.e.,* corpulent) person, a choppy and small pulse, shortness of breath, spontaneous sweating, and pain in every joint with inability to contract or stretch are all produced by sweating in a draft after drinking wine.

Suppose the *cun* opening pulse is deep and weak. The deepness rules the bones, while the

____

[1] The word moderate means lacking force and a little sluggish. However, there is a lapse in logic here. A freer translation would read: A moderate pulse is a revelation of slack or sluggish constructive qi, and, when the constructive is slack or sluggish... One should also note that the constructive and defensive stand in an internal/external relationship. Therefore, when they are spoken of, the internal and external are also implied.

[2] This implies internal heat due to food accumulation.

[3] This refers to the pulse at the point Great Ravine (*Tai Xi*, Ki 3).

weakness rules the sinews. The deepness rules the kidneys, while the weakness rules the liver.[4] If one plunges oneself into water with sweat on (their body), the water will damage the heart giving rise to pain in every joint and yellow sweating.[5] This is why what is called articular wind is produced.

The sour flavor damages the sinews. When damaged, the sinews become slack. This is called sluggishness (*xie*).[6] Saltiness damages the bones. When damaged, the bones become atonic. This is called withering. When withering and sluggishness mutually exacerbate each other, this is called deprivation sluggishness (*duan xie*). Since the constructive qi stops circulating, the defensive is unable to circulate by itself. (Then) the constructive and defensive both become faint and the triple burner is no longer able to control (water and essence transportation. As a result,) the four affiliates (*i.e.*, the limbs) are deprived (of supplies of nutrition). The body becomes markedly emaciated with the feet (read as knees) swollen and enlarged. There is yellow sweating and frigidity of the lower legs. If there is fever, this is articular wind. For the disease of articular wind with inability to contract and stretch (the joints), *Wu Tou Tang* (Wu Tou Aconite Decoction)[7] is the ruling formula.

For pain and aching in every limb joint, deformed limbs with emaciated muscles, feet (read as knees) swollen as if they were about to come off, dizziness, shortness of breath, and a distressing desire to vomit, *Gui Zhi Shao Yao Zhi Mu Tang* (Cinnamon Twig, Peony & Anemarrhena Decoction)[8] is the ruling formula.

---

[4] One should note the corresponding relationship that the bones are governed by the kidneys, while the sinews are governed by the liver. Therefore, this passage suggests that a deep pulse points to disease involving the bones and the kidneys, while a weak pulse reveals disease involving the sinews and the liver.

[5] Yellow sweating as a proper name refers to an illness characterized by a swollen face and limbs, fever, sticky yellow sweat, and other signs and symptoms of rheumatic arthritis. However, in this context, the term merely refers to sweat of a faint yellowish color.

[6] Because the Chinese ideogram *xie* is multivalent, the term may be also rendered as drain/drainage.

[7] This formula is composed of Herba Ephedrae (*Ma Huang*), Radix Aconiti (*Wu Tou*), Radix Glycyrrhizae (*Gan Cao*), Radix Paeoniae Lactiflorae (*Shao Yao*), and Radix Astragali Membranacei (*Huang Qi*).

[8] The ingredients in this formula are Ramulus Cinnamomi Cassiae (*Gui Zhi*), Rhizoma Anemarrhenae (*Zhi Mu*), Radix Ledebouriellae Divaricatae (*Fang Feng*), Radix Paeoniae Lactiflorae (*Shao Yao*), Radix Glycyrrhizae (*Gan Cao*), Herba Ephedrae (*Ma Huang*), Radix Praeparatus Aconiti Carmichaeli (*Fu Zi*), Rhizoma Zingiberis (*Jiang*), and Rhizoma Atractylodis Macrocephalae (*Bai Zhu*).

_________Chapter Six_________

A Discussion of the Pulse (& Other) Signs of Blood *Bi* & Vacuity Taxation

(The Yellow Emperor) asked:

How does blood *bi* arise?

The master answered:

Respectable and prestigious people (tend) to be weak in the bones and exuberant in the muscles and skin (*i.e.*, they tend to be fat). If, in addition, they sweat in fatigue and taxation or happen to be assaulted by slight draft when stirring in sleep, they will be taken with it. It resembles wind (stroke), but its pulse is faint and choppy and, in the *cun* and *guan*, small and tight. (To treat this,) it is appropriate to conduct yang qi with the needle. When the pulse is harmonized and is no longer tight, cure will ensue.

In the case of blood *bi*, yin and yang are both faint. The pulse is faint in the *cun* and *guan*, but small and tight in the *chi*. The external manifestation (of blood *bi*) is insensitivity of the body as in wind [*bi* is suspected to be left out here]. The ruling formula is *Huang Qi Gui Wu Wu Tang* (Astragalus & Cinnamon Five Materials Decoction).[1]

If one intends to treat a disease, one should first know what part is involved in the pattern before one attacks (the illness).

As for a normal[2] male, a large pulse reveals taxation, while a very vacuous pulse also reveals taxation, too.

---

[1] The ingredients in this formula include Ramulus Cinnamomi Cassiae (*Gui Zhi*), Radix Paeoniae Lactiflorae (*Shao Yao*), Radix Astragali Membranacei (*Huang Qi*), Fructus Zizyphi Jujubae (*Da Zao*), and Rhizoma Zingiberis (*Jiang*).

[2] The word normal should not be taken at face value here. Rather, it means that there is no serious disease observable from appearance or perceptible by the sick person himself.

The disease of taxation in males exhibits a floating and large pulse. The hands and feet are warm. It gets worse in spring and summer and is relieved in autumn and winter. There is cold in the genitals with seminal emission, aching and whittled [feet is suspected to be left out here] with inability to walk, and lower abdominal vacuity fullness.

As for persons aged fifty to sixty years, if the pulse is large, such diseases as numbness developing parallel to (the spine in) the back, tormenting rumbling in the interstices, and saber and pearl-string lumps are all produced by taxation.

If a normal male has a vacuous, weak, thin, and faint pulse, they will often (also) have thief sweating (*i.e.*, night sweats).

A pale face in a male rules thirst and blood collapse. Sudden dyspnea and palpitations with a floating pulse are due to internal vacuity.

Suppose a male has a vacuous, deep, and choppy pulse, suffers from no cold and heat, but has shortness of breath, abdominal urgency, inhibited urination, a white facial complexion, and, at times, heavy eyes. This person (must) suffer from frequent runny snivel nosebleeding and lower abdominal fullness. This is produced by taxation.

A male with a pulse which is faint and weak as well as choppy is infertile due to cold essence qi.

Suppose a person who has loss of essence (*i.e.*, seminal emission) suffers from hypertonicity of the lower abdomen, cold in the head of the penis, pain in the eyesockets [visual dizziness in another version], and loss of hair. If the pulse is very vacuous, scallion-stalk and slow, there (must) be clear grain (diarrhea), blood collapse, and loss of essence.

If the pulse feels scallion-stalk, stirring, faint, or tight, there is seminal emission in males or dreams of sexual intercourse in females. (To treat this,) *Gui Zhi Jia Long Gu Mu Li Tang* (Cinnamon Twig Plus Dragon Bone & Oyster Shell Decoction) is the ruling formula.

A deep, small, and slow pulse refers to desertion of qi. (With qi desertion,) the sick person suffers from rapid distressed dyspneic breathing in walking quickly, counterflow frigidity of hands and feet, abdominal fullness, and, in severe cases, duck-stool diarrhea with untransformed food in the stools.

There is a bowstring and large pulse. It is a moderate bowstring (as compared with a pure bowstring pulse), and it is not so large as scallion-stalk (as compared with a pure large pulse). A moderate (bowstring pulse) points to cold, and the scallion-stalk (quality) points to vacuity. When cold and vacuity act upon one another, a pulse named drumskin is produced. (With such a pulse,) a female suffers from miscarriage and dribbling vaginal bleeding, while a male suffers from blood collapse and seminal emission.

Chapter Seven
A Discussion of the Pulse (& Other) Signs of Wasting Thirst & Strangury

The master explained:

A *jue yin* disease is characterized by wasting thirst, qi surging up into the heart, pain and heat in the heart, hunger yet no desire for food, vomiting upon ingestion, and endless diarrhea following (treatment by) precipitation.

Suppose the *cun* opening pulse is floating and slow. In the presence of the floating, there is vacuity, and, in the presence of the slow, there is taxation. Vacuity is as good as insufficiency of the defensive qi, and the slow (pulse quality) is a reflection of exhausted constructive qi.

Suppose the instep pulse is floating and rapid. In the presence of the floating, there is (exuberance of) qi, and, in the presence of the rapidity, there is swift digestion with tight (defecation, *i.e.*, constipation). Exuberance of qi makes urination frequent, and frequent urination makes (defecation) tight. Tight (defecation) and frequent (urination) combine to produce wasting thirst.

For wasting thirst in males who suffer from frequent urination, voiding one *dou* after having drunk one *dou*, *Shen Qi Wan* (Kidney Qi Pills) is the ruling formula.

The master explained:

Heat in the lower burner gives rise to hematuria and also causes a person strangurious urinary block. The disease of strangury is characterized by grains in the urine (*i.e.*, turbid or cloudy urine) and hypertonicity of the lower abdomen with pain radiating to the umbilicus.

Suppose the *cun* opening pulse is thin and rapid. In the presence of the rapidity, there is heat, and, in the presence of the thinness, there is cold. The rapidity is a result of violent vomiting.

If the instep pulse is rapid, there is heat in the stomach. Thus there is swift digestion with a large food intake, the stool is inevitably hard, and urination is frequent.

If the *shao yin* pulse is rapid, there are sores in the genitals in females and qi strangury[1] in males.

A person who suffers from strangury should not be treated with diaphoresis since diaphoresis will inevitably produce hematuria.

---

[1]   Qi strangury is due to qi stagnation in the urinary bladder. This manifests as pain and swelling from the lower abdomen down to the scrotum, dribbling urination, and pain in the urethra following voiding.

——————————Chapter Eight——————————
A Discussion on the Pulse (& Other) Signs of Water Qi, Yellow Sweating & Qi Phase (Disease)

The master explained:

There are diseases of wind water, skin water, righteous water (*zheng shui*), stone water, and yellow sweating. In terms of wind water, the pulse is floating and its external manifestations are pain and aching in the bone joints. The sick person is averse to wind. As for skin water, the pulse is also floating and its external manifestations include inflated swelling which allows the pressing fingers to sink deep (into the flesh). There is no aversion to wind. The abdomen is (distended) like a drum. There is no thirst. This requires the promotion of sweating. In terms of righteous water, the pulse is deep and slow and its external manifestation is dyspnea. In terms of stone water, the pulse is deep and its external manifestations include abdominal fullness and no dyspnea. As for yellow sweating, the pulse is deep and slow and there is body heat, chest fullness, and swelling of the four limbs and the head and face. If this lasts for a long time, *yong* with purulence will inevitably develop.

Suppose the pulse is floating and surging. In the presence of the floating, there is wind, and, in the presence of the surging, there is (water) qi. Wind and (water) qi contend with each other. If wind prevails, there will be dormant papules with itching all over the body. Itching is due to discharging wind, and, over time, this will develop into a leprosy-like scarring disease. If (water) qi prevails, there will be water (illness) which makes it impossible to bend (the body) either forward or backward. If wind and (water) qi act upon one another, then there is spectacular swelling of the body. Diaphoresis can effect relief. Aversion to wind reveals vacuity. This is wind water. If there is no aversion to wind and urination is uninhibited, then there is cold in the upper burner and copious drooling from the mouth. This is yellow sweating.

If the *cun* opening pulse is deep and slippery, there is water qi in the center. The face and eyes are swollen and there is fever. This is named wind water. If the person is seen with slight swelling of the eyelids looking as in having just got up from bed, (visible) stirring of the pulse in the neck, occasional coughing, and depressions remaining in the hands or feet after pressure is relieved, this is wind water.

If a *tai yang* disease exhibits a floating and tight pulse, there ought to be pain in the bone joints. If, on the contrary, there is no pain but there is generalized heaviness and ache and the sick person feels no thirst, relief will follow diaphoresis. This is (a case of) wind water. If there is aversion to cold, this is due to excessive vacuity produced by diaphoresis. If there is thirst but no aversion to cold, this is ascribed to skin water. Generalized swelling with cold, migratory *bi* like (pain), a stuffy sensation in the chest, inability to take in food, gathering pain (in the stomach), and agitation causing sleeplessness in the night are (all characteristics of) yellow sweating. (In yellow sweating,) there is pain in the bone joints. Coughing, dyspnea, and no thirst are characteristic of spleen distention. It looks like swelling but diaphoresis results in relief. All the above diseases cannot be treated with diaphoresis if there is thirst, diarrhea, and frequent urination.

Suppose wind water exhibits a floating pulse. The floating shows that (the evil) is in the exterior. The sick person is able to take in food but suffers from headache and (spontaneous) sweating. (Other than these,) there are no other exterior diseases except that the sick person complains of heaviness of the lower body. If so, there is harmony from the lumbus up, but there ought to be swelling from the lumbus down to the genitals with difficulty in bending and stretching (the lumbus). The ruling formula is *Fang Ji Huang Qi Tang* (Stephania & Astragalus Decoction).[1]

For wind water manifesting as aversion to wind, swelling all over the body, a floating pulse, no thirst, continual spontaneous sweating, and no high fever, *Yue Bi Tang* (Keep Away the Maiden Decoction)[2] is the ruling formula.

The master explained:

Wrapped water (*i.e.*, skin water) may be characterized by spectacular swelling of the whole body including the face and eyes. The pulse is deep. Urination is inhibited and it is this which is responsible for this water disease. If urination becomes disinhibited by itself, collapse of fluids will arise. It follows that there will be thirst. (For wrapped water,) *Yue Bi Jia Zhu Tang* (Keep Away the Maiden Plus Atractylodes Decoction)[3] is the ruling formula.

For the disease of skin water characterized by swelling of the four limbs with water qi in the skin and twitching of the four limbs, *Fang Ji Fu Ling Tang* (Stephania & Poria Decoction)[4] is the ruling formula.

Suppose, when one expects the instep pulse to be hidden, it is now, on the contrary, tight. (This shows that) there was cold giving rise to *shan* conglomeration and abdominal pain but that the (attending) physician contrarily used precipitation. Precipitation has given rise to chest fullness and shortness of breath.

Suppose, when one expects the instep pulse to be hidden, it is now, on the contrary, rapid. (This shows that) there is heat giving rise to swift digestion and frequent urination. If now, on the contrary, urination is scanty, there is a tendency towards water (swelling).

---

[1] This formula is composed of Radix Stephaniae Tetrandrae (*Fang Ji*), Radix Astragali Membranacei (*Huang Qi*), Radix Glycyrrhizae (*Gan Cao*), and Rhizoma Atractylodis Macrocephalae (*Bai Zhu*).

[2] The ingredients in this formula include Herba Ephedrae (*Ma Huang*), Gypsum (*Shi Gao*), Rhizoma Zingiberis (*Jiang*), Radix Glycyrrhizae (*Gan Cao*), and Fructus Zizyphi Jujubae (*Da Zao*).

[3] This formula is the same as that in note 2 above only with Rhizoma Atractylodis Macrocephalae (*Bai Zhu*) added.

[4] The ingredients in this formula are Radix Stephaniae Tetrandrae (*Fang Ji*), Radix Astragali Membranacei (*Huang Qi*), Radix Glycyrrhizae (*Gan Cao*), and Sclerotium Poriae Cocos (*Fu Ling*).

Suppose the *cun* opening pulse is floating and slow. In the presence of the floating, there is heat, and, in presence of the slowness, there is hidden (yang).[5] The heat and hidden (yang) act upon one another, producing (a disease) named sinking (*chen*). Suppose the instep pulse is floating and rapid. In the presence of the floating, there is (external) heat, and, in the presence of the rapidity, there is arrested (heat internally. External) heat and arrested (internal heat) act upon one another, producing (a disease) named insidiousness. Sinking and insidious (heat) act upon one another, producing (a disease) named water. With sinking (of qi), the vessel networks becomes vacuous, and, with insidious (heat), urination becomes difficult. Vacuity (of the vessel networks) and difficult (urination) act upon one another, making water trespass within the skin. In consequence, water (swelling) arises.

Suppose the *cun* opening pulse is bowstring and tight. In the presence of the bowstring, there is stoppage of the defensive qi circulation. Since the defensive qi has stopped circulating, aversion to cold and inability of water to flow with the qi arises. (In consequence,) water trespasses between the intestines.

Suppose the *shao yin* pulse is tight and deep. In the presence of the tightness, there is pain, and, in presence of the deepness, there is water. (In this condition,) urination is difficult. The master explains that for the various types of deep pulse, water should be held responsible and that it is the producer of generalized swelling and heaviness. If the pulse of water disease is out (*i.e.*, floating), this is death.

The sick person of water may have sleeping silkworms beneath the eyes (*i.e.*, puffy bags beneath their eyes) and a bright, lustrous (*i.e.*, shiny) face. The pulse is hidden and the sick person suffers from wasting thirst. If the disease of water manifests as an enlarged abdomen and inhibited urination, there is water (internally) if the pulse is deep (and near to) expiry. This allows precipitation.

(The Yellow Emperor) asked:

If, following the disease of dysentery, there is thirst, (copious) drinking, inhibited urination, abdominal fullness, and swollen genitals, then what kind of disease is this?

---

[5] In the kidneys, there is true yin and true yang. This true yang is also sometimes known as hidden yang. The word hidden, therefore, simply refers to the true yang. However, in this context, it also does imply insufficiency of hidden or true yang.

.(The master) answered:

This is a disease of water. If urination becomes disinhibited by itself and sweat exits, it will heal by itself.

If the illness of water presents a deep, small pulse, it is ascribed to the *shao yin*. If the pulse is floating, (the illness) is wind (water). Vacuity distention with no water (contained) is ascribed to qi. If it is a water (illness), diaphoresis may effect a relief. If the pulse is deep, administer *Fu Zi Ma Huang Tang* (Aconite & Ephedra Decoction).[6] If the pulse is floating, administer *Xing Zi Tang* (Armeniaca Decoction).[7]

Heart water is characterized by generalized heaviness, diminished qi, insomnia, vexation, agitation, and swollen genitals.

Liver water is characterized by an enlarged abdomen, inability to turn over, and pain in the lateral costal region and abdomen. Fluids may be generated a little (in the mouth) at times, and urination may be disinhibited from time to time.

Lung water is characterized by generalized swelling, difficult urination, and occasional duck-stool diarrhea.

Spleen water is characterized by an enlarged abdomen, tormenting heaviness of the four limbs, no generation of fluids, tormenting diminished qi all the time, and difficult urination.

Kidney water is characterized by an enlarged abdomen, a swollen umbilicus, lumbago, inability to urinate, wet external genitals like the sweating nose of a cow, inversion frigidity of the feet, and an emaciated face.

The master explained:

For the various cases of water, it is necessary to disinhibit the urination if there is swelling from

---

[6] This formula is composed of Radix Glycyrrhizae (*Gan Cao*), Rhizoma Atractylodis Macrocephalae (*Bai Zhu*), Herba Ephedrae (*Ma Huang*), Radix Panacis Ginseng (*Ren Shen*), Rhizoma Zingiberis (*Jiang*), and Radix Praeparatus Aconiti Carmichaeli (*Fu Zi*).

[7] This formula is composed of Radix Panacis Ginseng (*Ren Shen*), Rhizoma Pinelliae Ternatae (*Ban Xia*), Sclerotium Poriae Cocos (*Fu Ling*), Radix Paeoniae Lactiflorae (*Shao Yao*), Cortex Tubiformis Cinnamomi Cassiae (*Guan Gui*), Rhizoma Zingiberis (*Jiang*), Radix Glycyrrhizae (*Gan Cao*), Herba Asari Cum Radice (*Xi Xin*), Fructus Schisandrae Chinensis (*Wu Wei Zi*), and Semen Pruni Armeniacae (*Xing Ren*).

the lumbus down, but it is necessary to promote sweating if there is swelling from the lumbus up. Then cure will follow (the treatment).

The master explained:

Suppose the *cun* opening pulse is deep and slow. In the presence of the deepness, there is water, and, in presence of the slowness, there is cold. Since cold and water act upon one another, the instep pulse is hidden and there is inability to transform water and grain. If the spleen qi is debilitated, there is duck-stool diarrhea. If the stomach qi is debilitated, there is generalized swelling. If the *shao yang* pulse is abject[8] and the *shao yin* pulse is thin, there will be inhibited urination in males and menstrual stoppage in females. Menstrual flow is blood. When blood (circulation) is inhibited, water (swelling) arises. This is called blood aspect (*shui fen*).

(The Yellow Emperor) asked:

There was a sick person who was tormented by water suffering from swelling all over the body, including the face and eyes and the four limbs, and whose urination was inhibited. While you, Sir, felt the pulse, (the sick person) did not mention water but talked about pain inside the chest and qi surging up into the throat with a sensation as if a piece of meat were stuck (in their throat). And (you determined that) there should be slight coughing and dyspnea. Your determination proved true, but what was the pulse like?

The master answered:

The *cun* opening pulse was deep and tight. In the presence of the deepness, there was water, and, in presence of the tightness, there was cold. The deepness and the tightness combined (showing cold and water) bound in the Origin Pass (*i.e.*, the lower burner). At its onset, (the condition) should have been slight and was not perceptible (while the sick person) was in the prime of his life. When yang began to become debilitated,[9] the constructive and defensive interfered with one another, and yang was reduced, while yin became exuberant. Then bound cold began to stir in a small way and tight [kidney is suspected to be instead of tight] qi surged upward. (As a result,) the throat became constricted and congested and there was hypertonicity and pain in the lateral costal regions. The (attending) physician assumed that there was retained rheum and carried out great (*i.e.*, drastic) precipitation. (However,) the attacking (cold) qi was not removed and the disease was not eliminated. Later, ejection was further carried out. (In consequence,) the stomach

---

[8] The *shao yang* pulse is located anterior to the auricle, while the *shao yin* is located around the point Great Ravine (*Tai Xi*, Ki 3). The word abject means faint and hidden.

[9] Yang qi begins to decline at the age of five times seven years in females (35) and at six times eight years (48) in males.

became vacuous and vexation, a dry throat, a desire to drink water, inhibited urination, inability to transform water and grain, and puffy swelling of the face and eyes and hands and feet arose. Then (the sick person) was administered *Ting Li Wan* (Lepidium Pills)[10] to precipitate water. At that time, there might have been relief to a small degree. (However,) because of overeating and overdrinking, the swelling came back as before. Then there arose tormenting pain in the chest and lateral costal regions as in running piglet. Then water flooded up, giving rise to floating cough and counterflow dyspnea. (In that case,) it was necessary to first thwart the surging qi. After (the surging qi) was suppressed, one could treat cough. After cough was checked, dyspnea would heal by itself. One should treat the new disease first and then later the (root) disease.

The disease of yellow sweating is characterized by spectacular generalized swelling, fever, (spontaneous) perspiration, and thirst. It looks like wind water. The sweat dyes the clothes a full yellow color like the sap of the cypress. The pulse is deep.

(The Yellow Emperor) asked:

How does the disease of yellow sweating arise?

The master answered:

If one plunges into water for a bath with sweat on (their body), water will penetrate (the body). Thus this disease arises. (To treat it,) *Huang Qi Shao Yao Gui Zhi Ku Jiu Tang* (Astragalus, Peony, Cinnamon Twig & Bitter Wine Decoction)[11] is the ruling formula.

In the disease of yellow sweating there is cold of the lower legs. If there is heat (in the legs), this falls under the category of articular wind. If there is perspiration upon ingestion of food in addition to frequent thief sweating (*i.e.*, night sweats) while asleep at night, this is (the illness of) taxed qi. If perspiration is followed contrarily by fever, over time, there will inevitably be scaling of the body. If there is ceaseless fever, malign sores will inevitably grow. If there is generalized heaviness which may be relieved (temporarily) after perspiration, over time, there will be twitching of the body. With this twitching, pain in the chest arises. In addition, there is invariably sweating from the lumbus upward which is absent from below. There is slackening and pain in the lumbus and hips and a sensation of something (foreign) within the skin. In severe cases, there are inability to take in food, generalized aching and heaviness, vexation, agitation, and inhibited

---

[10] This formula is composed of only two ingredients, namely, Semen Lepidii (*Ting Li Zi*) and Fructus Evodiae Rutecarpae (*Wu Zhu Yu*).

[11] The ingredients in this formula are Radix Astragali Membranacei (*Huang Qi*), Radix Paeoniae Lactiflorae (*Shao Yao*), Ramulus Cinnamomi Cassiae (*Gui Zhi*), and vinegar which was called bitter wine in olden times.

urination. This is yellow sweating. (For it,) *Gui Zhi Jia Huang Qi Tang* (Cinnamon Twig Plus Astragalus Decoction)[12] is the ruling formula.

Suppose the *cun* opening pulse is slow and choppy. In the presence of the slowness, there is cold, and, in the presence of the choppiness, there is insufficiency of blood. Suppose the instep pulse is faint and slow. In the presence of the faintness, there is qi (insufficiency), and, in the presence of the slowness, there is cold. With cold and qi insufficiency there is counterflow frigidity of the hands and feet. With counterflow frigidity of the hands and feet, the constructive and defensive are inhibited. When the constructive and the defensive are inhibited, abdominal and flank fullness and continual rumbling (in the intestines) arises. (Cold) qi turns about in the urinary bladder, and the constructive and the defensive are taxed. Because the yang qi is blocked, there is a cold body. Because the yin qi is blocked, there is pain in the bones. With the circulation of yang cut, there is aversion to cold. With the circulation of yin cut, there is *bi* insensitivity. Only when yin and yang coordinate can (the righteous) qi circulate, and only when the great qi (*i.e.,* the gathering, ancestral, or chest qi) resumes circulation can (the cold) qi be dispersed. In the case of repletion, there is flatus, and, in case of vacuity, there is urinary incontinence. (The above condition) is named qi phase (*qi fen*). Qi phase (disease) is characterized by a hard (mass) below the heart as large as a plate. Its edges are like that of a turning cup?????. This is a product of water rheum. (For it,) *Gui Zhi Qu Shao Jia Ma Huang Xi Xin Fu Zi Tang* (Cinnamon Twig Minus Peony Plus Ephedra, Asarum & Aconite Decoction)[13] is the ruling formula.

A hard (mass) below the heart as large as a plate whose edges are like that of a turning cup is a product of water rheum. (For it,) *Zhi Shi Zhu Tang* (Immature Aurantium & Atractylodes Decoction)[14] is the ruling formula.

---

[12] This formula is composed of Radix Astragali Membranacei (*Huang Qi*), Radix Paeoniae Lactiflorae (*Shao Yao*), Ramulus Cinnamomi Cassiae (*Gui Zhi*), Radix Glycyrrhizae (*Gan Cao*), Fructus Zizyphi Jujubae (*Da Zao*), and Rhizoma Zingiberis (*Jiang*).

[13] This formula is composed of Herba Ephedrae (*Ma Huang*), Herba Asari Cum Radice (*Xi Xin*), Ramulus Cinnamomi Cassiae (*Gui Zhi*), Radix Praeparatus Aconiti Carmichaeli (*Fu Zi*), Radix Glycyrrhizae (*Gan Cao*), Fructus Zizyphi Jujubae (*Da Zao*), and Rhizoma Zingiberis (*Jiang*).

[14] This formula is composed of only two ingredients: Fructus Immaturus Aurantii (*Zhi Shi*) and Rhizoma Atractylodis Macrocephalae (*Bai Zhu*).

Chapter Nine

A Discussion on the Pulse (& Other) Signs of Jaundice, Cold & Heat & Malaria

Such indications of jaundice as absence of the pulse from the *cun* near to the palm and cold of the mouth and nose demonstrate that it cannot be treated. If the pulse is deep and there is thirst with a desire to drink water and inhibited urination, then there will invariably be jaundice.

Abdominal fullness, a withered yellow complexion of the tongue [body is suspected instead of tongue], and agitation causing sleeplessness are characteristic of jaundice.

The master explained:

The disease of jaundice accompanied by fever, vexation, dyspnea, chest fullness, and a dry mouth is a result of the combination of two heats[1] caused by employing fire to force sweat out at the onset of a disease. However, a person is usually taken with jaundice due to dampness. If there is fever and yellowing all over the body with heat in the abdomen, then there is heat internally requiring precipitation.

The master explained:

In terms of the disease of jaundice, a course should be composed of eighteen days. After having been treated for more than ten days, it should be on the mend. If, on the contrary, it gets worse, this proves that (the case) is difficult to treat.

(The master) explained again:

Jaundice with thirst is difficult to treat, but jaundice with no thirst is curable. If (the disease) starts in the yin part (*i.e.*, internally), the sick person must suffer from vomiting. If (the disease) starts in the yang part, the sick person must suffer from cold shuddering and fever.

The master explained:

---

[1] Two heats refers to the internal heat and the heat from the fire attacking therapy.

For the various cases of jaundice, one can simply disinhibit urination. Suppose the pulse is floating and diaphoresis is required to effect a resolution, the appropriate (formula) is *Gui Zhi Jia Huang Qi Tang* (Cinnamon Twig with Added Astragalus Decoction).[2] Moreover, for jaundice in males with uninhibited urination, it is necessary to administer *Xiao Jian Zhong Tang* (Minor Fortify the Center Decoction).

If jaundice manifests abdominal fullness, inhibited voidings of reddish urine, and spontaneous sweating, this shows that the exterior is harmonious but there is a repletion of the interior. This requires precipitation, and the appropriate (formula) is *Da Huang Huang Bai Zhi Zi Mang Xiao Tang* (Rhubarb, Phellodendron, Gardenia & Mirabilitum Decoction).[3]

Jaundice with normal colored urine, a tendency to diarrhea, abdominal fullness, and dyspnea cannot be treated by means of removing heat. When heat is removed, retching will inevitably arise. If there is retching, *Xiao Ban Xia Tang* (Minor Pinellia Decoction)[4] is the ruling formula.

The disease of wine jaundice is invariably accompanied by inhibited urination. Its indications are heat within the heart and heat in the soles of the feet. These are its manifestations. A burning sensation and heat in the heart, inability to take in food, and occasional desire to vomit are named wine jaundice.

Wine jaundice may be characterized by absence of heat, serenity, normal speech, abdominal fullness, a desire to vomit, and a dry nose. If the pulse is floating, treat this first with ejection. If the pulse is deep, treat this first with precipitation. Wine jaundice with heat in the heart and a desire to vomit can be cured by ejection.

Wine jaundice may manifest as yellowing (of the body), bound heat below the heart, and vexation.

If treated with precipitation, wine jaundice may, over time, develop into black jaundice which is characterized by green-blue eyes, a black face, (a burning sensation) in the heart as after eating

---

[2] This formula is composed of Ramulus Cinnamomi Cassiae (*Gui Zhi*), Radix Paeoniae Lactiflorae (*Shao Yao*), Radix Glycyrrhizae (*Gan Cao*), Rhizoma Zingiberis (*Jiang*), Fructus Zizyphi Jujubae (*Da Zao*), and Radix Astragali Membranacei (*Huang Qi*).

[3] The ingredients in this formula are Radix Et Rhizoma Rhei (*Da Huang*), Cortex Phellodendri (*Huang Bai*), Fructus Gardeniae Jasminoidis (*Zhi Zi*), and Mirabilitum (*Mang Xiao*).

[4] This formula is composed of only two ingredients, namely, Rhizoma Pinelliae Ternatae (*Ban Xia*) and Rhizoma Zingiberis (*Jiang*).

garlic, completely black stools, insensitivity of the skin and nails, and a floating and weak pulse. Though black, (the complexion) is of a yellow shade. Therefore, it is known (to be transmuted from wine jaundice).

Suppose the *cun* opening pulse is faint and weak. In the presence of the faintness, there is aversion to cold, and, in the presence of the weakness, there is fever. When there should be but there is no fever, there is pain and aching in the bone joints. When there should be but there is no vexation, there is copious perspiration. Suppose the instep pulse is moderate and slow but the stomach qi is contrarily strong. If the *shao yin* pulse is faint, this faintness reveals damaged essence. (Therefore,) there is cold yin qi. Since there is an insufficiency of the *shao yin* (channel qi) while the grain qi is contrarily strong, vexation and fullness arise on surfeit. Following fullness, fever arises. Since guest (evil) heat disperses grain (quickly), following fever, hunger arises again. And fever gives rise to abdominal fullness. Because the faint (pulse quality) is the result of damaged essence, in spite of strong grain (qi), there is emaciation. This is called grain cold and heat.

If a *yang ming* disease exhibits a slow pulse, there is difficulty eating to the full. Once eating to the full, vexation will arise. If there is dizziness, there is invariably difficult urination. This shows a tendency towards grain jaundice. Even though precipitation is carried out, the abdomen will remain full as before. It is the slow pulse which accounts for this.

The master explained:

Suppose the *cun* opening pulse is floating and moderate. In the presence of the floating, there is wind, and, in the presence of the moderateness, there is *bi*. *Bi* is not wind stroke. (*Bi*) is characterized by a tormenting vexation in the four limbs and, invariably, yellowing spleen (skin is suspected instead of spleen [tr.]). This is the work of depressed heat.

Suppose the instep pulse is tight and rapid. In the presence of the rapidity, there is heat. Heat disperses grain (quickly). In the presence of the tightness, there is cold. (Cold) gives rise to (abdominal) fullness upon eating. The *chi* pulse is floating (in the *cun* opening) which points to damaged kidneys, while the tight instep pulse points to a damaged spleen. Since wind and cold act upon one another, dizziness arises upon eating, and the grain qi is unable to disperse (grain).[5] (As a result,) the stomach is tormented by turbidity. The turbid qi flows down causing urinary

---

[5] It says at the beginning of this passage that there is the ability to disperse grain. This refers to a large food intake because of a strong stomach. Later, it says that grain qi is not able to be dispersed. This implies that the spleen is damaged by cold and hence there is poor digestion.

block. While the (*tai*) *yin* is subjected to cold, heat flows into the urinary bladder. (In consequence,) the whole body is tinged with a yellow color. This is called grain jaundice.

A black complexion on the forehead, slight sweating, heat in the hands and feet, attacks arising towards evening, urgency of the urinary bladder, and uninhibited urination are (characteristic of the disease) known as sexual taxation jaundice. If the abdomen looks like water (swelling, the condition) is treatable.

If a person who is taken with jaundice suffers from fever in the late afternoon contrarily accompanied by aversion to cold, this is a product of sexual taxation. If there is urgency of the urinary bladder, lower abdominal fullness, generalized yellowing, a black complexion on the forehead, and heat in the soles of the feet, then black jaundice has developed. If the abdomen is distended like water (swelling), the stool is invariably black, and there is occasionally thin stool diarrhea, this is the disease of sexual taxation (jaundice) rather than water (disease). The case with abdominal fullness is difficult to treat. (To treat sexual taxation jaundice,) *Xiao Shi Fan Shi San* (Niter & Alumen Powder)[6] is the ruling formula.

The pulse of malaria is typically bowstring. A bowstring and rapid pulse points to abundant heat, while a bowstring and slow pulse points to abundant cold. If the pulse is bowstring, small, and tight, precipitation is allowed. If the pulse is tight and rapid, diaphoresis, needling, or moxibustion is allowed. If the pulse is floating and large, ejection is allowed. If the pulse is bowstring and rapid, (malaria) has been started by wind and can be checked by balancing the diet.

Concretions and conglomerations which develop in malaria are called mother of malaria (*nue mu*). The ruling formula (for this) is *Bei Jia Jian Wan* (Amyda Infusion Pills).[7]

Malaria where only heat is seen is warm malaria. The pulse is peaceful. Only heat with no cold, a vexing aching in the joints of the bones, occasional retching, and attacks occurring in the

---

[6] This formula is composed of Niter (*Xiao Shi*) and Alumen (*Fan Shi*).

[7] This formula is composed of Carapax Amydae Sinensis (*Bie Jia*), Rhizoma Belamcandae (*She Gan*), Radix Scutellariae Baicalensis (*Huang Qin*), Armadillidium Vulgarae (*Shu Fu*), Ramulus Cinnamomi Cassiae (*Gui Zhi*), Rhizoma Zingiberis (*Jiang*), Radix Et Rhizoma Rhei (*Da Huang*), Folium Pyrrosiae (*Shi Wei*), Cortex Magnoliae Officinalis (*Hou Po*), Flos Campsitis Grandiflorae (*Zi Rui*), Gelatinum Corii Asini (*E Jiao*), Radix Bupleuri (*Chai Hu*), Catharsius Molossus (*Qiang Lang*), Radix Paeoniae Lactiflorae (*Shao Yao*), Cortex Radicis Moutan (*Dan Pi*), Semen Lepidii (*Ting Li*), Rhizoma Pinelliae Ternatae (*Ban Xia*), Radix Panacis Ginseng (*Ren Shen*), Herba Dianthi (*Qu Mai*), Semen Pruni Persicae (*Tao Ren*), Niter (*Xiao*), and Nidius Vespae (*Feng Fang*).

morning and relieved in the evening are characteristic of warm malaria. The ruling (formula) is *Bai Hu Jia Gui Zhi Tang* (White Tiger Plus Cinnamon Twig Decoction).[8] Malaria with abundant cold is feminine malaria (*pin nue*. For it,) *Shu Qi San* (Dichroa Powder)[9] is the ruling formula.

---

[8] The ingredients in this formula include Rhizoma Anemarrhenae (*Zhi Mu*), Semen Oryzae Sativae (*Jing Mi*), Gypsum (*Shi Gao*), Radix Glycyrrhizae (*Gan Cao*), and Ramulus Cinnamomi Cassiae (*Gui Zhi*).

[9] This formula is composed of Herba Dichroae Febrifugae (*Shu Qi*), Os Draconis (*Long Gu*), and Muscovitum (*Yun Mu*).

Chapter Ten
A Discussion on the Pulse (& Other) Signs of Chest *Bi*, Heart Pain, Shortness of Breath & Running Piglet

The master explained:

Pulse (examination) should be focused on (finding) excess and insufficiency. If the pulse is faint in the yang (*i.e.*, the *cun*) and bowstring in the yin (*i.e.*, the *guan*), there is chest *bi* pain which should be due to severe vacuity. Since there is yang vacuity, it is known (that the trouble) is in the upper burner. It is (the fact that) the pulse is bowstring in the yin that makes chest *bi* heart pain known.

For the disease of chest *bi* manifesting as distressed rapid dyspneic breathing, coughing with (copious) sputum, pain in the chest and upper back, shortness of breath, and a pulse which is deep and slow in the *cun* and small, tight, and rapid in the *guan*, *Gua Lou Xie Bai Bai Jiu Tang* (Trichosanthes, Allium & Wine Decoction)[1] is the ruling formula.

---

[1] This formula is composed of Bulbus Allii (*Xie Bai*), Fructus Trichosanthis Kirlowii (*Gua Lou*), and white, *i.e.*, grain, alcohol (*Bai Jiu*).

If a normal person suffering from neither cold nor heat develops shortness of breath, then there is repletion.

The disease of running piglet is characterized by (qi) starting from the lower abdomen and surging up into the throat. During its attack, a desire to die will arise, but (all torment) disappears with the ending of the attack. This arises entirely from fright. If qi upsurging is accompanied by chest and abdominal pain and alternating cold and heat, *Ben Tun Tang* (Running Piglet Decoction)[2] is the ruling formula.

The master explained:

There are diseases of running piglet, ejection of pus, fright, and fire evil.[3] These four diseases all develop from fright.

---

[2] This formula is composed of Radix Glycyrrhizae (*Gan Cao*), Radix Scutellariae Baicalensis (*Huang Qin*), Radix Ligustici Wallichii (*Chuan Xiong*), Radix Paeoniae Lactiflorae (*Shao Yao*), Radix Angelicae Sinensis (*Dang Gui*), Rhizoma Pinelliae Ternatae (*Ban Xia*), Rhizoma Zingiberis (*Jiang*), Radix Puerariae (*Ge Gen*), and Cortex Radicis Pruni Salicinae (*Li Gen Bai Pi*).

[3] This implies problems caused by such fire therapies as red-hot needling, moxibustion, and fuming.

Chapter Eleven
A Discussion on the Pulse (& Other) Signs of Abdominal Fullness, Cold *Shan* & Food Retention

If the instep pulse is faint and bowstring, there ought to be abdominal fullness. If there is not, there must be block and congestion in the lower part (of the body) with difficult defecation and pain and aching in the subaxillary region. This is due to vacuity cold developing from the lower part to the upper. It requires taking warm medicinals.

Suppose a sick person suffers from fullness of the abdomen. If the abdomen feels no pain when pressed, there is vacuity. If the abdomen feels pain, there is repletion. (The latter condition) allows for precipitation. If the tongue is a yellow color and precipitation has not been used, apply precipitation and the yellow color will depart by itself. If abdominal fullness is less at one time but then comes back as it was before (at another), this is ascribed to cold and it requires taking warm medicinals.

Suppose the instep pulse is tight and floating. In the presence of the tightness, there is pain, and, in presence of the floating, there is vacuity. In the case of vacuity, there is rumbling in the intestines. In the case of a tight (pulse), there is tightness and fullness (in the abdomen).

If the pulse is bowstring and slow on both hands, there must be tightness below the heart. If the pulse is large and tight, there is yin within yang.[1] This can be treated with precipitation.

If the disease of abdominal fullness is accompanied by (abdominal) pain, there is repletion which requires precipitation.

Abdominal fullness which never gets better or whose improvement is beneath mentioning requires precipitation.

For the disease of abdominal fullness with fever for tens of [above ten is suspected] days running, a floating and rapid pulse, and normal food intake, *Hou Po San Wu Tang* (Magnolia Three Materials Decoction)[2] is the ruling formula.

For abdominal fullness and pain, *Hou Po Qi Wu Tang* (Magnolia Seven Materials Decoction)[3] is the ruling formula.

Suppose the *cun* opening pulse is slow and moderate. In the presence of the slowness, there is cold, and, in the presence of the moderateness, there is qi (stagnation). Qi (stagnation) and cold act upon one another giving rise to gripping pain.

Suppose the *cun* opening pulse is slow and choppy. In the presence of the slowness, there is cold, and in the presence of the choppiness, there is absence of blood.

---

[1] This is an internal or yin repletion case with the exterior or yang exuberant.

[2] This formula is composed of Cortex Magnoliae Officinalis (*Hou Po*), Radix Et Rhizoma Rhei (*Da Huang*), and Fructus Immaturus Aurantii (*Zhi Shi*).

[3] This formula is composed of Cortex Magnoliae Officinalis (*Hou Po*), Radix Glycyrrhizae (*Gan Cao*), Fructus Zizyphi Jujubae (*Da Zao*), Ramulus Cinnamomi Cassiae (*Gui Zhi*), Rhizoma Zingiberis (*Jiang*), Radix Et Rhizoma Rhei (*Da Huang*), and Fructus Immaturus Aurantii (*Zhi Shi*).

A sick person with cold in the center tends to yawn frequently. If the person has clear snivel running, fever, and a harmonious facial complexion, then there is frequent sneezing.

With cold in the center, a person will have diarrhea. This is because there is a vacuity internally. There is a desire but inability to sneeze. This is because there is cold in the belly.

If a thin person has periumbilical pain, there must be wind cold with blocked grain qi.[4] If one contrarily employs precipitation, the (cold) qi must surge (upward). If not, glomus below the heart will develop.

If the *cun* opening pulse is bowstring, there is hypertonicity and pain in the lateral costal region and the person is averse to cold as after a soaking.

If the *cun* opening pulse is floating and slippery, there is pain within the head. Suppose the instep pulse is moderate and slow. In the presence of the moderateness, there is cold, and, in the presence of the slowness, there is vacuity. When vacuity and cold act upon one another, there arises a desire for warm food. If cold food is taken, there will be pain in the throat.

Suppose the pulse is faint in the *cun* and tight and choppy in the *chi*. In the presence of the tightness, there is cold, in the presence of the faintness, there is vacuity, and, in the presence of the choppiness, there is insufficiency of blood. Therefore, it is known that diaphoresis and then precipitation was used. Since a tight (pulse) shows that (cold) is in the center; (therefore,) cold is known to still be there. Because this was originally (an illness of) cold qi, what could justify diaphoresis succeeded by precipitation?

Suppose the pulse is floating and tight, sort of bowstring, shaped like a string on a bow (which is so rigid that it does) not yield to pressure. If the pulse is rapid and bowstring, precipitation is required to remove cold. If there is one-sided pain in the lateral costal region and the pulse is tight and bowstring, this shows cold requiring warm medicinals to precipitate it. The appropriate (formula) is *Da Huang Fu Zi Tang* (Rhubarb & Aconite Decoction).[5]

Suppose the *cun* opening pulse is bowstring and tight. In the presence of the bowstring, there is stoppage of circulation of the defensive qi. When the defensive qi stops, there is aversion to cold.

---

[4] Blocked grain qi means stagnated digestion leading to constipation.

[5] This formula is composed of Radix Et Rhizoma Rhei (*Da Huang*), Radix Praeparatus Aconiti Carmichaeli (*Fu Zi*), and Herba Asari Cum Radice (*Xi Xin*).

In the presence of the tightness, there is no desire for food. The bowstring and the tightness combine, pointing to cold *shan*.

Suppose the instep pulse is floating and slow. In the presence of the floating, there is wind vacuity, and, in the presence of the slowness, there is cold *shan*. Cold *shan* is periumbilical pain. If, during an attack, there is spontaneous sweating and inversion frigidity of the hands and feet and the pulse is deep and bowstring, *Da Wu Tou Tang* (Major Wu Tou Aconite Decoction)[6] is the ruling formula.

(The Yellow Emperor) asked:

If a person suffers from the disease of food retention, how to diagnose it?

The master answered:

If the pulse is floating and large in the *cun*, turning choppy at a deeper level, and faint and choppy in the *chi* as well, then it is known that there is food retention.

If the *cun* opening pulse is as tight as a (fully) drawn rope and unpredictably changes on either hand, there is food retention.

If the *cun* opening pulse is tight, there is headache with cold and heat or there is retained untransformed food in the abdomen.

If the pulse is slippery and rapid, there is repletion. If there is food retention, it requires precipitation.

If diarrhea is accompanied by no desire for food, there is food retention which requires precipitation.

If, after great (*i.e.*, drastic) precipitation, there is absence of defecation for six or seven consecutive days, there (must) be persistent vexation and abdominal fullness and pain. This arises from the existence of dry stool. It is food retention which causes (the dry stool).

If food is retained in the upper venter, it is necessary to carry out ejection.

---

[6] This formula is the same as Wu Tou Aconite Decoction (*Wu Tou Tang*).

A Discussion on the Pulse (& Other) Signs of Accumulations & Gatherings of the Five Viscera

(The Yellow Emperor) asked:

There are diseases of accumulations and gatherings and grain qi. What are they?

The master answered:

Accumulation is a disease of the viscera. It never moves. Gathering is a disease of the bowels. It does not attack all the time. It gives a migratory pain. It is curable. Grain qi is lateral costal pain which is relieved by pressure. Grain qi is a recurrent (illness). After a disease is overcome, it should not relapse (so easily). If it relapses (easily), it is grain qi.

The great method of (determining) the various kinds of accumulation is, if the pulse is thin and sticking to the bone (*i.e.*, very deep), there are accumulations. If (this pulse) appears in the *cun*, the accumulation lies within the chest. If it out-reaches the *cun* a little, the accumulation lies in the throat. If it appears in the *guan,* the accumulation lies beside the umbilicus. If it upwardly out-reaches the *guan,* the accumulation lies below the heart. If it downwardly out-reaches the *guan*[1] a little, the accumulation lies in the lower abdomen. If it appears in the *chi*, the accumulation lies in the qi thoroughfare (*i.e.*, groins). If this pulse (image) appears on the left hand, the accumulation lies on the left side. If it appears on the right hand, the accumulation lies on the right side. If it appears on both (hands), the accumulation lies in the middle. (The accumulation) is located in accordance with the position (of this pulse image).

Suppose lung accumulation is ascertained. (Then) the pulse is floating and hair-like, eluding (detection) when pressure is applied. There is qi counterflow in the lateral costal region, contracting pain in the back, diminished qi, impaired memory, heavy eyes, and cold of the skin. (The accumulation) is relieved in autumn but gets worse in summer. Its ruling (characteristic) is oft-occurring pain in the skin like a louse bite. In severe cases, it is like needles pricking. There is occasional itching and the facial complexion is white.

---

[1] One should note the definition of up and down in respect to the wrist pulse. Up is distal, while down is proximal.

Suppose heart accumulation is ascertained. Then the pulse is deep and scallion-stalk. (The accumulation) goes up and down erratically. There are diseases of chest fullness, palpitations, heat within the abdomen, a red facial complexion, a dry throat, heart vexation, and heat in the palms. In severe cases, there is spitting of blood. Its ruling (characteristic) is tugging and slackening of the body. (Also) distinctive is blood inversion. It is relieved in summer and gets worse in winter. The facial complexion is red.

Suppose spleen accumulation is ascertained. (Then) the pulse is floating, large, and long. (The accumulation) lessens when hungry and becomes visible on eating to the full. The distention increases and lessens with (the amount) of grain (taken in). Below the heart, there is a string of masses shaped like peaches or plums which become visible on the exterior when standing up. There is abdominal fullness, retching, diarrhea, rumbling in the intestines, heaviness of the four limbs, swollen lower legs, and inversion (frigidity of the feet) causing sleeplessness. Its ruling (characteristic) is reduced muscles and flesh. The facial complexion is yellow.

Suppose liver accumulation is ascertained. (Then) the pulse is bowstring and thin. There is pain in the lateral costal regions which radiates obliquely to the infra-cardiac region. The feet are swollen and cold. There is lateral costal pain affecting the lower abdomen. In males, there is accumulation *shan*, and, in females, there are concretions and strangury. The body is lusterless and liable to cramps. The nails are dry and black. (This disease) is relieved in spring but gets worse in autumn. The facial complexion is green-blue.

Suppose kidney accumulation is ascertained. (Then) the pulse is deep and urgent. There is the bitterness of a dragging pain between the spine and loins. (The accumulation) is visible when hungry and lessens on eating to the full. There is urgency in the lower abdomen, a dry mouth, swollen throat with ulceration, blurred vision, and cold inside the bones. Its ruling (characteristics) are marrow inversion[2] and impaired memory. The facial complexion is black.

If the *cun* opening is deep yet rampant,[3] there is accumulation with pain lying transversely in the lateral costal region and abdomen. If the pulse is bowstring, there is acute abdominal pain, a dragging pain between the upper and lower back, cold in the abdomen, and *shan* concretion. If the pulse is bowstring and tight as well as faint and thin, there is conglomeration. Cold *bi*, concretions and conglomerations, and accumulations and gatherings all exhibit a bowstring and tight pulse. If they lie below the heart, the *cun* presents a bowstring and tight pulse. If they lie in

---

[2] This is collapse due to marrow vacuity.

[3] A rampant pulse is a forceful, tight pulse.

the venter, the *guan* presents a bowstring and tight pulse. If they lie below the umbilicus, the *chi* presents a bowstring and tight pulse.

Moreover, there is a method of (locating) concretions by the pulse. If the pulse appears rampant on the left hand, concretion lies in the left side; whereas if the pulse appears rampant on the right hand, concretion lies in the right side. If the pulse is larger at the head,[4] concretion lies in the upper. If the pulse is smaller at the head, concretion lies in the lower.

Moreover, there is another method (of diagnosing these conditions). If the pulse appears rampant on the left hand, accumulation lies in the right side. Whereas, if the pulse appears rampant on the right hand, accumulation lies in the left. If the pulse feels surging and replete as well as slippery on one hand, there is also accumulation. A bowstring and tight pulse also points to accumulation, cold *bi*, and *shan* pain. If there is accumulation but it gives no expression in the pulse, then it is difficult to treat. (However,) so long as one pulse (image) corresponding to (accumulation) is seen, it is easy to treat. If there is any kind of incongruity (between the pulse and the accumulation, the accumulation) is beyond cure.

Suppose the pulse is large on the left hand but small on the right. If there is a disease in the upper, it (must) be located in the left lateral costal region. If there is a disease in the lower, it (must) be located in the left foot. If the pulse is large on the right hand but small on the left hand, an upper disease is located in the right lateral costal region, but a lower disease is located in the right foot.

If the pulse is bowstring and hidden, there is unmovable concretion in the abdomen. It will inevitably cause death without a remedy.

If the pulse is thin and deep and, at times, rigid, there is *yong* swelling in the body or there is deep-hidden beam[5] in the abdomen.

If the pulse is not only small and deep but replete, there is accumulation gathering in the stomach giving rise to inability to take in food and vomiting upon eating.

---

[4] This section may be interpreted in either of two ways. First, when the pulse comes, it appears more forceful than when it retreats. Secondly, the pulse appears more forceful in the *cun* than in the *guan* and *chi*.

[5] Deep-hidden beam is the name of a mass which can be as long as an arm lying from the heart to the umbilicus.

_____Chapter Thirteen_____
A Discussion on the Pulse (& Other) Signs of Fright Palpitations, Ejection of Blood, Nosebleed, Hemafecia, Chest Fullness & Blood Stasis

Suppose the *cun* opening pulse is stirring and weak. In the presence of the stirring, there is susceptibility to fright, and, in the presence of the weakness, there is palpitation.

Suppose the instep pulse is faint and floating. In the presence of the floating, there is stomach qi vacuity, and, in presence of the faintness, there is inability to take in food. This is a pulse of susceptibility to fright caused by worry and oppression. In relation to the disease caused by fright, the pulse has pauses but is able to come again and the sick person is unable to roll their eyes or to breathe out.

If the *cun* opening pulse is tight while the instep pulse is floating, there is vacuity of the stomach qi.

If the *cun* opening pulse is tight, there is cold repletion. If the cold lies in the upper burner, there must be chest fullness with belching. In case of stomach qi vacuity, the instep pulse is floating and the *shao yang* pulse is tight. (And) there must (also) be palpitations below the heart. What accounts for this? When cold and water act upon one another, these two (evil) qi are locked in contention, thus giving rise to palpitations.

Any choppy, soggy, and weak pulse is (a sign of) blood collapse.

There is a bowstring and large *cun* opening pulse. It is a modulated bowstring (as compared to a purely bowstring pulse), and it is not as large as a scallion-stalk (compared to a purely large pulse). The modulated (bowstring quality) points to cold, and the scallion-stalk points to vacuity. Cold and vacuity act upon one another, giving rise to (a pulse) known as drumskin. (This pulse reveals) miscarriage and dribbling vaginal bleeding in females and blood collapse in males.

The person who suffers from blood collapse cannot be treated by means of attacking the exterior (*i.e.*, diaphoresis), for, following perspiration, cold shuddering will arise.

(The Yellow Emperor) asked:

If the disease of nosebleeding goes on for days on end, then what kind of pulse is there?

The master answered:

The pulse is light (*i.e.*, forceless) within the muscles and, in the *chi*, spilling [floating in another version]. Hazy vision without fail shows that nosebleeding is not yet at an end. When the hazy vision is gone and the eyes become clear, one knows that nosebleeding is now checked.

The master explained:

Nosebleeding occurring from spring to summer is ascribed to the *tai yang*. Nosebleeding occurring from autumn to winter is ascribed to the *yang ming*.[1]

Suppose the pulse is faint and weak in the *cun* and choppy in the *chi*. In presence of the weakness, there is fever, and, in presence of the choppiness, there is absence of blood. The person must suffer from inversion with mild retching. In inversion there should be dizziness. If there is not, but instead there is headache, the headache shows repletion. Since there is repletion above but vacuity below, nosebleeding will inevitably arise.

If the *tai yang* pulse[2] is large and floating, there is invariably nosebleeding and ejection of blood.

If the sick person's face is devoid of blood color but suffers from neither cold nor heat and the pulse is deep and bowstring, there is nosebleeding.

A sick person suffering from nosebleeding cannot be treated by diaphoresis since diaphoresis will inevitably produce a clamping (sensation) and tension of the forehead, eyes staring straight ahead with inability to roll (the eyes), and insomnia.

If the pulse is floating and weak and expires (*i.e.*, becomes intangible) under pressure, there is hemafecia. If there is vexation and cough, there must be ejection of blood.

———————————————————————————

[1] The *tai yang* refers to the exterior and the *yang ming* refers to the interior. Therefore, this section tells us that nosebleeding may be due to external heat or internal heat.

[2] This pulse might be located in the *cun* on the left hand. However, it is also possible that this refers to a pulse in the temple.

If the *cun* opening pulse is faint and weak, there is vacuity of both the qi and blood. In males, there is ejection of blood, and, in females, hemafecia. If there is retching and vomiting and sweating, (the condition) is treatable.

Suppose the instep pulse is faint and weak. In the spring, the stomach qi is the root (of the body). Vomiting with diarrhea is treatable. If there is no (vomiting or diarrhea), this shows that there is water qi and that there must be abdominal fullness and difficult urination.

If a sick person suffers from body heat (*i.e.*, generalized fever) and the pulse is small and expiring, there is ejection of blood or hemafecia and, in females, absence of menstruation. This is a cold (pattern). If the pulse is slow, there is cold in the chest with belching and frequent spitting.

There are cases where the yin-yang (*i.e.*, the pulses throughout the *cun* opening), the instep, and the *shao yin* pulse are all faint but the sick person suffers from neither vomiting nor diarrhea. (In that case,) there is invariably blood collapse.

A deep pulse points to the internal (or rather to) the constructive and defensive bound internally. If there is chest fullness, ejection of blood will inevitably arise.

If a male is exuberant and bulky and his yin-yang pulse (at the superficial and deep levels of the *cun* opening) is faint, and if the instep pulse is also faint but the *shao yin* pulse alone is floating and large, he must have suffered from hemafecia and seminal emission. Suppose there is strangury, urination ought to be inhibited.

If the instep pulse is bowstring, there must be hemorrhoids with blood in the stool.

Suppose a sick person suffers from chest fullness, withered lips, a green-blue tongue, and a dry mouth. The sick person has a desire to rinse their mouth but not to swallow the water. There is no cold and heat. The pulse is slightly large and slow. If this person complains of abdominal fullness when the abdomen is not full, there is blood stasis. If sweat refuses to exit when it is expected to, there is internal binding also giving rise to blood stasis. If a sick person looks as if running a fever, suffering from vexation, fullness, a dry mouth, and thirst, but the pulse reflects, contrarily, no fever, there is hidden yin[3] and there is blood stasis. This requires precipitation.

In connection with hemafecia, blood appearing before the stool is proximal bleeding, whereas stool appearing before the blood is distal bleeding.

---

[3] This means that yin blood is depressed so as to generate heat.

A Discussion on the Pulse (& Other) Signs of Retching, Vomiting, Dry Retching & Diarrhea

Suppose vomiting is accompanied by a weak pulse, uninhibited urination, and slight fever. If inversion appears, (the condition) is difficult to treat.

If the instep pulse is floating, there is stomach qi vacuity with cold qi above and warm qi below. Because the two qi contend, there is exiting but no entrance. That is to say, the sick person simply vomits without the ability to take in food. Those who are frightened (by the disease) will die. Those who keep relaxed and undisturbed may recover.

If a sick person who suffers from vomiting has *yong* purulence, one should not treat vomiting. When purulence runs out, healing will occur by itself.

If vomiting is followed by thirst, this is a tendency towards resolution. If thirst goes before vomiting, there is water collected below the heart. This is a case of rheum. A person who suffers from vomiting ought to be thirsty. If now, on the contrary, there is no thirst, this is because there is propping rheum below the heart.

(The Yellow Emperor) asked:

Suppose the sick person has a rapid pulse. Since a rapid (pulse) points to heat, there ought to be swift digestion with large food intake. If, instead, there is vomiting, then why?

The master answered:

This is because diaphoresis has been carried out. It has made yang faint. Since the diaphragm qi[1] is vacuous, the pulse has become rapid. This rapidity points to guest heat[2] which is not able to disperse grain. Because there is vacuity cold in the stomach, vomiting arises.

---

[1] Diaphragm qi is often used as the equivalent of righteous qi or gathering qi.

[2] In this context, guest heat refers to vacuity or false heat.

If the pulse is tight in the yang (*i.e.*, the *cun*) and rapid in the yin (*i.e.*, the *guan* and *chi*), the person vomits upon ingestion. If the pulse is floating and rapid in the yang, there is also vomiting.

If the pulse is tight in the *cun* and choppy in the *chi*, the person suffers from chest fullness, inability to take in food, and vomiting. Vomiting may be arrested by precipitation. As a consequence, (however,) there will be inability to take in food. Suppose vomiting is not arrested (by precipitation), this is stomach reflux that makes the pulse faint and choppy in the *chi*.

Suppose the *cun* opening pulse is tight and scallion-stalk. In the presence of the tightness, there is cold, and, in the presence of the scallion-stalk (quality), there is vacuity. Since vacuity and cold act upon one another, the pulse becomes slow because of bound yin (cold). Then the person suffers from upper esophageal constriction. If the pulse is rapid in the *guan*, the person suffers from vomiting.

If the pulse is bowstring, there is vacuity. For lack of stomach qi, food taken in the morning is vomited out in the evening. This is transmuted stomach reflux. When cold lies in the upper (part of the body) but the (attending) physician contrarily employs precipitation, the pulse will become bowstring. Therefore, one speaks of vacuity.

Suppose the instep pulse is faint and choppy. In the presence of the faintness, there is diarrhea, and, in the presence of the choppiness, there is counterflow vomiting with no grain able to enter.

Suppose the *cun* opening pulse is faint and rapid. In the presence of the faintness, there is absence of qi. When there is no qi, the constructive becomes vacuous. When the constructive is vacuous, blood becomes insufficient. When blood is insufficient, there is cold in the chest. The instep pulse is floating and choppy. In the presence of the floating, there is vacuity, and, in the presence of the choppiness, there is a damaged spleen. When damaged, the spleen will not grind (grain). Then food taken in the morning is vomited in the evening or food taken in the evening is vomited the next morning. (The spleen) is unable to transform the retained food. This is called stomach reflux. If the pulse is tight and choppy, the disease is difficult to treat.

If a person suffers from vomiting, the pulse will feel (flaccid) like (one feels) when one has just risen from bed.

A person with a desire to vomit cannot be treated with precipitation.

Suppose there is retching and vomiting with the trouble lying above the diaphragm. If, following (vomiting), a desire for water arises, a resolution will come. One should give water (to the sick person) without delay. For those who have a desire for water, *Zhu Ling San* (Polyporous Powder) is the ruling formula.

In regard to dry retching with abdominal fullness, one should examine urination and defecation to determine which is inhibited. Then (proper) disinhibition will effect recovery.

When the qi of the six bowels expires externally, there are cold hands and feet, qi ascent, and foot contraction. When the qi of the five viscera expires internally, there is uncheckable diarrhea. If diarrhea is severe, there will be insensitivity of the hands and feet.

If diarrhea exhibits a deep and bowstring pulse, there is pressure in the rectum. So long as the pulse is large, diarrhea is not checked. If the pulse is faint, weak, and rapid, diarrhea will tend to resolve itself. Even though there is fever, it will not end in death.

If the pulse is slippery but turns vacuous and expires (*i.e.*, becomes intangible) under pressure, the person must suffer from diarrhea.

Suppose diarrhea is accompanied by slight fever. If the sick person is thirsty and the pulse is weak, recovery is now coming by itself.

Suppose diarrhea exhibits a rapid pulse. If slight fever and spontaneous sweating arise, recovery will come by itself. If the pulse is also tight, resolution has yet to occur.

If diarrhea exhibits a pulse which is contrarily floating and rapid in the *cun* and choppy in the *chi*, the sick person must have pus and blood in their stool.

Suppose inversion frigidity of the hands and feet with no pulse arises in diarrhea. If moxibustion not only fails to restore warmth (to the hands and feet) and recover the pulse but is followed by slight dyspnea, this is death.

A *shao yin* (pulse) which is inferior to the instep (pulse in force) is a favorable (sign).

If diarrhea exhibits a pulse which is rapid and floating, recovery is now coming by itself. If relief does not come, the sick person will inevitably have pus and blood in their stool since there is heat (internally).

Suppose, following diarrhea, the pulse expires with inversion frigidity of the hands and feet. If, one day later, the pulse restores (itself) and the hands and feet become warm, there is life (*i.e.*, there is hope of survival). If the pulse does not come back, this is death.

Suppose diarrhea exhibits a bowstring pulse. If there is fever and spontaneous sweating, relief will come by itself.

Diarrhea with flatus requires disinhibiting urination.

Diarrhea of clear grain (in the stools) prohibits attacking the exterior since perspiration would be followed by (abdominal) distention and fullness. If the viscera are cold, it is necessary to warm them.

Suppose diarrhea exhibits a deep and slow pulse. If the sick person has a slightly red face, there is slight heat in the body.

Clear-grain diarrhea will invariably be resolved by diaphoresis if it is accompanied by faintness and dizziness. The sick person (must) have slight inversion frigidity (of the extremities). What accounts for this is the face wearing yang.[3] This is produced by vacuity below.

Diarrhea with abdominal distention and fullness and generalized pain and aching should be treated first through warming the interior before attacking the exterior.

If diarrhea exhibits a slow and slippery pulse, (this shows that) there is repletion and that diarrhea is not tending to stop. (To treat this,) precipitation is required.

If diarrhea exhibits contrarily a slippery pulse, there must be something retained requiring removal. Relief will follow precipitation.

If, after having been overcome, diarrhea relapses at the watch, the day, the month, and the year (when it first happened),[4] this is because the disease is not yet (totally) exterminated. It requires precipitation once more.

Diarrhea with delirious speech is due to dry stool, indicating precipitation.

---

[3] Face wearing yang refers to a red or bright facial complexion due to vacuity cold in the lower burner. This term, however, is often rendered as capping yang. It is a result of upborne yang qi, a sign of true cold below with false heat above.

[4] This section seems illogical. The translator speculates that diarrhea recurs at the same watch, etc. of the *next year(s)* as it first occurred. However, the apparent lack of logic may be remedied by another interpretation. In this case, the illness recurs at a time when the Heaven Stem and Earthly Branch combination falls on the same combination as when the disease first occurred.

Diarrhea with abdominal pain and fullness is due to cold repletion, requiring precipitation.

Diarrhea with tightness in the abdomen requires precipitation.

Suppose, following diarrhea, vexation becomes more serious. If the region below the heart feels soft when palpated, this is vacuity vexation.

Suppose, following diarrhea, the pulse becomes peaceful in all the three positions. If the region below the heart feels tight when palpated, precipitation is allowed.

If, following diarrhea, the pulse becomes floating and large, there is vacuity which is a result of forced (*i.e.*, wrong employment of) precipitation. Suppose the pulse is floating and drumskin and subsequently there is rumbling in the intestines, this requires warming.

If a sick person with a withered yellow facial complexion suffers from agitation, no thirst, cold repletion in the stomach, and incessant diarrhea, this is death.

Cold wind accompanied by diarrhea cannot be treated with precipitation since, following precipitation, tightness and pain below the heart will arise. If the pulse is slow, there is cold. This requires warming. If the pulse is deep and tight, precipitation will bring about the same (consequences as above). If the pulse is large, floating, and bowstring, precipitation will effect recovery.

_______________Chapter Fifteen_______________

A Discussion on the Pulse (& Other) Signs of Lung Atony, Lung *Yong*, Counterflow Cough, Qi Ascent & Phlegm Rheum

(The Yellow Emperor) asked:

When there is heat in the upper burner, cough may lead to lung atony. How does this disease of lung atony arise?

The master answered:

It may arise from sweating, retching and vomiting, wasting thirst, or frequent, uninhibited urination. It may (also) arise from difficult defecation when it is treated with drastic medicinals to loosen the bowel movements. (These medicinals) add to loss of fluids, thus producing (lung atony).

When the *cun* opening pulse is not out (*i.e.*, not floating) but diaphoresis is contrarily employed, the pulse will become scattered at the yang (*i.e.*, superficial level) but not choppy at the yin (*i.e.*, deep level) and the triple burner will become faltering. (The yang qi) only submerges but does not emerge.[1] If the pulse is not choppy in the yin but there is contrarily vexation internally, copious sputum, dry lips, and difficult urination, this is lung atony. It is due to damaged fluids. The stool looks like rotten melon or pig's brain. (All this) is entirely produced by diaphoresis.

Taken with lung atony, the sick person may suffer from a desire but inability to cough and discharge of a dry (*i.e.*, sticky), foamy substance with coughing. In due time, urination will become inhibited, and, in severe cases, the pulse will become floating and weak.

Suppose lung atony manifests spitting of foamy substance but no coughing. If the sick person does not suffer from thirst, there will invariably be urinary incontinence or frequent voiding of urine. This is because the upper (burner) is too vacuous to control (water) in the lower. This is ascribed to cold in the lungs. Invariably, there is dizziness and copious sputum. (To treat this,) administer *Gan Cao Gan Jiang Tang* (Licorice & Dry Ginger Decoction) to warm the lung viscus.

The master explained:

In connection with lung atony, those who suffer from coughing of sputum will heal by themselves if their mouths are dry with a desire to drink water. Those whose mouths are open are short of breath.

If coughing is with fluids automatically generated in the mouth and the tongue fur is glossy, it is (an indication of) floating cold rather than lung atony.

(The Yellow Emperor) asked:

The *cun* opening pulse is rapid and the sick person who is taken with cough has turbid saliva in the mouth and foamy sputum. What kind (of disease) is this?

The master answered:

---

[1] In other words, the yang qi is sunken internally.

This is the disease of lung atony. If there is cracking dryness of the mouth, dull pain arises in the chest when coughing, and the pulse is contrarily slippery and rapid, this is lung *yong*.

Coughing with ejection of pus and blood is lung atony if the pulse is rapid and vacuous. If the pulse is rapid and replete, it is lung *yong*.

(The Yellow Emperor) asked:

What kind of pulse shows that the disease of counterflow cough is lung *yong*? Suppose (lung *yong*) ought to develop pus and blood and ought to end in death when (pus and blood) is vomited. It turns out that death does eventually come following vomiting of pus. Then what kind of pulse is there?

The master answered:

The *cun* opening pulse is faint and rapid. The faintness points to wind, and the rapidity to heat. The faintness points to sweating, and the rapidity to aversion to cold. When struck by wind, the defensive follows exhalation, not submerging. When penetrated by heat, the constructive follows inhalation, not emerging. (Therefore,) wind damages the skin and hair, and heat damages the blood vessels. When wind lodges in the lungs, the sick person suffers from cough, a dry mouth, dyspnea with (chest) fullness, dry throat, no thirst, spitting of copious turbid, foamy substance, and frequent cold shuddering. As heat penetrates, blood congeals and stagnates, accumulating and condensing into *yong* pus which looks like rice gruel after being spit out. At its onset, (this disease) is treatable, but once purulence has developed, this is death.

Cough accompanied by chest fullness, cold shuddering, a rapid pulse, a dry throat, no thirst, and frequent discharge of turbid sputum with a foul fishy smell is lung *yong* when the pus ejected is like rice gruel. (For this,) *Jie Geng Tang* (Platycodon Decoction)[2] is the ruling formula.

For lung *yong* with chest distention and fullness, puffy swelling of the whole body including the face and eyes, nasal congestion with clear snivel, inability to tell fragrance from fetor, sourness or acridity, counterflow cough with qi ascent, dyspnea with rales, oppression and congestion (of the chest), *Ting Li Da Zao Xie Fei Tang* (Lepidium & Red Dates Drain the Lungs Decoction)[3] is the ruling formula.

---

[2] This formula is composed of Radix Platycodi Grandiflori (*Jie Geng*) and Radix Glycyrrhizae (*Gan Cao*).

[3] There are only two ingredients in this formula, namely, Semen Lepidii (*Ting Li*) and Fructus Zizyphi Jujubae (*Da Zao*).

When the *cun* opening pulse is rapid and the instep pulse is tight, cold and heat are contending with one another and, consequently, cold shuddering and cough occur. If the instep pulse is floating and moderate with the stomach qi normal, this points to lung *yong*.

(The Yellow Emperor) asked:

If there is cold shuddering with fever, the *cun* opening pulse is slippery and rapid, and the sick person eats, drinks, gets up, and sleeps in a normal way, this is a disease of *yong* swelling. If the (attending) physician is ignorant and treats this as cold damage, (of course) no cure can be effected. Then how can one know if there is purulence? How can one determine the location of purulence?

The master answered:

Suppose there is pus inside the chest and lung *yong* has developed. The sick person will have a rapid pulse and suffers from coughing and ejection of pus and blood. Suppose purulence has not (well) developed. The pulse (then) is tight and rapid. If the tightness is gone but the rapidity is left, purulence has developed.

The disease of ejection of blood, dyspnea, cough, and qi ascent will end in death if the pulse is rapid and there is fever and insomnia. (The disease of) qi ascent, puffy swelling of the face, and shrugging the shoulders to facilitate breathing is hardly curable if the pulse is floating and large. If there is diarrhea in addition, (the case) is more serious. Qi ascent with agitation and dyspnea is ascribed to lung distention which tends to wind water. Promotion of sweating may effect a cure.

An alcoholic who suffers from cough will invariably develop ejection of blood. This is a result of excessive drinking.

A sick person suffering from cough has water (qi) if the pulse is bowstring. One may administer *Shi Zao Tang* (Ten Dates Decoction)[4] to precipitate (water qi). If cough exhibits a floating pulse and the sick person suffers from no cough [thirst is suspected] but inability to take in food, relief will not be realized till forty days later. Cough frequently accompanied by fever is not due to vacuity if the pulse (is capable of) suddenly becoming bowstring. It is a result of cold repletion in the chest requiring ejection. Suppose a sick person suffers from cough and the pulse is bowstring. Before prescribing emetics, one should take into account whether the person is strong or weak. One should not employ ejection when there is heat. If the pulse is deep, one cannot employ

---

[4] This formula is composed of Flos Daphnis Genkwae (*Yuan Hua*), Herba Circii Japonici (*Da Ji*), Radix Euphorbiae Kansui (*Gan Sui*), and Fructus Zizyphi Jujubae (*Da Zao*).

diaphoresis. Years long enduring cough is curable if the pulse is weak, but incurable if the pulse is replete, large, and rapid. If the pulse is vacuous, it is certain that there is tormenting dizziness, the cause of which is propping rheum in the chest of the sick person. The treatment is the same as for rheum.

(The Yellow Emperor) asked:

There are four categories of rheum. What are they?

The master answered:

They are phlegm rheum [lodged rheum in another version], suspended rheum, spillage rheum, and propping rheum.

(The Yellow Emperor) asked:

How are the four categories of rheum differentiated?

The master answered:

If a person was exuberant in the past but now is thin with water traveling in their intestines with a gurgling sound, this is known as phlegm rheum. If, upon drinking, water flows down into the lateral costal regions and causes coughing and spitting provoking a contracting (chest) pain, this is known as suspended rheum. If the water drunk flows (wildly), gathering in the four limbs, causing refusal of sweat to exit when it should and generalized pain and aching, this is known as spillage rheum. Counterflow cough with having to lean against something to facilitate breathing, such shortness of breath as to cause inability to lie down, and seeming swelling of the body are characteristic of propping rheum.

Lodged rheum is characterized by lateral costal pain which radiates to the supraclavicular fossa and becomes worse when coughing. If there is lodged rheum in the chest, the sick person will suffer from shortness of breath, thirst, and pain in every limb joint. The deep pulse is an indication of lodged rheum. If there is lodged rheum below the heart, there will be a cold area in the back the size of the palm.

Suppose a sick person has a deep pulse and is liable to diarrhea. If diarrhea leads to comfort and if, in spite of diarrhea, tightness and fullness remains the same below the heart, this shows that lodged rheum is about to leave. (In this case,) *Gan Sui Ban Xia Tang* (Kansui & Pinellia Decoction)[5] is the ruling formula.

The disease of phlegm rheum should be treated by harmonizing with warm medicinals. If there is phlegm rheum below the heart with propping fullness of the chest and lateral costal region and visual dizziness, *Gan Cao* [*Gan Sui* in another version] *Tang* (Licorice [or Kansui] Decoction)[6] is the ruling formula.

The disease of spillage rheum should be treated by diaphoresis. The ruling formula is *Xiao Qing Long Tang* (Minor Blue-green Dragon Decoction).

Propping rheum is also characterized by dyspnea and inability to lie down in addition to shortness of breath, but the pulse is level (*i.e.*, peaceful, normal).

With propping rheum around the diaphragm, the sick person will suffer from dyspnea with (chest) fullness, glomus and tightness below the heart, and a soot black facial complexion. The pulse is deep and tight. Ten days after contraction, if the (attending) physician uses ejection and precipitation but achieves no cure, then *Mu Fang Ji Tang* (Cocculus Decoction)[7] is the ruling formula.

If there is propping rheum below the heart and the sick person suffers from oppression and dizziness, *Ze Xie Tang* (Alisma Decoction)[8] is the ruling formula.

A sick person who suffers from vomiting should be thirsty. Thirst shows a tendency towards resolution. If now, on the contrary, there is no thirst, this is because there is propping rheum below the heart. (For this case,) *Xiao Ban Xia Tang* (Minor Pinellia Decoction)[9] is the ruling formula.

---

[5] The ingredients in this formula are Radix Euphorbiae Kansui (*Gan Sui*), Radix Paeoniae Lactiflorae (*Shao Yao*), Rhizoma Pinelliae Ternatae (*Ban Xia*), and Radix Glycyrrhizae (*Gan Cao*).

[6] *Gan Cao Tang* (Licorice Decoction) is composed of only Radix Glycyrrhizae (*Gan Cao*). *Gan Sui Tang* (Kansui Decoction) is also composed of only one ingredient, *i.e.*, Radix Euphorbiae Kansui (*Gan Sui*).

[7] This formula is composed of Radix Cocculi (*Mu Fang Ji*), Gypsum (*Shi Gao*), Ramulus Cinnamomi Cassiae (*Gui Zhi*), and Radix Panacis Ginseng (*Ren Shen*).

[8] The ingredients in this formula are Rhizoma Alismatis (*Ze Xie*) and Rhizoma Atractylodis Macrocephalae (*Bai Zhu*).

[9] This formula is composed of Rhizoma Pinelliae Ternatae (*Ban Xia*) and Rhizoma Zingiberis (*Jiang*).

A sick person with propping rheum who suffers from cough, vexation, and pain in the chest will not sustain sudden death. (The condition) may last one hundred days to one year. (To treat this case,) one may administer *Shi Zao Tang* (Ten Dates Decoction).

Disease above the diaphragm may manifest (chest) fullness, dyspnea, coughing, and spitting. During an attack, cold and heat, pain in the upper and lower back, and tearing [dizziness in another version] may arise. If, (in addition,) the sick person suffers from severe trembling and jerking of the body, it is certain that there is hidden rheum.

If a sick person drinks quantities of water, there must arise sudden dyspnea and (chest) fullness. With low food intake and copious drinking, water collected below the heart will give rise to palpitations in severe cases and shortness of breath in mild ones.

If the pulse is bowstring on both hands, there is cold. This is invariably a result of subjection to vacuity caused by drastic precipitation. If the pulse is bowstring on one hand, there is rheum. Lung rheum, (however,) presents no bowstring pulse but is disposed to give rise to dyspnea and shortness of breath.

If a sick person suffers from paralysis of one arm and sometimes of the other arm, this is not wind (disease) if the pulse is deep and thin. There must be rheum in the upper burner. If the pulse is vacuous, this is slight taxation. It is the result of failure of the constructive and defensive to circulate throughout the body. It will heal in due time.

Abdominal fullness with a bitter taste and dryness in the mouth is due to water qi in the intestines. (In this case,) *Fang Ji Jiao Mu Ting Li Da Huang Wan* (Stephania, Sophora, Lepidium & Rhubarb Pills)[10] are the ruling formula.

If a thin person suffers from palpitations below the umbilicus, vomiting of foamy substances, and dizziness, this is due to water. The ruling formula (for this) is *Wu Ling San* (Five [Ingredients] Poria Powder).

Thirst preceding retching is due to water collecting below the heart. This is a case of rheum, and the ruling formula is *Ban Xia Jia Fu Ling Tang* (Pinellia Plus Poria Decoction).[11]

---

[10] This formula is composed of Radix Stephaniae Tetrandrae (*Fang Ji*), Fructus Sophorae Japonicae (*Jiao Mu*), Semen Lepidii (*Ting Li*), and Radix Et Rhizoma Rhei (*Da Huang*).

[11] The ingredients in this formula include Rhizoma Pinelliae Ternatae (*Ban Xia*), Sclerotium Poriae Cocos (*Fu Ling*), Radix Rehmanniae (*Di Huang*), Pericarpium Citri Reticulatae (*Chen Pi*), Herba Asari Cum Radice (*Xi Xin*), Radix Panacis Ginseng (*Ren Shen*), Radix Paeoniae Lactiflorae (*Shao Yao*), Flos Inulae (*Xuan Fu*), Radix Ligustici Wallichii (*Chuan Xiong*), Radix Platycodi Grandiflori (*Jie Geng*), Radix Glycyrrhizae (*Gan Cao*), and Rhizoma Zingiberis (*Jiang*).

If water lies in the heart, there is tightness and palpitations below the heart, shortness of breath, and aversion to water with no desire to drink. If water lies in the lungs, there is vomiting of foamy substances and a desire to drink water. If water lies in the spleen, there is diminished qi with generalized heaviness. If water lies in the liver, there is propping fullness in the lateral costal region with pain and sneezing. If water lies in the kidneys, there are palpitations below the heart.

_______________Chapter Sixteen_______________
A Discussion on the Pulse (& Other) Signs of *Yong* Swelling, Intestinal *Yong*, Incised Wounds & Sapping Sores

If the pulse is rapid but there is no fever, there must be *yong* internally.

Any floating and rapid pulse should be accompanied by fever. If, on the contrary, there is cold shuddering as after a soaking and there is a painful place, *yong* should develop there. A faint and slow pulse invariably points to fever.[1] If the pulse is weak and rapid, there is cold shuddering and *yong* swelling should develop.

If the pulse is floating and rapid and there is no heat but there is taciturnity, slight agitation in the chest [stomach in another version], and a pain baffling location, this person will develop *yong* swelling.

Suppose the pulse is slippery and rapid. In the presence of the rapidity, there is heat, and, in presence of the slipperiness, there is repletion. The slipperiness rules the constructive, and the rapidity rules the defensive. When (repletion of) the constructive and (heat of) the defensive meet, they will combine, giving rise to *yong*. Where the heat penetrates, there will be purulence.

The master explained:

In terms of various categories of *yong* swelling, if one intends to determine whether there is pus

____

[1] If the pulse is floating and rapid, there is usually external heat or fever. If the pulse is weak and slow, there is also heat or fever. In the latter case, however, the heat is generated internally by vacuity.

or not, one may lay the hand over the swelling. If it feels hot, there is purulence. If it is not hot, there is no purulence.

(The Yellow Emperor) asked:

Suppose the wife of a Plumage Forest[2] is ill. How can a physician determine whether there is purulence in the intestines by examining the pulse and whether it will be cured through precipitation?

The master answered:

The *cun* opening pulse is slippery and rapid. In the presence of the slipperiness, there is repletion, and, in presence of the rapidity, there is heat. The slipperiness rules the constructive, and the rapidity rules the defensive. The defensive, if rapid (*i.e.*, hot), descends, while the constructive, if slippery (*i.e.*, replete), ascends. (Thus) the constructive and defensive interfere with one another, and, (in consequence,) blood becomes turbid and decayed. Then glomus and tightness in the lower abdomen with inhibited urination or occasional (spontaneous) sweating arise. In addition, there is aversion to cold. Now purulence has developed. Suppose the pulse is slow and tight, then static blood gathers. After the (static blood) is precipitated, healing will ensue.

Intestinal *yong* is characterized by rough skin of the body and tense abdominal skin which feels soft when palpated and which looks as if swollen.

Intestinal *yong* manifests as lower abdominal swelling giving pain when pressed, strangury-like frequent urination, occasional fever, and spontaneous sweating. In addition, there is aversion to cold. If the pulse is slow and tight, purulence has not yet developed. (This) allows precipitation. Then blood will be discharged (by precipitation). If the pulse is surging and rapid, purulence has developed and precipitation is not allowed. The ruling formula is *Da Huang Mu Dan Tang* (Rhubarb & Moutan Decoction).[3]

(The Yellow Emperor) asked:

———————————————————————

2 The Plumage Forest is the bodyguard of the emperor. In this context, it refers to lords and nobles in general.

3 This formula is composed of Radix Et Rhizoma Rhei (*Da Huang*), Cortex Radicis Moutan (*Dan Pi*), Mirabilitum (*Mang Xiao*), Semen Pruni Persicae (*Tao Ren*), and Semen Benincasae Hispidae (*Gua Zi*).

If the *cun* opening pulse is faint and choppy, there should be blood collapse or sweating. Suppose there is no sweating; what accounts for this?

(The master) answered:

There are sores in the body or incised wounds. Blood collapse accounts (for absence of sweating).

Sapping sore (*jin yin chuang*)[4] is treatable if it spreads from the mouth to the limbs but is incurable if it spreads from the four limbs to the mouth.

———————————————

[4] This is impetigo.

BOOK NINE

Collated & Edited by Honorary Minister Without Portfolio,
Curator of the Imperial Library,
Imperial Courier and Senior Army Protector,
Lin Yi *et al.*

A Discussion of the Signs of Pregnancy, Difference in the Sex (of the Fetus) & Various Diseases (Occurring) Before Birth

A level (*i.e.*, peaceful) but vacuous pulse is the norm for breast-feeding. It is said in the classic that beating yin and distinct yang[1] tells baby-carrying (*i.e.*, pregnancy). This shows harmonious blood and qi and that yang has donated and yin is transforming.[2] On examination, if the hand *shao yin* pulse stirs in a big way, pregnancy is determined. The *shao yin* is the pulse of the heart. The heart governs the blood vessels. In addition, the kidneys are named the uterine gate and infant's door. The pulse in the *chi* is that of the kidneys. If the pulse in the *chi* does not expire (*i.e.*, yield) under pressure, this should indicate pregnancy. If the pulse remains quite the same in the superficial and deep levels in the three positions, not yielding to pressure, there is pregnancy. In the initial stage of pregnancy, the pulse is slightly small in the *cun*, beating five times for one respiration. In the third month, the pulse is rapid in the *chi*. If the pulse is slippery and racing but scattered under heavy pressure of the fingers, the fetus is in its third month. If the pulse is not scattered under heavy pressure of the fingers and it is racing but not slippery, the fetus is in its fifth month.

When a woman is in the fourth month of pregnancy, the method of determining the sex (of the fetus) is that a racing pulse on the left hand tells a male, while a racing pulse on the right tells a female. If the pulses are racing on both hands, this tells that two babies will be born.

Another method is that perception of the *tai yin* pulse shows a male, while perception of a *tai yang* pulse shows a female. The *tai yin* pulse is a deep pulse, while a *tai yang* pulse is a floating pulse.

Another method is that a deep and replete pulse on the left hand shows a male, while a floating and large pulse on the right hand shows a female. If the pulse is deep and replete on both the left

---

1   This is an image of a pulse beating vigorously in the *chi* (yin) while being conspicuously slippery in the *cun* (yang).

2   Yang means the male (husband), while yin, the female (wife). Thus, this phrase implies successful copulation and development of a fetus. However, yang may also mean qi and yin may mean blood. From this point of view, a somewhat different interpretation arises that qi and blood coordinate well, qi exerting itself to maintain normal physical activities, while blood is being transformed into the fetus.

and right hands, as a rule, male twins will be born. If the pulse is floating and large on both the left and right hands, as a rule, female twins will be born.

Another method is that, if the pulse is large in the *chi* on the left hand alone, a male is indicated. If the pulse is large in the *chi* on the right hand alone, a female is indicated. If the pulse is large on both the left and right hands, twins will be born. This large pulse is similar to a replete pulse.

Another method is that, if the pulse is floating in the *chi* on both the left and right hands, a male twin will be born. If not, the female sex will be born in place of the male.[3] If the pulse is deep in the *chi* on both the left and right hands, female twins will be born. If not, males will be born in place of the females.

Another method is to instruct the pregnant woman to walk southward and then call her. If she turns left, a male (fetus) is suggested. If she turns right, a female is suggested.

Another method is to call her suddenly while she is seen walking to the latrine. If she turns left, a male is suggested. If she turns right, a female is suggested.

Another method is that, if, during the pregnancy, the husband of the woman develops a tubercle on his left breast, a male (fetus) is suggested. If he develops a tubercle on his right breast, a female is suggested.

In pregnancy, the woman may have channel aberration,[4] (*e.g.*, a floating pulse). Suppose there is abdominal pain radiating to the lumbar spine. Birth is imminent. Mere channel aberration suggests no disease.

Another method (of determining labor) is this: Towards labor the woman has a pulse of channel aberration. If she feels (abdominal pain) at midnight, then she will give birth at midday (the next day).

---

[3] Given a free translation this sentence might be rendered as follows: If a female twin is given birth to this time, then next time when the pulse suggests a female, a male will be given birth to instead. This implies the possibility of unusual pulse indications.

[4] Channel aberration means chaotic channel qi. In reference to the pulse, however, it often means the sudden appearance of abnormal pulse images.

320

A Discussion of the Diseases of Stirring Fetus, Blood Aspect, Water Aspect, Vomiting, Diarrhea & Abdominal Pain in Pregnancy

During a woman's first month of pregnancy, the fetus is nourished by the foot *jue yin* vessel. During the second month, it is nourished by the foot *shao yang* vessel. During the third month, it is nourished by the hand heart-governor vessel. During the fourth month, it is nourished by the hand *shao yang* vessel. During the fifth month, it is nourished by the foot *tai yin* vessel. During the sixth month, it is nourished by the foot *yang ming* vessel. During the seventh month, it is nourished by the hand *tai yin* vessel. During the eighth month, it is nourished by the hand *yang ming* vessel. During the ninth month, it is nourished by the foot *shao yin* vessel. During the tenth month, it is nourished by the foot *tai yang* vessel. The above yin and yang (vessels) each provide nourishment for thirty days in order that the baby (*i.e.*, the fetus) lives on. The reason why the hand *tai yang* and *shao yin* do not provide nourishment (to the fetus) is that they govern the menstrual flow below and produce breast milk above to keep the baby alive and to nurture the mother. A pregnant woman cannot be treated by means of moxibustion or needling the channels.[1] Otherwise, miscarriage is unavoidable.

If, in the third month of pregnancy, the woman suffers from thirst and the pulse is contrarily slow, this is a tendency toward water aspect (disease).[2] If there is abdominal pain in addition, miscarriage is unavoidable.

If the pulse is floating and there is sweating, it is certain that there is blocked (heat). If the pulse is rapid, *yong* purulence will inevitably develop. If, in the fifth or sixth month (of pregnancy), the pulse is rapid, there must be an obnoxious tendency. If the pulse is tight, there must be uterine

---

[1] There can be at least two interpretations of this section. One says that one should not moxa or needle the channel in a month when it is the turn of this channel to provide nourishment for the fetus. Another interpretation, which is more consistent with the context, is that one should not moxa or needle the hand *tai yang* and *shao yin*.

[2] See below in this chapter.

leaking (*bao lou*).[3] If the pulse is slow, there must be abdominal fullness and dyspnea. If the pulse is floating, water will invariably become obnoxious, developing into swelling.

(The Yellow Emperor) asked:

Suppose there is a woman aged twenty years or so. Her pulse is floating and rapid (and she suffers from) fever, retching, cough, occasional diarrhea, and no desire for food. Then her pulse becomes floating and her menses stop. What problem is this?

The master answered:

She should be pregnant. What justifies (this diagnosis)? This woman is vacuous and should have a faint and weak pulse. On the contrary, however, the pulse is floating and rapid. This is capping yang.[4] Since yin and yang are in harmony, she should be pregnant. When the Beginning of Autumn comes, fever will leave by itself. What justifies the prediction? A rapid pulse points to heat, and heat is fire. Fire is the child of wood. It becomes dead in the last month (of summer) which is the sixth month. (This month) is ascribed to earth. (In this month,) earth is king, while wood is at an end and has abdicated. Further, yin qi begins to engender. (Therefore,) when the qi of the autumn season arrives, fire qi should be concluded and heat is eliminated automatically. Then the disease will heal.

The master explained:

After the (first) three months of breast-feeding, (the menses) reappear. If, three months later, the pulse reveals absence (of menstruation), this shows a (new) body (*i.e.,* pregnancy). The breast-feeding mother ought to protect the baby for fear that it should be taken with diarrhea. What underlies (this fear)? In pregnancy, yang qi has to nourish (the fetus) internally and, (consequently,) the breasts become vacuous and cold so that the baby may be taken with diarrhea.

In the sixth or seventh month of pregnancy, the woman may have a bowstring pulse, suffering from fever, the fetus out-reaching (the right position) in the abdomen, and abdominal pain and aversion to cold. This cold (sensation) is as if the lower abdomen were being fanned. What

---

3   *I.e.,* constant bleeding in pregnancy.

4   See note 3, Ch.14, the present book. In this context, this specifically refers to floating vacuity yang, implying that yin blood gathers below because of pregnancy, leaving the upper part vacuous. Thus yang qi is upborn. This manifests as fever. Since this is a physiological rather than a pathological change *per se,* yin and yang, or qi and blood, do not interfere with one another.

accounts for this is the opening of the uterus. (To treat it,) it is necessary to warm the uterus with *Fu Zi Tang* (Aconite Decoction).

In the seventh month of pregnancy, if the woman has a replete, large, firm, and strong pulse, (the fetus) will survive. If she has a deep, thin pulse, (the fetus) will die.

In the eighth month of pregnancy, if the woman has a replete, large, firm, strong, bowstring, and tight pulse, (the fetus) will survive. If she has a deep and thin pulse, (the fetus) will die.

If, in the sixth or seventh month of pregnancy, the woman abruptly discharges one *dou* (= 10 liters) or more of fluid, the fetus will inevitably abort since the discharge of amniotic fluid is untimely.

The master explained:

Suppose the *cun* opening pulse is surging and choppy. In the presence of the surging, there is qi (exuberance), and, in the presence of the choppiness, there is blood (insufficiency). When qi is dynamic in the Cinnabar Field, the form (of the fetus) is warm. If a choppy (pulse image) is felt in the lower (*i.e.*, the *chi*), the fetus will be ice-cold. Yang qi keeps the fetus alive, while (exuberant) yin invariably puts an end to it. To tell yang from yin, the pulse remains strong (even) under heavy pressure. Suppose yang is at an end. There will be an accumulation shaped like a cup (in the lower abdomen).

(The Yellow Emperor) asked:

Suppose a pregnant woman is ill. How can you, Master, determine whether the woman has twin fetuses and whether one of the twins is dead, while the other is alive? If the dead one is precipitated, the woman may be rid of the disease and deliver a (living) baby. (In this case,) what kind of pulse is there and how to identify it?

The master answered:

If the *cun* opening pulse suggests balanced and harmonious defensive qi and relaxed and moderate constructive qi, then yang is donating and yin is transforming. The essence is exuberant and has a surplus, while yin and yang are both exuberant. Therefore, two bodies have developed (in the womb). If now the *shao yin* (pulse) is faint and tight, blood is turbid and congealed. Since the channels are unable to provide nourishment to both fetuses, one perishes. Lower abdominal cold and fullness, pain and aching in the kneecaps, and heaviness of the lumbus and difficulty in rising, these show blood blockage. If it is not removed early enough, it will bring damage to the mother and cause loss of the fetus.

The master explained:

Suppose a pregnant woman suffers from abdominal pain and restlessness and the fetus is diseased and stops growing. If one intends to know whether (the fetus) is alive or dead, one may have someone else palpate (the abdomen of the woman).[5] If (the fetus thus felt) is shaped like an inverted cup, the fetus is a male. If it is shaped like the rugged end of the elbow, the fetus is a female. Then what does a cold (feeling) signify? A cold (feeling) is a dead (fetus), while a warm (feeling) is a living (one).

The master explained:

Women may have dribbling uterine bleeding, post-miscarriage incessant uterine bleeding, or bleeding during pregnancy. If there is abdominal pain in pregnancy, this shows uterine leaking. (For it,) *Jiao Ai Tang* (Gelatin & Mugwort Decoction)[6] is the ruling formula.

Suppose a pregnant woman's menses have been stopped for three months when she develops dribbling uterine bleeding. The bleeding lasts forty days and the fetus is (felt) stirring above the umbilicus. This is a bitterness wrought by enduring concretion. Suppose there is a stirring (sensation in the abdomen) in the sixth month of (supposed) pregnancy. If menstrual flow continues uninhibited for three months before pregnancy, this is (the fetus) that stirs. If, three months before the cessation of menstruation, there was uterine bleeding, this is coagulated blood (rather than pregnancy). The cause of incessant bleeding is persistent concretion. This concretion requires precipitation. The appropriate (formula) is *Gui Zhi Fu Ling Wan* (Cinnamon Twig & Poria Pills).[7]

---

5   In old China, physicians were almost exclusively males, and males were not allowed to have any form of physical contact with a woman. Therefore, during examination when palpation was necessary, the attending physician had to have a woman do the palpating.

6   This formula is composed of Radix Ligustici Wallichii (*Chuan Xiong*), Gelatinum Corii Asini (*E Jiao*), Radix Glycyrrhizae (*Gan Cao*), Folium Artemisiae Argyii (*Ai Ye*), Radix Angelicae Sinensis (*Dang Gui*), Radix Rehmanniae (*Di Huang*), Radix Paeoniae Lactiflorae (*Shao Yao*), and wine.

7   The ingredients in this formula are Ramulus Cinnamomi Cassiae (*Gui Zhi*), Sclerotium Poriae Cocos (*Fu Ling*), Cortex Radicis Moutan (*Dan Pi*), Semen Pruni Persicae (*Tao Ren*), and Radix Paeoniae Lactiflorae (*Shao Yao*).

(The Yellow Emperor) asked:

Suppose a woman has a disease of cessation of menstruation for one or two months. Contrarily, menstruation comes again. Now the pulse is faint and choppy. What (kind of problem) is this?

The master answered:

In the month prior (to the cessation of menstruation), there should have been diarrhea. (Diarrhea) interfered with the menses. After the diarrhea is checked, menstruation will come by itself. There is no pregnancy involved.

Suppose a woman has absence of menses and has conceived a body (*i.e.*, is pregnant). If the pulse is bowstring, there is a fear that there will be profuse vaginal bleeding and the (fetus) cannot take shape.

Suppose a woman has conceived a body for seven months, yet she is still not certain of it. If there is frequent nose bleeding accompanied by cramps, this is pregnancy. If nose bleeding is accompanied by sneezing and a stirring (sensation in the abdomen), this is not pregnancy.

If the pulse arrives forcefully but retreats feebly, this points to an anomaly. It may lead to the assumption that there is a fetus. And (the menses is really) at a stop. This is a result of existence of yin with absence of yang.

A woman had her menstruation every month, even though it was scanty. You, Master, examined the pulse but contrarily declared that there was a fetus. Later, (your words) proved true. What kind of pulse was it? And how to identify it?

The master answered:

The *cun* opening pulse was level (*i.e.*, peaceful or normal) both at the yin and at the yang (*i.e.*, the *cun* and *chi*). The constructive and defensive were in harmony. (The pulse) was slippery in the deep level and less so in the superficial. Either the *yang ming* or the *shao yin* (pulse) was compatible to the (relevant) channel. However, there were cold shivering as after a soaking, no desire for food or drink, headache, upset heart, and retching with desire to vomit. With breathing out, (the pulse) was slightly rapid, but, with breathing in, (the pulse) was not disconcerted. When yang is abundant, qi will spill.[8] What the yin slipperiness suggested was qi exuberance.[9] In the presence of the slippery (pulse quality), there is usually repletion which is the result of (abundant) nourishment by the six channels. The reason why (the menses) appeared monthly was that, after yin met with yang essence, the condensed juice might be ruptured with the placenta.[10] This rupture might lead to reduction or miscarriage. Suppose yang had been (very) exuberant, there might have developed two fetuses. (However, in this case,) yang was not (so) exuberant and there appeared incited menstruation (ji jing).[11]

For pregnant women who suffer from difficult urination with normal food intake, *Dang Gui Bei Mu Ku Shen Wan* (Dang Gui, Fritillaria & Sophora Pills)[12] is the ruling formula.

For pregnant women who, taken with water qi, suffer from generalized heaviness, inhibited urination, quivering with cold as after a soaking, and dizziness occurring on attempt to rise, *Kui Zi Fu Ling San* (Malva Seed & Poria Powder)[13] is the ruling formula.

For a pregnant woman, it is appropriate to take *Dang Gui San* (Dang Gui Powder)[14] since this will bring to pass a smooth delivery without any trouble.

The master said:

Suppose a woman comes for an examination complaining of cessation of menstruation.

---

[8] This passage implies that, in the initial stages of pregnancy, yin blood gathers below to nourish the fetus, while yang becomes exuberant, and that this exuberant yang qi surges upward. This upsurging yang qi may provoke the liver qi to offend the stomach qi, thus giving rise to the disorders described in the text. This, however, is normal.

[9] A free translation of this section would read as follows: When the pulse feels slippery at the yin or the deep level, there is exuberance...

[10] Condensed juice means the fetus.

[11] This refers to monthly scanty uterine bleeding in pregnancy. This is an unusual but harmless phenomenon.

[12] This formula is composed of Radix Angelicae Sinensis (*Dang Gui*), Radix Sophorae Flavescentis (*Ku Shen*), and Bulbus Fritillariae Cirrhosae (*Chuan Bei Mu*). For male patients, add Talcum (*Hua Shi*).

[13] The ingredients in this formula include Semen Malvae Verticillatae (*Dong Kui Zi*) and Sclerotium Poriae Cocos (*Fu Ling*).

[14] This formula is composed of Radix Angelicae Sinensis (*Dang Gui*), Radix Scutellariae Baicalensis (*Huang Qin*), Radix Paeoniae Lactiflorae (*Shao Yao*), Rhizoma Atractylodis Macrocephalae (*Bai Zhu*), and Radix Ligustici Wallichii (*Chuan Xiong*).

The master explained:

(Cessation of menstruation) for one month is due to coagulated blood. (Cessation of menstruation) for two months is due to blood (aspect disease. Cessation of menstruation) for three months is respited menstruation. Whether there is a fetus developing or (merely) blood accumulating, this is likened to a hen incubating an egg. Heat is the producer (of a fetus), while cold usually leads to turbidity (of the egg). Moreover, this also depends on whether the menses will come again the next month. The menstrual period should be figured out. Suppose it begins on the seventh day of the month. Then one may bid (the woman) not to come for an answer till around the tenth day of the next month. Suppose (menstrual flow or, practically speaking, vaginal bleeding) comes again. One should examine the pulse. If the pulse is contrarily deep and choppy and if it is ascertained that (the woman) has had miscarriage in the past or dribbling uterine bleeding causing blood collapse, then pregnancy can be diagnosed. If the woman confirms it, it is necessary to (take precautions to) protect (the fetus). Since the channels are faint and weak, there is a fear that (the fetus) will be restless. Then what should be done about (such a case)? It is necessary to compose an (appropriate) formula to treat it.

The master said:

A woman came for an examination saying that her menstruation had ceased and that this had occurred recently.

The master explained:

(Cessation of menstruation) for one month is blood block. (Cessation of menstruation) for two months may or may not point to (pregnancy. Cessation of menstruation) for three months is blood accumulation.

(A woman having conceived a child) is like a hen incubating an egg. If it gets cold, (the egg) becomes turbid, but if it obtains heat, (the egg) will produce a fetus. In order to keep the fetus alive, one should treat the mother. Cold contained in pregnancy will make the (new) life short. This is likened to the hen incubating an egg. Take a hen. If one plucks off all her feathers, then she can no longer cover over (the egg). Getting cold, (the egg) becomes turbid.

Now the lady had a fetus, but she suffered from cold in the lower abdomen and counterflow frigidity of the palms. Then how could she have a fetus (develop)? Subsequently the lady asked what to do. The master said that it was necessary to administer *Wen Jing Tang* (Warm the Channels Decoction).[15]

Suppose the lady came along with a relative of her husband. Then she would have had a fetus (*i.e.*, be pregnant). If she came with a relative of her parents, she would say nothing but of abundant cold and would not have a fetus even though (her menses had ceased) for a long time.

The master explained:

Suppose a woman comes for an examination, saying that her yin and yang are both harmonious. (However, the pulse) qi is long in the yang (*i.e.*, the *cun*) and short in the yin (*i.e.*, the *chi*), emerging all the time without submerging,[16] retreating forcefully but arriving feebly. Therefore, this points to an anomaly, (possibly) leading to a diagnosis of pregnancy. It so happens that she has menstrual stoppage which occurred only a few days ago. If (pregnancy) is certain, (the physician) should pronounce that it is necessary to treat without delay for fear that menstrual flow will resume. Suppose the woman is a palace lady[17] or a widow. She may have had dreams of sexual intercourse with an evil qi during sleep or have harbored oppressed emotions for a long time. Consequently, concretions and conglomerations have developed requiring immediate treatment through precipitation by means of administering two decoctions.[18] If no cure is effected, (the physician) may declare that the *Fa Tang* (Hair Decoction)[19] will strike (the disease). If thetreatment of precipitation fails to precipitate the (false) fetus, then what kind of spiritual evil is this?[20] One may read the red bird.[21]

---

[15] This formula is composed of Radix Ligustici Wallichii (*Chuan Xiong*), Radix Angelicae Sinensis (*Dang Gui*), Radix Paeoniae Lactiflorae (*Shao Yao*), Ramulus Cinnamomi Cassiae (*Gui Zhi*), Cortex Radicis Moutan (*Dan Pi*), Gelatinum Corii Asini (*E Jiao*), Radix Panacis Ginseng (*Ren Shen*), Rhizoma Zingiberis (*Jiang*), Rhizoma Pinelliae Ternatae (*Ban Xia*), Fructus Evodiae Rutecarpae (*Wu Zhu Yu*), and Tuber Ophiopogonis Japonici (*Mai Dong*).

[16] This is a description of a floating pulse image.

[17] One should note that in feudal China, the majority of palace ladies were virgins. They rarely if ever had the chance to come into contact with males.

[18] The translator has not been able to identify these two decoctions.

[19] The translator has not been able to identify the so-called Hair Decoction.

[20] This passage may also be interpreted in another way: Then what does this mean?

[21] This was an imaginary divine bird which was capable of telling fortunes. Therefore, this passage implies that life hangs in the balance.

The master explained:

If the palace lady Zhang has not recovered and comes to ask [The humble subject (Lin) Yi and his fellows find that lacunae here make the text dangling. With no other versions at hand to cross-reference, (we can only) show our suspicions of lacunae here. Similarly hereinafter.]

The master explained:

Suppose, on examination of a woman, her pulse is found to be level (*i.e.*, peaceful or normal. Only) it is small and weak in the yin (*i.e.*, the *chi*). The woman suffers from thirst, inability to take in food, but no cold or heat. This can be diagnosed as pregnancy. The ruling formula is *Gui Zhi Tang* (Cinnamon Twig Decoction). Sixty days later, there should appear (a pulse) typical of pregnancy. Suppose a physician gives an erroneous treatment, and one month later (the woman) therefore suffers from vomiting and diarrhea in addition. Then one should not administer *Gui Zhi Tang* (Cinnamon Twig Decoction). The formula is contained in the *Shang Han (Lun) ([Treatise on] Cold Damage)*.

A level (*i.e.*, peaceful) yet vacuous pulse in a woman is normal while breast-feeding. A level (*i.e.*, peaceful, normal) yet slightly replete pulse is normal after pregnancy (in breast-feeding). Suppose the pulse is contrarily faint and choppy. If the woman does not suffer from blood collapse or diarrhea but the pulse contrarily becomes (even) more vacuous, this is a result of simultaneously breast-feeding a baby and feeding a fetus. This is a normal pulse. (However, one should be careful) not to make the woman too vacuous and exhausted. This condition is like blood collapse and vacuity. It is invariably accompanied by dizziness and shortness of breath.

The master explained:

Suppose a woman likes to dress up when she comes for examination. If her pulse feels choppy; she should accordingly be asked whether she is breast-feeding or suffers from diarrhea. These conditions should present such a pulse. So should miscarriage or dribbling uterine bleeding. If there is no such disorder, then the menses should have been absent for three to six months. Given breast-feeding or dribbling uterine bleeding, a succeeding pregnancy (while still breast-feeding) is possible. (In that case, bid her) to wean the baby from the breast, wait for the diarrhea to stop, and then come for confirmation (of pregnancy). One should (then) examine the pulse.

The master explained:

Suppose the *cun* opening pulse is faint and slow, fainter in the *chi* than in the *cun*. A slow pulse in the *cun* points to cold lying in the upper burner. This requires ejection. Now, (however,) the pulse is vacuous in the *chi*. If one employs forced (*i.e.,* wrongful) precipitation, this will give rise to chest fullness and pain and ejection of blood will invariably arise. If lower abdominal pain and pain in the lumbar spine arise, there will invariably be hemafecia.

The master explained:

If the *cun* opening pulse is faint and weak, there is vacuity of both the qi and blood. There may be hemafecia, retching and vomiting, or sweating (with such a pulse). If there are no (such disorders,) the instep pulse will be faint and weak. In spring, since the stomach qi is the root, vomiting and diarrhea may present (such a pulse). If there is no (vomiting and diarrhea,) there is water qi, and (thus) there is (also) invariably abdominal distention and difficult urination.

Suppose a woman suffers from frequent retching and vomiting or frequent dyspnea. She has menstrual block. Even though her menses resume, their quantity must be scant.

The master explained:

There is a woman aged sixty or so who often menstruates. Suppose she is taken with an enduring disease of diarrhea. If there is lower abdominal tightness and fullness, (she) is difficult to treat.

The master said:

Suppose a woman comes for examination complaining that her menstrual flow is less than before (in quantity). What is the cause?

The master explained:

Diarrhea, sweating, or disinhibited urination may cause (such a condition). Why?

The master explained:

Loss of fluids makes menses decrease. If, on the contrary, there is more menstrual flow than before, there should be some (other) afflictions, say, difficult defecation and absence of sweat.

The master explained:

Suppose the *cun* opening pulse is deep and slow. In the presence of the deepness, there is water, and, in the presence of the slowness, there is cold. Since cold and water act upon one another, the instep pulse is hidden and there is inability to transform water and grain. When the spleen qi is debilitated, there is duck-stool (diarrhea). When the stomach qi is debilitated, there is generalized swelling. If the *shao yang* pulse (*i.e*, the pulse at *He Liao*, TB 22) is abject, while the *shao yin* pulse (*i.e.*, the pulse at *Tai Xi*, Ki 3) is thin, there will be inhibited urination in males and menstrual block in females. The menses are blood. When blood is inhibited, it gives rise to water (disease). This is known as blood aspect (disease) [water aspect in another version].

The master explained:

Suppose the *cun* opening pulse is deep and rapid. The rapidity is the same as emerging, while the deepness is submerging.[22] Emerging means yang repletion, while submerging means bound yin. The instep pulse is faint and bowstring. In the presence of the faintness, there is absence of stomach qi, and, in the presence of the bowstring, there is gasping for breath. The *shao yin* pulse is deep and slippery. In the presence of the deepness, there are internal (evils), and, in the presence of the slipperiness, there is repletion. The deepness and the slipperiness combine to show that blood is bound in the uterine gate. The viscera are no longer able to drain, and the channels and their vessel networks are blocked. This is known as blood aspect (disease).

(The Yellow Emperor) asked:

There is blood aspect disease. What is this?

The master answered:

Cessation of menstruation preceding water disease is called blood aspect (disease). This disease is difficult to treat.

(The Yellow Emperor) asked:

There is water aspect disease. What is it?

The master answered:

Water disease preceding cessation of menstruation is called water aspect (disease). This disease is easy to treat. Why? When water is removed, the menses will resume by themselves.

---

[22] See note 5, Book 1, Ch.3. One should note that submerging, which is yin, is an equivalent to internal, while emerging, which is yang, implies external.

Suppose the pulse is soggy and weak, weak contrarily in the *guan* and soggy contrarily in the upper (*i.e.*, the *cun*). The pulse is also slow in the upper (*i.e.*, the *cun*) and tight in the lower (*i.e.*, the *chi*). In the presence of the slowness, there is cold which results in what is called muddiness.[23] When yang is turbid, dampness arises which results in what is called fog.[24] In the presence of the tightness, there is yin qi (*i.e.*, exuberance giving rise to) shuddering. Since the pulse is soggy and weak, the sogginess points to dampness in the center, and the weakness to cold in the center. Cold and dampness act upon one another, resulting in what is called *bi*. Tormenting pain and aching of the joints of the lumbar spine and insensitivity of the muscles are the characteristics of *bi*. This may be contrarily determined as pregnancy because of retarded menstrual flow. Generalized heaviness, puffy, swollen lower legs and feet whose (surface) allows the fingers to sink in, and cold and insensitivity of the lumbus, these are the characteristics of pregnancy of water. Having to lean against something to facilitate breathing once dyspnea arises, urinary block, a tight pulse showing retching, and no surplus (*i.e.*, insufficiency) of blood and qi, these are ascribed to the water phase. (In water phase disease,) the constructive and defensive are in conflict and collapsing. This is not pregnancy.

---

[23] This section implies that, when the pulse is slow in the *chi*, there is cold. Cold brings damage to yang qi. If yang qi is damaged, qi and blood become static. The author refers to static as muddy.

[24] When cold yang qi becomes turbid or static, it is no longer able to move water. Consequently, water gathers and develops into damp disease.

_________Chapter Three_________

A Discussion of the Various Postpartum Diseases (Including) Faintness & Dizziness, Wind Stroke, Fever, Vexation, Retching & Diarrhea

(The Yellow Emperor) asked:

There are three (common) diseases in newly birthed women. The first is the illness of tetany, the second is faintness and dizziness, and the third is difficult defecation. How do they arise? The master answered:

Newly birthed (women) have blood collapse and vacuity and copious perspiration and are subject to wind stroke. Therefore, the disease of tetany is produced.

How does faintness and dizziness arise?

The master explained:

Blood collapse followed by sweating and abundant cold is the cause of faintness and dizziness.

How does difficult defecation arise?

The master explained:

Collapse of fluids resulting in dryness in the stomach makes defecation difficult. The reason why birthing women are faint and dizzy with a faint, weak pulse, suffer from retching, are unable to take in food, and have hard stools and sweating confined to the head is blood vacuity and inversion. Inversion is invariably accompanied by (faintness and) dizziness. When a sick person suffering from (faintness and) dizziness tends towards a resolution, there is invariably copious perspiration. With blood vacuity and inversion (frigidity of) the lower limbs, solitary yang strays upward. As a result sweat exits only on the head. The tendency of birthing women to perspire is due to collapse of yin with blood vacuity and exuberance of solitary yang. Therefore, only when sweat exits can yin and yang be restored to normal. Hard stool is due to retching and inability to take in food. (In this case,) *Xiao Chai Hu Tang* (Minor Bupleurum Decoction) is the ruling formula. If fever recurs seven or eight days after the (above) diseases are resolved and ability to take in food is restored, this shows that there is stomach heat and qi repletion. (For this,) *Cheng Qi Tang* (Support the Qi Decoction) is the ruling formula. This formula is contained in the *Shang Han (Lun) ([Treatise on]) Cold Damage*.

If a woman is hit by wind during labor, (wind evils) may remain unresolved for tens of days, giving rise to slight headache, aversion to cold, occasional fever, tightness below the heart, dry retching, and (spontaneous) sweating. Even though (the disease) has persisted for a long time, so long as the manifestations indicating *Yang Dan* (Yang Dawn) stay, one may administer Yang Dawn. This formula is contained in the *Shang Han (Lun) ([Treatise on] Cold Damage)*. (Yang Dawn) is nothing but *Gui Zhi Tang* (Cinnamon Twig Decoction).

If a woman who is taken with postpartum wind stroke suffers from fever, a full red facial complexion, dyspnea, and headache, *Zhu Ye Tang* (Bamboo Leaf Decoction) is the ruling formula.

If a woman suffers from postpartum continual dull pain in the abdomen, one may administer *Dang Gui Yang Rou Tang* (Dang Gui & Mutton Decoction).[1]

The master explained:

For a birthing woman who suffers from abdominal pain, vexation, fullness, and insomnia, *Zhi Shi Shao Yao San* (Immature Aurantium & Peony Powder)[2] should be the ruling formula. If it fails to bring about a cure, there is dried blood fixed to the region below the umbilicus inside the abdomen. (In this case,) one may administer *Xia Yu Xue Tang* (Precipitate Static Blood Decoction).[3]

Seven or eight days after delivery, if a woman not displaying a *tai yang* disease suffers from lower abdominal tightness and pain, this is due to persistent flow of lochia. If there has been no defecation for four or five days, the instep pulse is slightly replete, and the woman suffers from worse fever, vexation, and agitation in the late afternoon, cure may be effected by disinhibition if there is inability to take in food and delirious speech. The appropriate formula is *Cheng Qi Tang* (Support the Qi Decoction). The reason (for this treatment) is that there is internal binding in the urinary bladder. The formula is contained in the *Shang Han (Lun) ([Treatise on] Cold Damage)*.

If, during labor, the woman suffers from vexation, restlessness, and counterflow retching, (it is necessary to) calm the center and boost the qi. The ruling formula is *Zhu Pi Da Wan* (Bamboo Peel Big Pills).[4]

For women who suffer from heat diarrhea, pressure in the rectum, and postpartum excessive vacuity, *Bai Tou Weng Jia Gan Cao Tang* (Pulsatilla with Added Licorice Decoction)[5] is the ruling formula.

---

[1] This formula is composed of Radix Angelicae Sinensis (*Dang Gui*), Mutton (*Yang Rou*), Radix Astragali Membranacei (*Huang Qi*), Radix Panacis Ginseng (*Ren Shen*), and Rhizoma Zingiberis (*Jiang*).

[2] The ingredients in this formula are Fructus Immaturus Aurantii (*Zhi Shi*) and Radix Paeoniae Lactiflorae (*Shao Yao*).

[3] This formula is composed of Radix Et Rhizoma Rhei (*Da Huang*), Semen Pruni Persicae (*Tao Ren*), and Eupolyphaga Seu Opisthoplatia (*Zhe Chong*).

[4] This formula is composed of Caulis Bambusae In Taeniis (*Zhu Ru*), Gypsum (*Shi Gao*), Radix Cynanchi Atrati (*Bai Wei*), Ramulus Cinnamomi Cassiae (*Gui Zhi*), Radix Glycyrrhizae (*Gan Cao*), and Fructus Zizyphi Jujubae (*Da Zao*).

[5] This formula is composed of Radix Pulsatillae Sinensis (*Bai Tou Weng*), Radix Glycyrrhizae (*Gan Cao*), Cortex Phellodendri (*Huang Bai*), Rhizoma Coptidis Chinensis (*Huang Lian*), and Cortex Fraxini (*Qin Pi*).

A Discussion of the *Dai Xia* Diseases, Sterilization,[1] Infertility, Blood Collapse & Respited Menses

The master explained:

In connection with the women's diseases of vaginal discharge and the six extremes (*liu ji*),[2] a floating pulse points to rumbling in the intestines and abdominal fullness, a tight pulse to abdominal pain, a rapid pulse to itching inside the genitals, a surging pulse to growth of sores, and a bowstring pulse to contracting pain in the genitals.

The master explained:

There are three categories of vaginal discharge. The first is known as uterine gate, the second as dragon gate, and the third as jade gate.[3] In (a woman) who has given birth, (vaginal discharge) is classified as uterine gate. In (a married woman) who has not given birth, it is classified as dragon gate. In an unmarried woman, it is classified as jade gate.

(The Yellow Emperor) asked:

There are three (common) kinds of diseases in unmarried women. What are they?

The master answered:

The first disease is heat in the genitals at the beginning of menstruation. This is caused by being caught in a draft or being fanned (during menstruation). The second disease is due to washing

---

1. Literally, the Chinese for this term is cutting off of birth or expiring of the capability of reproduction. In modern English, sterilization implies a surgical procedure which this term does not imply here.

2. The six extremes refer to severe vacuity detriment and taxation damage of the qi, blood, sinews, bones, muscles, and essence.

3. Of the three gates, the last two are usually the same in most cases, *i.e.*, the vaginal meatus. But in this context, the classification of three gates is intended to show the degree of depth of the evils. The uterine gate is the deepest, the jade gate the least deep, and the dragon gate lies in-between.

in cold water (during menstruation). The third disease is discharging cinnabar (*i.e.*, a red colored fluid discharge). This disease is produced by fright and falls within the category of vaginal discharge.

The master explained:

Vaginal discharge in women is among the troubles of the nine repletions.[4] When accompanied by the disease of rat's breast (*shu ru*), (vaginal discharge) may easily become worse. This exacerbation happens on a certain date. The date is the *geng* or *xin* day. In connection with other (illnesses), the date can be inferred in the same way.

(The Yellow Emperor) asked:

There is a woman aged fifty or so who complains of a tormenting pain in the back all the time, abdominal pain from time to time, low food intake, constantly feeling fed up, and frequent abdominal distention. Her pulse is faint in the yang (*i.e.*, the *cun*) and small and tight in the *guan* and *chi*. There is incongruity between the form and the pulse. I would like to hear what you would say about this.

The master answered:

It is necessary (first) to inquire about what the sick person feels about food and drink. If the sick person says, "I have no desire for food and drink and have a foul smell of grain qi," the disease lies in the upper burner. If the sick person says, "I have more or less a desire for food and drink, but it is (also) alright if I have nothing to take in," then the disease lies in the middle burner. If the sick person says, "I have normal food intake as before," then the disease lies in the lower burner. The (last) disease belongs to the category of *dai xia*[5] and should be treated as such.

---

4 The translator suspects that the nine repletions are nine kinds of pain which include: pain in the genitals due to injury, strangury with pain, pain on urination, abdominal cold pain, abdominal pain in menstruation, abdominal qi fullness with pain, vaginal discharge and pain, pain in the lateral costal skin, and pain in the lumbus.

5 One should note that, at the time this book was compiled, the term *dai xia* meant not only abnormal vaginal discharge but also other conditions in women occurring "below the belt." Thus this term was used as a synonym for gynecological diseases in general, including but not necessarily limited to, abnormal vaginal discharge..

For women who suffer from vaginal discharge, inhibited menstrual flow, lower abdominal fullness and pain, and menstruation appearing twice in a month, *Tu Gua Gen San* (Trichosanthes Root Powder)[6] is the ruling formula.

If a woman with vaginal discharge has a floating pulse, aversion to cold, and dribbling uterine bleeding, there is no cure.

The master explained:

Once a woman brought with her a girl of fifteen years for an examination, saying that the girl began her menses at the age of fourteen but now it had strangely stopped. The mother expressed fear and worry. The master asked, "Is this girl your Lady's own daughter? If so, I'll go on." The lady replied, "Yes, she is." The master continued, "When I raised the question, I meant nothing special. You, Lady, also began to have your menses at the age of fourteen. Right? Therefore, I decide (your daughter's) cessation of menstruation is (nothing but) annual evasion.[7] Do not worry. Her menstruation will come again by itself."

Suppose a woman suffers from cold in the lower abdomen and enduring aversion to cold. If this is contracted at a young age, it will cause infertility. If it occurs at an older age, it will cause sterilization.

The master explained:

Suppose the pulse is not only faint and weak but choppy. If this pulse appears at a young age, it is an indication of infertility. If it appears during middle age, it is an indication of sterilization.

The master explained:

Suppose the *shao yin* pulse is floating and tight. In the presence of the tightness, there are *shan* conglomeration, abdominal pain, miscarriage, and injury due to falling, and, in the presence of the floating, there is blood collapse, sterilization, and aversion to cold.

---

6   This formula is composed of Radix Trichosanthis Cucumeroidis (*Tu Gua Gen*), Radix Paeoniae Lactiflorae (*Shao Yao*), Ramulus Cinnamomi Cassiae (*Gui Zhi*), and Eupolyphaga Seu Opisthoplatia (*Zhe Chong*).

7   Annual evasion is menstruation that appears only once in a year. Though rarely seen, this is not pathologic. Its key distinguishing feature from menstrual block or amenorrhea is that the menses do come at the same time every year cyclically.

The master explained:

If a fat person has a thin pulse, there is cold in the uterus. As a result, (she) has few (if any) children. If the facial complexion is yellow, there is cold in the chest.

If a woman suffers from a lower abdominal gripping, rolling pain which is relieved by itself but attacks unpredictably, and, if cessation of menstruation and hard binding in the urinary bladder with hypertonicity radiating down to the genitals and Qi Thoroughfare (*i.e.,* the groins) arise, in due time, hypertonicity will inevitably develop in the lateral costal regions.

(The Yellow Emperor) asked:

Suppose a woman of fifty years or so suffers from the disease of diarrhea [hemafecia is suspected instead] which has persisted for tens of days without a break. She has fever in the evening, lower abdominal urgency and pain, abdominal fullness, heat in the palms, and a dry mouth and lips. Then what kind of disease is this?

The master answered:

This disease falls within the category of *dai xia* (*i.e.,* gynecological disease).

What is its cause?

There has been miscarriage and, (consequently,) blood stasis is lingering in the lower abdomen.

Then what is the indication (of this blood stasis)?

The sign of dry mouth and lips is its revelation. (To treat this case,) it is necessary to administer *Wen Jing Tang* (Warm the Channels Decoction).

(The Yellow Emperor) asked:

Why does the menstrual flow stop when a woman is taken with the disease of diarrhea?

The master answered:

Only if diarrhea is checked will the menstrual flow come back by itself. There is no need to worry. The menstrual flow ought to stop as long as diarrhea does not stop because diarrhea depletes fluids. When the diarrhea stops, fluids will be restored and the menstrual flow will come by itself.

If a woman suffers from hemafecia and a dry throat but there is no thirst, her menses must be at a stop. This is due to insufficiency of the constructive. Since there is slight cold, there is no (desire) to drink. When the sick person is thirsty and drinks, then fluids will be freed, the constructive and defensive will become harmonious by themselves, and the menstruation will certainly be restored.

The master explained:

Suppose the *cun* opening pulse is faint and choppy. In the presence of the faintness, there is an insufficiency of the defensive qi. In the presence of the choppiness, there is no surplus (*i.e.*, there is a lack) of blood and qi. Insufficient defensive (qi) leads to shortness of breath and dry form. Insufficient blood leads to abnormality of the form. Vacuity of both the constructive and defensive produces confused speech. The instep pulse is floating and choppy. In the presence of the choppiness, there is a vacuity of the stomach qi. Vacuity (of the stomach qi) results in shortness of breath, a dry throat, and a bitter taste in the mouth. The choppy (*i.e.*, vacuous) stomach qi means loss of fluids (in the stomach). The *shao yin* pulse is faint and slow. In the presence of the faintness, there is absence of essence. In the presence of the slowness there is cold in the genitals. In the presence of the choppiness, blood is kept from coming. Then there is respited menses. (This means) a menstrual flow which comes every three months.

The master explained:

If the pulse is faint, there is a vacuity of both blood and qi. A young woman will suffer from blood collapse. Breast-feeding or diarrhea may present such a pulse. Otherwise, this shows respited menses, (or, in other words,) menstrual flow coming every three months.

(The Yellow Emperor) asked:

A woman had (allegedly) been pregnant for three months. After examination of her pulse, the master determined that this woman was not pregnant and that that very month she would have her menses. Then what kind of pulse was hers and how to identify it?

The master answered:

The *cun* opening pulse was floating and large at the defensive (*i.e.*, the superficial level) but weak contrarily at the constructive (*i.e.*, the deep level). In the presence of the floating and largeness, there is strong qi (*i.e.*, yang), and, in the presence of the weakness, there is diminished blood.

Solitary yang kept exhaling, while yin was unable to inhale.[8] The two qi were not in concord. The defensive was downborne, while the constructive was exhausted. Yin was turning into accumulated cold and yang into accumulated heat. Yang exuberance made moisture nil. (The qi) of the channels and the vessel networks became insufficient. Yin was vacuous, while yang went unrestrained. As a result, shortness of blood arose. (Therefore,) there was cold shuddering as after a soaking, a dry throat, and (spontaneous) sweating or frequent voiding of thick urine and frequent spitting of foamy substance. This added to vacuity (of yin) and (deteriorated into) leaking and draining of fluids. All this showed lack of pregnancy. If (blood) accumulates and is propagated to fill the ditches (on time), the menstrual flow will come once a month. (A menstrual flow) which comes once every three months is due to (blood) not draining till yin becomes exuberant. This is called respited menses.

(The Yellow Emperor) asked:

Suppose a woman aged fifty years or so one day suddenly begins to clear blood and (the uterine bleeding) runs for two or three days on end. Then how can one treat her?

The master answered:

This woman is infertile and has had no menstruation (for a certain period of time). Now blood is contrarily cleared. This is respited menses. It does not need treatment. It will come to a stop of itself. If she usually had a menstrual period of five days, then she will recover in five days.

Suppose a woman has menstrual flow twice a month. During menstruation, her pulse has been normal. If now, on the contrary, her pulse is faint and there is no diarrhea or sweating, she must have menses the next month.

---

[8] This sentence implies that solitary yang qi is exuberant and continues outwards, while yin blood is unable to penetrate internally.

_______________Chapter Five_______________
A Discussion of Faintness & Dizziness,
the Five Categories of Flooding & Leaking,
Menstrual Block, Inhibited Menses,
& Various Abdominal Diseases

(The Yellow Emperor) asked:

If a woman happens to fall ill in the course of menstruation and is treated with diaphoresis, then she may suffer from faintness and dizziness with an inability to recognize people. What is the reason?

The master answered:

During the menstrual flow, the internal becomes vacuous. If sweating is promoted, the exterior may become vacuous in addition. This is vacuity of both the exterior and interior. Thus faintness and dizziness result.

(The Yellow Emperor) asked:

A woman had a disease like epilepsy. There were more than twenty attacks of faintness and dizziness in a day. You, Master, examined her pulse and contrarily determined it to be a case of *dai xia* (*i.e.*, a gynecological disease), and your words proved true. What kind of pulse was it? And how to identify it?

The master answered:

The *cun* opening pulse was soggy and tight. In the presence of the sogginess, yang qi was faint, and, in the presence of the tightness, there was cold in the constructive (*i.e.*, the blood). Faint yang meant vacuity of the defensive qi. Blood was exhausted and congealed by the cold. Since yin and yang were not in harmony, the evil qi lodged in the constructive and defensive. This trouble starts at a young age. If one is engaged in sexual intercourse in the course of menstruation and continues this for a long time and beyond measure, essence will be so stirred that it forces the life gate open. Then the menses are discharged so (massively) that blood becomes vacuous and the hundreds of vessels are lax. At the Central Pole (*i.e.*, somewhere around *Zhong Ji*, CV 3), yang is felt stirring, and the slightest waft of breeze will evoke a cold (feeling). Taking advantage of vacuity, cold lodges in the constructive and defensive and accumulates in the Cinnabar Field (*i.e.*, the lower abdomen). It starts up, surging upward, trespassing in the chest and diaphragm. (As a result,) fluid regurgitation and swallowing, gushing and spilling drool, inversion-like dizziness, and heat in the Qi Thoroughfare (*i.e.*, groins) and the upper thigh arise. An inferior physician may diagnose this as epilepsy and (accordingly) treat with moxibustion. In consequence, (the condition) will be greatly exacerbated.

(The Yellow Emperor) asked:

A woman had a disease of tormenting qi surging up into the chest with dizziness, foamy drool, and heat in the upper thigh and qi thoroughfare. After examining her pulse, you, Master, diagnosed it to be not *dai xia* (*i.e.*, not a gynecological disease). What kind of pulse was hers, and how to identify it?

The master answered:

The *cun* opening pulse was deep and faint. In the presence of the deepness, the defensive qi was hidden, and, in the presence of the faintness, the constructive qi had expired. Hidden yang resulted in febrile disease, and expired yin meant blood collapse. The disease ought to have included inhibited urination and blocked fluids. Now, on the contrary, urination was uninhibited and there was slight sweating. (In that case,) it was cold that was revealed by the deep (pulse quality). Counterflow cough and retching of foamy substances showed that the lungs had become atonic. Fluids were exhausted and scanty. Blood collapse damaged the channels and the vessel works. From cold developed blood inversion,[1] giving rise to tormenting insensitivity of the hands and feet. Qi started from the Cinnabar Field, surging upward into the chest and the lateral costal region. Deep cold was accumulated and depressed above. There was suffocation and congestion in the chest. This qi visited the yang portions, tinging the face with a red color as in intoxication. The formal body seemed to be fat, but this was vacuity puffiness. The (attending) physician, however, treated (her) with precipitation and used a long needle so as to add to the vacuity of the constructive and defensive. In due time, dizziness arose. For (all these) reasons, (I) arrived at the diagnosis of blood inversion.

(The Yellow Emperor) asked:

---

[1] *I.e.*, inversion due to blood vacuity.

What are the five categories of flooding like?

The master answered:

White flooding is like snivel. Red flooding is like crimson saliva. Yellow flooding is like mashed melon. Green-blue flooding is bluish. Black flooding is like coagulated blood.

The master explained:

Once a woman came for examination. Her pulse was faint and choppy. By reason, she should have been suffering from vomiting or diarrhea. However, she said not. Subsequently, (I) asked the lady her age. The lady was seven times seven (or, in other words,) forty-nine. (By this age,) the menses should have stopped but they continued up to then. It was this that accounted for her vacuity.

There is a *cun* opening pulse which is bowstring and large. It is modulated bowstring (compared with the pure bowstring pulse), and it is not so large as scallion-stalk (compared with the purely large pulse). The modulated (bowstring quality) points to cold, and the scallion-stalk (pulse) to vacuity. Because vacuity and cold act upon one another, the pulse becomes drumskin. (With such a pulse,) women will miscarry or have leaking (*i.e.*, dribbling uterine bleeding. For this,) *Xuan Fu Hua Tang* (Inula Decoction)[2] is the ruling formula.

For women who suffer from sunken channel[3] leaking which is black in color and which remains unresolved (for a long time), *Jiao Jiang Tang* (Gelatin & Ginger Decoction)[4] is the ruling formula. For women who suffer from inhibited menstrual flow, *Di Dang Tang* (Flushing Decoction) is the ruling formula. This formula is contained in the *Shang Han (Lun)* (*[Treatise on] Cold Damage*).

If a woman suffers from menstrual block or inhibited menses with persistent hard glomus in the viscus (*i.e.*, the uterus), this is due to dried blood. If what is discharged is white, *Fan Shi Wan* (Alumen Pills)[5] are the ruling formula.

---

[2] There are only two ingredients in this formula: Flos Inulae (*Xuan Fu Hua*) and Bulbus Allii Fistulosi (*Cong Bai*).

[3] This refers to channel qi sunken below leading to uterine bleeding.

[4] The translator suspects that this formula is the same as *Jiao Ai Tang* (Gelatin & Mugwort Decoction).

[5] This formula is composed of Alumen (*Fan Shi*) and Semen Pruni Armeniacae (*Xing Ren*).

For various kinds of abdominal pain in women, *Dang Gui Shao Yao San* (Dang Gui & Peony Powder)[6] is the ruling formula.

For abdominal pain in women, *Xiao Jian Zhong Tang* (Minor Fortify the Center Decoction) is the ruling formula. This formula is contained in the *Shang Han (Lun) ([Treatise on] Cold Damage)*.

____

[6] This formula is composed of Radix Angelicae Sinensis (*Dang Gui*), Radix Paeoniae Lactiflorae (*Shao Yao*), Radix Rehmanniae (*Di Huang*), Radix Panacis Ginseng (*Ren Shen*), Cortex Cinnamomi Cassiae (*Gui Xin*), Radix Glycyrrhizae (*Gan Cao*), Rhizoma Zingiberis (*Jiang*), and Fructus Zizyphi Jujubae (*Da Zao*).

_________________________Chapter Six_________________

A Discussion of the Diseases of a Sensation of Something Like Roasted Meat Stuck in the Throat, Susceptibility to Sorrow, Heat Penetrating the Blood Chamber & Abdominal Fullness

For women who suffer from a feeling of something like a piece of roasted meat stuck in the throat, *Ban Xia Hou Po Tang* (Pinellia & Magnolia Decoction)[1] is the ruling formula.

For visceral agitation in women characterized by susceptibility to sorrow, desire to cry, acting as if possessed by a spirit or ghost, and frequent yawning, *Gan Cao Xiao Mai Tang* (Licorice & Wheat Decoction)[2] is the ruling formula.

Suppose, in the course of menstruation, a woman is taken with wind stroke, (suffering from) fever and aversion to cold. On the seventh or eighth day of contraction, fever is eliminated and the

____

[1] This formula is composed of Rhizoma Pinelliae Ternatae (*Ban Xia*), Cortex Magnoliae Officinalis (*Hou Po*), Sclerotium Poriae Cocos (*Fu Ling*), Rhizome Zingiberis (*Jiang*), and Folium Perillae Frutescentis (*Su Ye*).

[2] This formula is composed of Radix Glycyrrhizae (*Gan Cao*), Fructus Tritici Aestivi (*Xiao Mai*), and Fructus Zizyphi Jujubae (*Da Zao*).

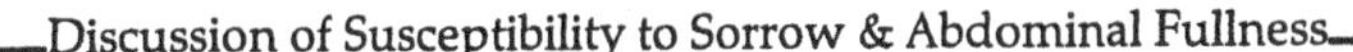

binding, and delirious speech. This is heat penetrating the blood chamber, requiring needling Cycle Gate (*Qi Men*, Liv 14), (supplementing or drainage) depending on vacuity or repletion.

Suppose, on the seventh or eighth day of wind stroke, the woman suffers again from cold and heat which gives attacks at regular intervals. If (now) her menstrual flow happens to come to a stop, this is heat penetrating the blood chamber. There must be binding in the blood that produces a malaria-like (disease) attacking at regular intervals. (For this,) *Xiao Chai Hu Tang* (Minor Bupleurum Decoction) is the ruling formula. This formula is contained in the *Shang Han (Lun)* (*[Treatise on] Cold Damage*).

If a woman happens to be taken with cold damage with fever in the course of menstruation and she is serene at day but raves at night as if seeing ghosts, this is heat penetrating the blood chamber. (To treat this,) one should avoid offending the stomach qi and the two upper burners, and then it will certainly heal by itself [the last three words challenge suspicion].

If a *yang ming* disease is accompanied by hemafecia and raving, this is heat penetrating the blood chamber. If there is sweat exiting only from the head, it is necessary to needle Cycle Gate (*Qi Men*, Liv 14), draining repletion. After moderate sweating has been promoted, a cure will ensue.

Suppose a woman suffers from fullness of the lower abdomen which looks like a ball with slightly difficult urination but no thirst. If this happens postpartum [this phrase challenges suspicion], this is water and blood bound together in the blood chamber. (For this case,) *Da Huang Gan Sui Tang* (Rhubarb & Kansui Decoction)[3] is the ruling formula.

---

[3] This formula is composed of Radix Et Rhizoma Rhei (*Da Huang*), Radix Euphorbiae Kansui (*Gan Sui*), and Gelatinum Corii Asini (*E Jiao*).

A Discussion of Cold in the Genitals, Shifted Bladder, Vaginal Flatulence, Genital Sores & Vaginal Protrusion

For cold genitals in women, warm the center with a suppository. The ruling formula is *She Chuang Zi San* (Cnidium Powder).[1]

If a woman has a suppository (inserted) to force the discharge of her menses, pain in the eye sockets, inability of the heels to touch on the ground, and (a sensation of) the heart as if being suspended will arise.

(The Yellow Emperor) asked:

Suppose a woman is ill but has normal food intake. There is vexation, fever, insomnia, and having to lean against something to facilitate breathing. What kind of disease is this?

The master answered:

This is the disease of shifted bladder (*zhuan bao*) giving rise to inability to void urine.

What causes it?

The master explained:

In the past, this woman had exuberant muscles with head erect and body full, but now, on the contrary, she is markedly emaciated, having an empty sensation in the center (of her head) when she raises her head. This disease is due to the entanglement and twisting of the bladder ligation. Mere disinhibition of urination will result in a cure. It is appropriate to administer *Shen Qi Wan* (Kidney Qi Pills) since there is Sclerotium Poriae Cocos (*Fu Ling*) in the pills. This formula is contained in "Vacuity Taxation" (see Bk. 8, Ch.7, present work).

The master explained:

---

[1]   This formula is composed of only one ingredient: Fructus Cnidii Monnieri (*She Chuang Zi*).

If the pulse is floating and tight, by reason, there should be generalized pain and aching. If there is not, then what supposition can be made about it? A hypothesis should be made in accordance with the complaints (given by the sick person). If there is intestinal pain, rumbling in the abdomen, and cough, this is due to failure to defecate (*i.e.*, constipation). If a woman has such a pulse, by reason, there should be genital flatulence.

The master explained:

Suppose the *cun* opening pulse is floating and weak. In the presence of the floating, there is vacuity, and, in presence of the weakness, there is absence of blood. In the presence of the floating, there is shortness of breath, and, in presence of the weakness, there is fever with spontaneous sweating. The instep pulse is floating and choppy. In the presence of the floating, there is qi fullness, and, in the presence of the choppiness, there is cold giving rise to frequent belching and acid regurgitation. Since (cold) qi descends, there is cold in the lower abdomen. The *shao yin* pulse is weak and faint. In the presence of the faintness, there is shortage of blood, and, in the presence of the weakness, wind (*i.e.*, flatulence) is generated. The faintness and the weakness combine revealing that the genitals are averse to cold, and the stomach qi is drained out from below, giving rise to boisterous vaginal flatulence.

The master explained:

If the stomach qi is drained from below with boisterous vaginal flatulence, this shows repletion of the grain qi. It should be conducted with *Gao Fa Jian* (Lard & Hair Infusion).[2]

If the *shao yin* pulse is slippery and rapid, sores grow in the genitals. If the *shao yin* pulse is rapid, there is qi strangury with sores in the genitals. If a woman has ulcerating sores in the genitals, wash the genitals with *Lang Yu Tang* (Potentilla Decoction).[3]

---

[2] This formula is composed of lard and human hair. The hair is boiled in the lard until it dissolves. It is divided into two doses which are taken two times each day.

[3] This formula is identified as Potentilla Decoction in *Chin Kuei Yao Lue, Prescriptions from the Golden Chamber* translated by Hong-yen Hsu & Su-yen Wang, Oriental Healing Arts Institute, Taiwan, 1983. However, Hong-yen Hsu's *Oriental Materia Medica: A Concise Guide*, Oriental Healing Arts Institute, Long Beach, CA, 1986, does not give *Lang Ya* as an alternative name for Potentilla Chinensis (*Fan Bai Cao*). Since Rhizoma Alocasiae Seu Euphorbiae Pallasii Seu Radix Stellerae (*Lang Du*) is used in contemporary Chinese formulas for vaginal sores, it is a good guess that this is the ingredient which comprises this formula.

If a woman suffers from a swollen viscus (*i.e.*, uterus) which becomes as large as a melon with genital pain initiating lumbago, *Xing Ren Tang* (Armeniaca Decoction)[4] is the ruling formula.

If the *shao yin* pulse is bowstring, it is certain that the white intestine (*i.e.*, the rectum) prolapses looking like a walnut.

Suppose the *shao yin* pulse is floating and stirring. In the presence of the floating, there is vacuity, and, in the presence of the stirring, there is pain. In women, there is vaginal protrusion.

---

[4] The translator has failed to identify this formula.

_________________Chapter Eight_________________
A Discussion of Life & Death (Signs) in Women's Diseases

Suppose a woman has downward leaking which is colored red and white, discharging several *sheng* of blood a day. If the pulse is urgent and racing, death is a certainty. If the pulse is slow, there is life (*i.e.*, hope of survival).

Suppose a woman has incessant red and white downward leaking. If the pulse is vacuous and slippery, there is life. If the pulse is large, tight, replete, and rapid, this is death.

When examining a newly birthed woman who is breast-feeding, there is life if the pulse is deep, small, and slippery, but death if the pulse is replete, large, hard, bowstring, and urgent.

Suppose a woman has *shan* conglomeration, accumulations and gatherings. If the pulse is bowstring and urgent, there is life. If the pulse is vacuous, weak, and small, this is death.

Suppose a newly birthed woman who is breast-feeding has a suspended, small pulse due to febrile disease. If the four limbs are warm, there is life. If the four limbs are cold and frigid, this is death.

Suppose, in the process of labor, a woman suffers from dyspnea with rales and shrugging of her shoulders to facilitate breathing due to wind stroke, cold damage, or febrile disease. If the pulse is replete, large, floating, and moderate, there is life. If the pulse is small and urgent, this is death.

When examining postpartum, if the woman has an inharmonious *cun* opening pulse which is spark-like and racing, this is death. If the pulse is deep, sticking nearly to the bone but not expiring, there is life.

Suppose there is an incised wound in the genitals with incessant bleeding. If the yin pulse fails to reach the yang,[1] this is death. If the (yin) pulse emerges, tangible throughout the yang, there is life.

---

[1]   Yin means the *chi* position, while yang refers to the *cun* position. This passage says that the pulse can be felt in the *chi* but cannot be felt in the *cun*.

_________Chapter Nine_________

A Discussion of Miscellaneous Children's Diseases

If the child's pulse beats eight times for one respiration, this is normal. If it beats nine times, there is damage. If it beats ten times, there is (great) trouble.

When examining children, their pulse often displays (an image of) bird's fighting.[1] The rule is to take the three positions of the pulse as a whole. If the pulse is taut, there is wind leprosy.[2] If the pulse is deep, there is untransformed milk. If the pulse is bowstring and urgent, there is visiting unruliness qi.[3]

---

[1]   This describes a quick and forcefully beating pulse.

[2]   Wind leprosy in this context means tugging and slackening due to invasion of wind.

[3]   This is a disease which manifests as a green-blue facial complexion, vomiting, diarrhea, abdominal pain, and convulsions due to fright from a strange sound, sight, or person.

On the day of transmutation steaming[4] the infant may have fever and a chaotic pulse. There is no sweating, no desire for food, and vomiting of milk upon ingestion. Although the pulse is chaotic, there is no (real) bitterness (*i.e.*, suffering or affliction).

If a child's pulse is deep and rapid, there is heat in the bones with a desire to have the abdomen stroked by something cool and cold.

When a child has reddish stools mixed with green-blue curds, (*i.e.*, swill diarrhea), this is difficult to treat if the pulse is small and the hands and feet are cold but is easy to treat if the pulse is small and the hands and feet are warm.

If a child is afflicted by some disease with sweat exiting like pearls, sticking to the body without flowing down, this is death.

A sick child whose head hair all is standing on end is bound to die. If there are protruding green-blue veins around the auricles, there are cramps and pain.

In connection with a sick child, a sunken fontanel, a dry mouth and lips, out-turned eyelids, cold breath coming from the mouth, (the body so flaccid that) the feet may meet the head, inability to sit up from the lying position, dangling hands and feet from the four limbs, lying straight as if bound up, and cold in the palms are all death (signs. Leave these untreated) for ten days and there will be no hope of curing them.

---

[4] In Chinese medicine, it is believed that young children grow in stages and not necessarily steadily in a smooth progression. Thus every 32 days there is a stage called transmutation, while every 64 days there is a bigger stage called steaming. On the first day of transmutation and steaming, because growth is essentially a process of warm transformation, various transient conditions like fever, restlessness, irritability, and crying may manifest due to the increase in righteous heat in the baby's body. For instance, fever due to teething would be an example of transmutation and fuming. Since this is a normal physiological process, it typically does not require treatment and the symptoms will abate on their own.

BOOK TEN

Hand Diagram of the Thirty-One Positions[1]

**Collated & Edited by Honorary Minister Without Portfolio,
Curator of the Imperial Library,
Imperial Courier and Senior Army Protector,
Lin Yi *et al.***

It is said in the classics that the lungs are the canopy of the five viscera in the human body. Analogous to heaven above, they manage tens of thousands of affairs, governing the movement of essence and qi, going by the five phases and the four seasons, and detecting the five flavors. The *cun* opening is the place where yin and yang meet. (The *cun* opening) is divided into five portions. The distal and the proximal (positions), the left and the right (sides), each rules something. Based on the upper (*i.e.*, the *cun*), the lower (*i.e.*, the *chi*), and the middle (*i.e.*, the *guan*), there is a division of nine portions.[2] The floating, deep, bound, and dissipated (images) make known the location of evils. What is the *dao* (to this knowledge)?

Qi Bo explained:

If the pulse is large but weak, there is qi repletion and blood vacuity. If the pulse is large and long, the disease is shown to lie below. If the pulse is floating and straight, fluent from the upper to the

---

[1] One should note that this section does not include the pulses of the governing, conception, and penetrating vessels which are described in Book 2, Ch.4. There is no description of the pulse of the hand *shao yang* channel, etc. However, even if these pulses are transferred to this section, there would still be far less than 31 pulses. This has remained a controversial issue for centuries.
One should also note that the pulse locations are concerned with the channels and vessels rather than the viscera and bowels. Centering around Book1, Ch.7, there are illustrations of the pulse locations concerning the viscera and bowels. Also see Book 2, Ch.4.

[2] The nine portions include the center, the radial, and ulnar sides of each of the three positions, the *cun*, *guan*, and *chi*. These are not the same as the nine indicators. See chart on page 360.

lower, this is a yang pulse. The hard (quality) reveals kidney (disease). The urgent reveals liver (disease), and the replete reveals lung (disease).

At the outer (*i.e.*, radial) side of the distal position beats the foot *tai yang* pulse. At the outer side of the middle position beats the foot *yang ming* pulse. At the outer side of the proximal position beats the foot *shao yang* pulse. At the center of the distal position beats the hand *shao yin* pulse. At the center of the middle position beats the hand heart-governor pulse. At the center of the proximal position beats the hand *tai yin* pulse. At the inner (ulnar) side of the distal position beats the foot *jue yin* pulse. At the inner side of the middle position beats the foot *tai yin* pulse. At the inner side of the proximal position beats the foot *shao yin*. Striking (forcefully) at both the left and right (*i.e.*, outer and inner) side of the distal position is the yang motility (vessel pulse). Striking (forcefully) at both the left and right (*i.e.*, outer and inner) side of the middle position is the girdling (*dai*) vessel pulse. Striking (forcefully) at both the left and right (*i.e.*, outer and inner) side of the proximal position is the yin motility pulse. From the (foot) *shao yang* to the (foot) *jue yin*[3] beats the yin linking (vessel). From the (foot) *shao yin* to the (foot) *tai yang* beats the yang linking (vessel. A pulse) which arrives large but becomes gradually small is of the yin vessel network. (A pulse) arriving small but becoming gradually large is of the yang vessel network.

At the outer side of the distal position beats the foot *tai yang* pulse. If (this channel) is affected, there will be the bitterness of headache and pain in the nape (to) the lumbus. If this pulse is floating, there is wind. If it is choppy, there is cold and heat. If it is tight, there is food retention.

At the outer side of the distal position beats the foot *tai yang* pulse. If (this channel) is affected, there will be the bitterness of visual dizziness and pain in and stiffness of the head, the nape of the neck, and the upper and lower back. In males, there is dampness in the (external) genitals, and, in females, there is inhibited menstrual flow and lower abdominal pain radiating to the life gate (*i.e.*, the loins) and genitals. (This is due to) blocked uterus. If this pulse is floating, there is wind. If it is choppy, there is cold blood. If it is slippery, there is taxation heat. If it is tight, there is food retention. (To treat these disorders), insert the needle to the depth of nine *fen* and then retract it to a depth of six *fen*.[4]

At the outer side of the middle position beats the foot *yang ming* pulse. If (this channel) is affected, there will be the bitterness of headache and a red facial complexion. If this pulse is faint and

---

[3] This pulse travels from the outer (radial) side of the *chi* position corresponding to the foot *shao yang* obliquely to the inner (ulnar) side of the *cun* corresponding to the foot *jue yin*. Similar descriptions of other pulse locations that follow in this part can be interpreted in the same way.

[4] In this section, when no points are specified, then the relevant channel or vessel is meant.

slippery, there is the bitterness of difficult defecation, rumbling in the intestines, inability to take in food, and *bi* in the lower leg.

At the outer side of the middle position beats the foot *yang ming* pulse. If (this channel) is affected, there will be the bitterness of headache with a red hot face. If this pulse is floating, faint, and slippery, there is the bitterness of difficult defecation and frequent qi fullness. If it is slippery, there is rheum. If it is choppy, there is somnolence, rumbling in the intestines, inability to take in food, and *bi* in the lower leg. (To treat these disorders,) insert the needle to the depth of nine *fen* and then retract it to a depth of six *fen*.

At the outer side of the proximal position beats the foot *shao yang* pulse. If (this channel) is affected, there will be the bitterness of pain in the upper and lower back, the thigh, the lower leg, and the joints of the limbs.

At the outer side of the proximal position beats the foot *shao yang* pulse. If it is floating, there is inhibited qi. If it is choppy, there is wind and blood (disease). If it is urgent, there are cramps. If it is bowstring, there is taxation. Insert the needle to the depth of nine *fen* and then retract it to a depth of six *fen*.

The above are the three foot yang vessels.

At the inner side of the distal position beats the foot *jue yin* pulse. If (this channel) is affected, there will be the bitterness of lower abdominal pain and inhibited menstrual flow. (This is due to) blocked uterus.

At the inner side of the distal position beats the foot *jue yin* pulse. If (this channel) is affected, there will be the bitterness of lower abdominal pain involving the lower back, difficult defecation, difficult urination, and pain in the penis. In females, there is inhibited menstrual flow, cold in the genitals, congested and shut infant's door (*i.e.*, the vaginal meatus), and lower abdominal urgency. In males, there is *shan* qi with the testicles retracted and strangury. Insert the needle to the depth of six *fen* and then retract it to a depth of three *fen*.

At the inner side of the middle position beats the foot *tai yin* pulse. If (this channel) is affected, there will be the bitterness of pain in the stomach, inability to take in food, coughing and spitting of blood, cold of the lower legs, diminished qi, generalized heaviness, and (a sensation of) the part from the lower back above as if dipped in water.

At the inner side of the middle position beats the foot *tai yin* pulse. If (this channel) is affected, there will be the bitterness of abdominal fullness, cold in the upper venter, and failure of food to descend. The disease arises from drink and food. If (this pulse) is deep and choppy, there is the bitterness of generalized heaviness, inability to move the four limbs, inability to transform food, vexation and fullness, insomnia, pain in the lower leg with tormenting cold, occasional coughing of blood, and diarrhea of yellow stools. Insert the needle to the depth of six *fen* and then retract it to a depth of three *fen*.

At the inner side of the proximal position beats the foot *shao yin* pulse. If (this channel) is affected, there will be the bitterness of lower abdominal pain, a contracting pain between the heart and upper back, and strangury. In the case of fall causing injury internally, there will be blood in the urine.

At the inner side of the proximal position beats the foot *shao yin* pulse. If (this channel) is affected, there will be the bitterness of lower abdominal pain, a contracting pain between the heart and upper back, and strangury. In the case of fall causing injury to the coccyx, there will be hemafecia and abdominal urgency. During menstruation, qi will surge up into the heart giving rise to fullness and hypertonicity of the chest and lateral costal region and hypertonicity of the medial aspect of the thigh. Insert the needle to the depth of six *fen* and then retract it to a depth of three *fen*.

The above is the three foot yin vessels.

Forcefully striking at the outer and inner sides of the distal position is the yang motility pulse. If (this vessel) is affected, there will be the bitterness of pain in the upper and lower back. If this pulse is faint and choppy, there is wind epilepsy. (For these disorders,) treat the yang motility.

Forcefully striking at the outer and inner side of the distal position is the yang motility pulse. If (this vessel) is affected, there will be the bitterness of pain in the lower back, epilepsy, aversion to wind, hemilateral withering, sudden collapse with bleating, insensitivity of the extremities, and stiffness and insensitivity of the skin and the body. (For this,) promptly treat the yang motility at (the point) located parallel to Severed Bone (*Jue Gu*, GB 39)[5] three *cun* above the lateral malleolus.

Forcefully striking at the outer and inner side of the middle position is the girdling vessel pulse. If (this vessel) is affected, there will be the bitterness of lower abdominal pain radiating to the life gate. In females, there is absence of menstruation or postmenopausal recommencement of the

---

[5] This point is Yang Attachment (*Fu Yang*, Bl 59).

periods, genital (pain) as if being slashed, and genital cold and infertility. In males, there is tormenting hypertonicity of the lower abdomen or seminal emission.

Forcefully striking at the outer and inner side of the proximal position is the yin motility pulse. If (this vessel) is affected, there will be the bitterness of epilepsy, cold and heat, and stiffness and insensitivity of the skin.

Forcefully striking at the outer and inner side of the proximal position is the yin motility pulse. If (this vessel) is affected, there will be the bitterness of lower abdominal pain, abdominal urgency, and pain in the lower back and the pelvis down to the genitals. In males, there is yin *shan*,[6] and, in females, there is incessant downward leaking.

The above is the yang motility, yin motility, and girdling vessel.

At the center of the distal position beats the hand *shao yin* pulse. If (this channel) is affected, there will be the bitterness of heart pain. If this pulse is faint and hard, there is hypertonicity of the abdomen and lateral costal region. If it is replete and hard, there is the experience of frustration. If it is purely vacuous, there is diarrhea with rumbling in the intestines. If it is slippery, there may be pregnancy and itching and pain in the female's genitals. The pain is located one *fen* above the jade gate (*i.e.*, the vaginal meatus).

At the center of the middle position beats the hand heart-governor pulse. If (this channel) is affected, there will be the bitterness of heart pain, a red face, a bitter taste to food, copious saliva, and irascibility. If (this pulse) is faint and floating, there is the bitterness of sentimentality, abstraction, and susceptibility to sorrow. If it is choppy, there is cold below the heart. If it is deep, there is apprehension as if fearing arrest. If there is occasional cold and heat, there is (still) blood and qi.

At the center of the proximal position beats the hand *tai yin* pulse. If (this channel) is affected, there will be the bitterness of counterflow cough and gasping for breath. If (this pulse) is floating, there is internal wind. If it is tight and choppy, there is accumulated heat in the chest with occasional coughing of blood. There is deeply hidden heat.

The above is the three hand yin vessels.

---

[6] This refers to acute pain and swelling of the external genitals due to invasion by cold.

From the (foot) *shao yin* obliquely to the (foot) *tai yang* beats the yang linking pulse. If (this vessel) is affected, there will be the bitterness of *bi* and itching of the muscles and flesh.

From the (foot) *shao yin* obliquely to the (foot) *tai yang* beats the yang linking pulse. If (this vessel) is affected, there will be the bitterness of epilepsy of sudden collapse with bleating and contracted hands and feet. In severe cases, there is loss of voice and inability to speak. (For epilepsy,) treat promptly Guest Host Person (*Ke Zhu Ren*, GB 3) and treat the yang linking vessel bilaterally at (the point) located two *cun* below Severed Bone (*Jue Gu*, GB 39) above the lateral malleolus.

From the (foot) *shao yang* obliquely to the (foot) *jue yin* beats the yin linking pulse. If (this vessel) is affected, there will be the bitterness of epilepsy of sudden collapse with bleating.

From the (foot) *shao yang* obliquely to the (foot) *jue yin* beats the yin linking pulse. If (this vessel) is affected, there will be the bitterness of sudden collapse, loss of voice, extensive itching and *bi* of the muscles and flesh, and aversion to wind in sweating.

The pulse abruptly gong from large to small is of the yin network vessels. If (these network vessels) are affected, there will be the bitterness of flesh *bi* which starts in (bad) weather, causing cold shuddering as after a cold bath.

The pulse abruptly going from small to large is of the yang vessel network. If (these network vessels) is affected, there will be the bitterness of pain in the skin, insensitivity of the lower part (of the body), and sweating with aversion to cold.

If the lung pulse feels like stroking an elm leaf, this is normal. If it feels like hair being blown in the wind, this indicates disease. If it feels like a string of pearls (fused together), this is death. Death is expected to fall at the outlying region watch (9-11 a.m.) and midday watch (11 a.m.-1 p.m.) on the *bing* and *ding* days.

If the heart pulse is large like an upside down bamboo shoot[7] and (tender) like cattail, this is normal. If it is like a string of pearls (fused together), this indicates disease. If it is first crooked and then straight, giving the sensation of holding the crook of a girdle, this is death. (Death) is expected to fall at the serenity watch (9-11 p.m.) and midnight watch (11 p.m.-1 a.m.) on the *ren* and *gui* days.

---

[7] The bamboo shoot is cone-shaped. Therefore, an inverted bamboo shoot is a description of a pulse image which is large in the superficial level but small in the deep.

If the liver pulse is striking but weakly, this is normal. If it is like a fully drawn bowstring, this indicates disease. If it is like a cock letting its feet down on the ground,[8] this is death. (Death) is expected to fall at the late afternoon watch (3-5 p.m.) and sundown watch (5-7 p.m.) on the *geng* and *xin* days.

If the spleen pulse beats gracefully moderate, this is normal. If it is like a cock lifting its feet,[9] this indicates disease. If it is like a bird pecking[10] or like a leak in the roof,[11] this is death. (Death) is expected to fall at the calm dawn watch (3-5 a.m.) and sunrise watch (5-7 a.m.) on the *jia* and *yi* days.

If the kidney pulse is faint, fine, and long, this is normal. If it is (hard) like a pellet, this indicates disease. If it is like an entangled rope,[12] this is death. (Death) is expected to fall at the breakfast watch (7-9 a.m.), sun's descent watch (1-3 p.m.), dusk watch (7-9 p.m.), and cockcrow watch (1-3 a.m.) on the *wu* and *ji* days.

If the pulse is agitated in the *cun*, reaches the *guan*, but fails to appear in the *chi*, this is yang interfering with yin. The affection (thus suggested) will give rise to the bitterness of pain in the upper and lower back and abdomen, the genitals (painful) as if being cut, and cold feet. (To treat this,) needle the foot *tai yang* and *shao yin* and (the point) parallel to Severed Bone (*Jue Gu*, GB 39), to a depth of nine *fen* and moxa the (foot) *tai yin* (i.e., *San Yin Jiao*, Three Yin Intersection, Sp 6) with five cones.

If the pulse is hard and replete in the *chi*, reaches the *guan*, but fails to appear in the *cun*, this is yin interfering with yang. The affection (thus suggested) will give rise to the bitterness of heaviness of the two lower legs and lumbus, lower abdominal pain, and troubles involving the head. (To treat this,) needle the point of the foot *tai yin* three *cun* above the malleolus, inserting the needle to a depth of five *fen*. In addition, moxa the (foot) *tai yang* and the yang motility (at the point) three *cun* above the lateral malleolus parallel to Severed Bone (*Jue Gu*, GB 39).

If the *cun* opening pulse is tight, out-reaching down to the fish border, and, at the slightest touch, gives a sensation of holding a (taut) rope or a bamboo pole, then there are the diseases of

---

[8]   This is a description of a leisurely and soft pulse.

[9]   This is a rapid, abrupt pulse.

[10]   This is a swift, irregular pulse.

[11]   This pulse beats at very long intervals.

[12]   This is a scattered and chaotic pulse.

rumbling in the intestines, *bi* pain and aching in the feet, abdominal fullness, and inability to take in food. This arises from cold dampness. Needle the yang linking (vessel) at the point three *cun* above the lateral malleolus, inserting the needle to a depth of five *fen*. This pulse out-reaches the fish border.

If the *cun* opening pulse is deep, sticking to the bone, and intangible unless the palm (of the sick person) is placed downward, this is a pulse of kidney (disease). The affection (thus suggested) will give rise to the bitterness of lower abdominal pain, aching of the loins, and troubles involving the head. (To treat these disorders,) needle Kidney Shu (*Shen Shu*, Bl 23), inserting the needle to a depth of seven *fen*. In addition, needle the yin linking (vessel, *i.e.*, *Yin Wei*, Ki 12), inserting the needle to a depth of five *fen*.

If the *cun* opening pulse appears thin and hard at first and then feels large and deep after a long hold, the affection (thus suggested) will give rise to the bitterness of cold below the heart, tormenting pain in the chest and lateral costal region, pain in the genitals, and no desire to approach the husband. This is yin (qi) counterflow. (To treat this,) needle Cycle Gate (*Qi Men*, Liv 14), inserting the needle to a depth of six *fen*. In addition, needle Kidney Shu (*Shen Shu*, Bl 23), inserting the needle to a depth of five *fen*. One may moxa Stomach Venter (*Wei Guan*, CV 12) with seven cones (at the same time).

If the *cun* opening pulse seems agitated, surging and large at first but then feels thin, firm, and hard after a long hold, the affection (thus suggested) will give rise to the bitterness of a contracting pain between the lower back and abdomen, heaviness from the lower back to the feet, and inability to take in food. (To treat this,) needle Kidney Shu (*Shen Shu*, Bl 23), inserting the needle to a depth of four to five *fen*. One may instead moxa Stomach Venter (*Wei Guan*, CV 12) with seven cones.

If the pulse is deep in both the *chi* and *cun* but present (at the superficial level, *i.e.*, practically, floating) in the *guan*, the bitterness is cold, and pain below the heart.

If the pulse is deep in both the *chi* and *cun* and absent from the *guan* (even at the deep level), the affliction is (qi counterflow) below the heart giving rise to dyspnea.

If the pulse is rapid in both the *chi* and *cun*,[13] there is heat. If it is slow in both positions, there is cold.

---

[13] The *chi* and *cun* in this context refer to all the three positions of the pulse.

If the pulse is faint in both the *chi* and *cun*, there is inversion due to insufficiency of blood and qi. The sick person suffers from diminished qi.

If the pulse is soggy and weak in both the *chi* and *cun*, there is fever, aversion to cold, and (spontaneous) sweating.

If the pulse is deep in the *cun*, there is pain in the chest radiating to the back. If the pulse is deep in the *guan*, there are heart pain and acid swallowing. If the pulse is deep in the *chi*, there is a contracting pain in the back.

If the pulse is hidden in the *cun*, there is counterflow qi inside the chest. If the pulse is hidden in the *guan*, there are water qi and duck-stool diarrhea. If the pulse is hidden in the *chi*, there is inability to disperse water and grain.

If the pulse is bowstring in the *cun*, there is hypertonicity of the stomach. If the pulse is bowstring in the *guan*, there is cold in the stomach giving rise to hypertonicity of the infra-cardiac region. If the pulse is bowstring in the *chi*, there is hypertonicity of the lower abdomen below the umbilicus.

If the pulse is taut in the *cun*, there is headache and qi counterflow. If the pulse is taut in the *guan*, there is pain below the heart. If the pulse is taut in the *chi*, there is pain below the umbilicus in the lower abdomen.

If the pulse is choppy in the *cun*, there are absence of yang and diminished qi. If the pulse is choppy in the *guan*, there is absence of blood and inversion frigidity (of the four limbs). If the pulse is choppy in the *chi*, there is absence of yin and inversion frigidity (of the limbs).

If the pulse is faint in the *cun*, there is absence of yang with cold in the exterior. If the pulse is faint in the *guan*, there is repletion in the center [absence of the stomach qi in another version] (yet) with ability to take in food. Thus, this leads to abdominal urgency. If the pulse is faint in the *chi*, there is absence of yin, inversion frigidity (of the limbs), and hypertonicity within the abdomen.

If the pulse is slippery in the *cun*, there is fullness in the chest due to (qi) counterflow. If the pulse is slippery in the *guan*, there is repletion in the center with (stomach qi) counterflow. If the pulse is slippery in the *chi*, there is diarrhea and diminished qi.

If the pulse is rapid in the *cun*, there is vomiting. If the pulse is rapid in the *guan*, there is heat in the stomach. If the pulse is rapid in the *chi*, there are aversion to cold and reddish or yellow urine.

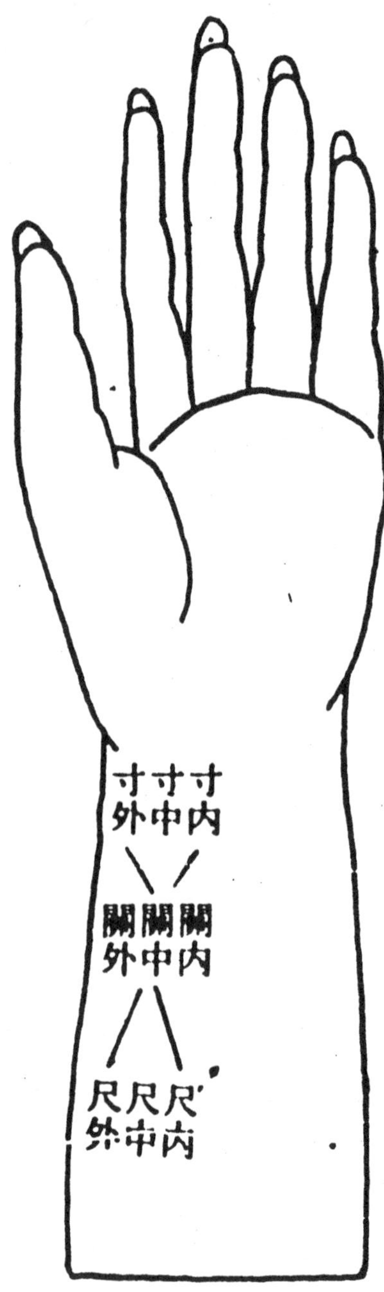

This diagram shows the nine portions which are arranged from
lateral to medial on each wrist.

If the pulse is replete in the *cun*, there is generation of heat. If it is vacuous, there is generation of cold. If the pulse is replete in the *guan*, there is pain. If it is vacuous, there is distention and fullness.

If the pulse is replete in the *chi*, there is difficult urination with tightness and pain in the lower abdomen. If it is vacuous, there is inhibited or blocked (urination).

If the pulse is scallion-stalk in the *cun*, there is ejection of blood. If it is slightly scallion-stalk, there is runny snivel nosebleeding. If the pulse is scallion-stalk in the *guan*, there is vacuity of the stomach. If the pulse is scallion-stalk in the *chi*, there is hemafecia. If it is slightly scallion-stalk, there is hematuria.

If the pulse is floating in the *cun*, the sick person suffers from wind stroke with fever and headache. If the pulse is floating in the *guan*, there is abdominal pain and fullness below the heart. If the pulse is floating in the *chi*, there is difficult urination.

If the pulse is slow in the *cun*, there is cold in the upper burner. If the pulse is slow in the *guan*, there is cold in the stomach. If the pulse is slow in the *chi*, there are cold in the lower burner and pain in the back.

If the pulse is soggy in the *cun*, there is a weakness of yang with spontaneous sweating. If the pulse is soggy in the *guan*, there is pressure in the rectum. If the pulse is soggy in the *chi*, there is a shortage of blood with fever and aversion to cold.

If the pulse is weak in the *cun*, there is diminished yang qi. If the pulse is weak in the *guan*, there is no stomach qi. If the pulse is weak in the *chi*, there is a shortage of blood.

Postscript to Wang's *Pulse Classic*

As the Confucians look upon the six prototypes[1] as the root (of philosophy), so do medical students look upon the seven classics[2] as the root of medicine. None of the seven classics, however, give a more detailed elucidation of the essentials and subtleties of the pulse theories than Wang's *Pulse Classic* does. It is well outlined and well organized. Its words are clear, yet their meanings are profound. For that reason, this work has been handed down together with the books by the Yellow Emperor and Lu Bian,[3] and all medical students from the Western Jin[4] to this day have been learning it as the archetype (of all study of the pulse).

Since the southward movement,[5] a good edition of this classic has been a rarity. All the versions available abound in mistakes and typographical errors. Da-ren often felt pain about (this situation. Accidentally,) in the collection of my family, there was a copy of the edition published by the Supervision[6] in the reign of Shao Sheng.[7] This copy, old of age, was worn out and abraded, and it was impossible that there were not any miswritten characters in it. However, since it had undergone collation by past sages, this edition must have been true to the original. For quite a long time, I cherished a desire to collate and edit it, but I was always too busy. It happened that I was once again given the position of teaching medicine and that I made acquaintances with those experienced and knowledgeable colleagues Elder-born Mao Sheng, Elder-born Li Bang-yan,

---

1   The six prototypes are the *Shi Jing (Classic of Poetry)*, *Shang Shu (Anthology of Ancient Literature)*, *Li Ji (The Records of Rites)*, *Yue Jing (The Classic of Music)* , *Yi Jing (The Classic of Change)*, and *Chun Qiu (Spring & Autumn)*.

2   The seven classics include the *Huang Di Nei Jing (Yellow Emperor's Inner Classic)*, the *Huang Di Wai Jing (Yellow Emperor's Outer Classic)*, *Bian Que Nei Jing (Bian Que's Inner Classic)*, *Bian Que Wai Jing (Bian Que's Outer Classic)*, *Bai Shi Nei Jing (Master Bai's Inner Classic)*, *Bai Shi Wai Jing (Master Bai's Outer Classic)*, and *Bai Shi Pang Jing (Master Bai's Companion to the Classics)*.

3   I.e., Bian Que, one of whose style names was Lu Sheng. The book that is supposed to be written by him is the *Nan Jing (Classic of Difficulties)*.

4   This dynasty lasted from 265-316 CE.

5   As a result of invasion by northern minorities, the Song court was forced to move its capital southward to the present Hangzhou in 1127 CE. Accordingly, the dynasty was renamed the Southern Song.

6   This is a shortened name for the National Board of Supervision of Youth, an organization in charge of education and imperial examination in some of the dynasties.

7   1094-98 CE

Elder-born Wang Bang-zuo, and Elder-born Gao Zong-qing. After they were informed of this intention of mine, together with me they made reference to a wealth of books and toiled for months, correcting as many as over a thousand typographical errors. Then we had some workers print this newly edited copy in our Board in hope that it might be shared by the public. As to the lacunae and doubtful places in the old version, we have not ventured to add new annotations. This is left to later sages to do.

Written by He Da-ren of Haoliang[8]
on the full moon day, midsummer month, *ding chou* year,[9] in the reign of Jia Qing[10]

---

[8] This was an old county situated in the present Fengyang county, Anhui Province.

[9] *I.e.*, the fifteenth of the fifth month, 1217 CE

[10] 1208-1224 CE

General Index

A

Formula Index

CURING ARTHRITIS NATURALLY WITH CHINESE
MEDICINE by Douglas Frank & Bob Flaws
ISBN 0-936185-87-2
ISBN 978-0-936185-87-3

CURING DEPRESSION NATURALLY WITH
CHINESE MEDICINE by Rosa Schnyer & Bob Flaws
ISBN 0-936185-94-5
ISBN 978-0-936185-94-1

CURING FIBROMYALGIA NATURALLY WITH
CHINESE MEDICINE by Bob Flaws
ISBN 1-891845-09-8
ISBN 978-1-891845-09-3

CURING HAY FEVER NATURALLY WITH
CHINESE MEDICINE by Bob Flaws
ISBN 0-936185-91-0
ISBN 978-0-936185-91-0

CURING HEADACHES NATURALLY WITH
CHINESE MEDICINE by Bob Flaws
ISBN 0-936185-95-3
ISBN 978-0-936185-95-8

CURING IBS NATURALLY WITH CHINESE
MEDICINE by Jane Bean Oberski
ISBN 1-891845-11-X
ISBN 978-1-891845-11-6

CURING INSOMNIA NATURALLY WITH
CHINESE MEDICINE by Bob Flaws
ISBN 0-936185-86-4
ISBN 978-0-936185-86-6

CURING PMS NATURALLY WITH
CHINESE MEDICINE by Bob Flaws
ISBN 0-936185-85-6
ISBN 978-0-936185-85-9

DISEASES OF THE KIDNEY & BLADDER
by Hoy Ping Yee Chan, et al.
ISBN 1-891845-37-3
ISBN 978-1-891845-35-6

THE DIVINE FARMER'S MATERIA MEDICA:
A Translation of the Shen Nong Ben Cao
translation by Yang Shouz-zhong
ISBN 0-936185-96-1
ISBN 978-0-936185-96-5

DUI YAO: THE ART OF COMBINING CHINESE
HERBAL MEDICINALS by Philippe Sionneau
ISBN 0-936185-81-3
ISBN 978-0-936185-81-1

ENDOMETRIOSIS, INFERTILITY AND TRADITION-
AL CHINESE MEDICINE: A Layperson's Guide
by Bob Flaws
ISBN 0-936185-14-7
ISBN 978-0-936185-14-9

THE ESSENCE OF LIU FENG-WU'S GYNECOLOGY
by Liu Feng-wu, translated by Yang Shou-zhong
ISBN 0-936185-88-0
ISBN 978-0-936185-88-0

EXTRA TREATISES BASED ON INVESTIGATION &
INQUIRY: A Translation of Zhu Dan-xi's Ge Zhi Yu
Lun translation by Yang Shou-zhong
ISBN 0-936185-53-8
ISBN 978-0-936185-53-8

FIRE IN THE VALLEY: TCM Diagnosis & Treatment
of Vaginal Diseases by Bob Flaws
ISBN 0-936185-25-2
ISBN 978-0-936185-25-5

FULFILLING THE ESSENCE: A Handbook of
Traditional & Contemporary Treatments for Female
Infertility by Bob Flaws
ISBN 0-936185-48-1
ISBN 978-0-936185-48-4

FU QING-ZHU'S GYNECOLOGY
trans. by Yang Shou-zhong and Liu Da-wei
ISBN 0-936185-35-X
ISBN 978-0-936185-35-4

GOLDEN NEEDLE WANG LE-TING: A 20th Century
Master's Approach to Acupuncture by Yu Hui-chan
and Han Fu-ru, trans. by Shuai Xue-zhong
ISBN 0-936185-78-3
ISBN 978-0-936185-78-1

A HANDBOOK OF CHINESE HEMATOLOGY
by Simon Becker
ISBN 1-891845-16-0
ISBN 978-1-891845-16-1

A HANDBOOK OF TCM PATTERNS
& THEIR TREATMENTS   Second Edition
by Bob Flaws & Daniel Finney
ISBN 0-936185-70-8
ISBN 978-0-936185-70-5

A HANDBOOK OF TRADITIONAL CHINESE
DERMATOLOGY by Liang Jian-hui, trans. by Zhang
Ting-liang & Bob Flaws
ISBN 0-936185-46-5
ISBN 978-0-936185-46-0

A HANDBOOK OF TRADITIONAL CHINESE
GYNECOLOGY by Zhejiang College of TCM,
trans. by Zhang Ting-liang & Bob Flaws
ISBN 0-936185-06-6 (4th edit.)
ISBN 978-0-936185-06-4

A HANDBOOK of TCM PEDIATRICS by Bob Flaws
ISBN 0-936185-72-4
ISBN 978-0-936185-72-9

THE HEART & ESSENCE OF DAN-XI'S METHODS
OF TREATMENT
by Xu Dan-xi, trans. by Yang Shou-zhong
ISBN 0-926185-50-3
ISBN 978-0-936185-50-7

HERB TOXICITIES & DRUG INTERACTIONS:
A Formula Approach by Fred Jennes with Bob Flaws
ISBN 1-891845-26-8
ISBN 978-1-891845-26-0

IMPERIAL SECRETS OF HEALTH & LONGEVITY
by Bob Flaws
ISBN 0-936185-51-1
ISBN 978-0-936185-51-4

INSIGHTS OF A SENIOR ACUPUNCTURIST
by Miriam Lee
ISBN 0-936185-33-3
ISBN 978-0-936185-33-0

INTEGRATED PHARMACOLOGY: Combining
Modern Pharmacology with Chinese Medicine
by Dr. Greg Sperber with Bob Flaws
ISBN 1-891845-41-1
ISBN 978-0-936185-41-3

INTEGRATIVE PHARMACOLOGY: Combining
Modern Pharmacology with Integrative Medicine
Second Edition by Dr. Greg Sperber with Bob Flaws
ISBN 1-891845-69-1
ISBN 978-0-936185-69-7

INTRODUCTION TO THE USE OF PROCESSED
CHINESE MEDICINALS by Philippe Sionneau
ISBN 0-936185-62-7
ISBN 978-0-936185-62-0

KEEPING YOUR CHILD HEALTHY WITH
CHINESE MEDICINE by Bob Flaws
ISBN 0-936185-71-6
ISBN 978-0-936185-71-2

THE LAKESIDE MASTER'S STUDY OF THE PULSE
by Li Shi-zhen, trans. by Bob Flaws
ISBN 1-891845-01-2
ISBN 978-1-891845-01-7

MANAGING MENOPAUSE NATURALLY WITH
CHINESE MEDICINE by Honora Lee Wolfe
ISBN 0-936185-98-8
ISBN 978-0-936185-98-9

MASTER HUA'S CLASSIC OF THE CENTRAL
VISCERA by Hua Tuo, trans. by Yang Shou-zhong
ISBN 0-936185-43-0
ISBN 978-0-936185-43-9

THE MEDICAL I CHING: Oracle of the Healer Within
by Miki Shima
ISBN 0-936185-38-4
ISBN 978-0-936185-38-5

MENOPAIUSE & CHINESE MEDICINE
by Bob Flaws
ISBN 1-891845-40-3
ISBN 978-1-891845-40-6

MOXIBUSTION: A MODERN CLINICAL HANDBOOK
by Lorraine Wilcox
ISBN 1-891845-49-7
ISBN 978-1-891845-49-9

MOXIBUSTION: THE POWER OF MUGWORT FIRE
by Lorraine Wilcox
ISBN 1-891845-46-2
ISBN 978-1-891845-46-8

A NEW AMERICAN ACUPUNTURE By Mark Seem
ISBN 0-936185-44-9
ISBN 978-0-936185-44-6

PLAYING THE GAME: A Step-by-Step Approach to
Accepting Insurance as an Acupuncturist
by Greg Sperber & Tiffany Anderson-Hefner
ISBN 3-131416-11-7
ISBN 978-3-131416-11-7

POCKET ATLAS OF CHINESE MEDICINE
Edited by Marne and Kevin Ergil
ISBN 1-891-845-59-4
ISBN 978-1-891845-59-8

POINTS FOR PROFIT: The Essential Guide to
Practice Success for Acupuncturists   5th Fully
Edited Edition
by Honora Wolfe with Marilyn Allen
ISBN 1-891845-64-0
ISBN 978-1-891845-64-2

PRINCIPLES OF CHINESE MEDICAL ANDROLOGY:
An Integrated Approach to Male Reproductive and
Urological Health by Bob Damone
ISBN 1-891845-45-4
ISBN 978-1-891845-45-1

PRINCE WEN HUI's COOK: Chinese Dietary
Therapy by Bob Flaws & Honora Wolfe
ISBN 0-912111-05-4
ISBN 978-0-912111-05-6

THE PULSE CLASSIC: A Translation of the Mai Jing
by Wang Shu-he, trans. by Yang Shou-zhong
ISBN 0-936185-75-9
ISBN 978-0-936185-75-0

THE SECRET OF CHINESE PULSE DIAGNOSIS
by Bob Flaws
ISBN 0-936185-67-8
ISBN 978-0-936185-67-5

SECRET SHAOLIN FORMULAS FOR THE
TREATMENT OF EXTERNAL INJURY
by De Chan, trans. by Zhang Ting-liang & Bob Flaws
ISBN 0-936185-08-2
ISBN 978-0-936185-08-8

STATEMENTS OF FACT IN TRADITIONAL CHINESE
MEDICINE by Bob Flaws   Revised & Expanded
ISBN 0-936185-52-X
ISBN 978-0-936185-52-1

STICKING TO THE POINT: A Step-by-Step Approach
to TCM Acupuncture Therapy
by Bob Flaws & Honora Wolfe (2 Condensed Books)
ISBN 1-891845-47-0
ISBN 978-1-891845-47-5

A STUDY OF DAOIST ACUPUNCTURE
by Liu Zheng-cai
ISBN 1-891845-08-X
ISBN 978-1-891845-08-6

THE SUCCESSFUL CHINESE HERBALIST
by Bob Flaws and Honora Lee Wolfe
ISBN 1-891845-29-2
ISBN 978-1-891845-29-1

THE SYSTEMATIC CLASSIC OF ACUPUNCTURE
& MOXIBUSTION: A translation of the Jia Yi Jing
by Huang-fu Mi, trans. by Yang Shou-zhong &
Charles Chace
ISBN 0-936185-29-5
ISBN 978-0-936185-29-3

THE TAO OF HEALTHY EATING: DIETARY
WISDOM ACCORDING TO CHINESE MEDICINE
by Bob Flaws Second Edition
ISBN 0-936185-92-9
ISBN 978-0-936185-92-7

TEACH YOURSELF TO READ MODERN MEDICAL
CHINESE by Bob Flaws
ISBN 0-936185-99-6
ISBN 978-0-936185-99-6

TEST PREP WORKBOOK FOR BASIC TCM THEORY
by Zhong Bai-song
ISBN 1-891845-43-8
ISBN 978-1-891845-43-7

TEST PREP WORKBOOK FOR THE NCCAOM
BIOMEDICINE MODULE: Exam Preparation & Study
Guide by Zhong Bai-song
ISBN 1-891845-34-9
ISBN 978-1-891845-34-5

TREATING PEDIATRIC BED-WETTING WITH
ACUPUNCTURE & CHINESE MEDICINE
by Robert Helmer
ISBN 1-891845-33-0
ISBN 978-1-891845-33-8

TREATISE on the SPLEEN & STOMACH: A
Translation and annotation of Li Dong-yuan's Pi Wei
Lun by Bob Flaws
ISBN 0-936185-41-4
ISBN 978-0-936185-41-5